THE ANNA FREUD TRADITION

LINES OF DEVELOPMENT
Evolution of Theory and Practice over the Decades

Series Editors: Norka T. Malberg and Joan Raphael-Leff

THE ANNA FREUD TRADITION

Lines of Development—Evolution of Theory and Practice over the Decades

Edited by

Norka T. Malberg and Joan Raphael-Leff

Routledge
Taylor & Francis Group
LONDON AND NEW YORK

First published 2012 by Karnac Books Ltd.

Published 2022 by Routledge
2 Park Square, Milton Park, Abingdon, Oxon OX14 4RN
605 Third Avenue, New York, NY 10017

Routledge is an imprint of the Taylor & Francis Group, an informa business

First issued in paperback 2019

British Library Cataloguing in Publication Data

A C.I.P. for this book is available from the British Library

ISBN-13: 978-1-78049-021-2 (pbk)
ISBN-13: 978-0-367-32746-0 (hbk)

Typeset by Vikatan Publishing Solutions (P) Ltd., Chennai, India

To all who have been touched in one way or another by the work of Anna Freud, especially children and their families.
And to our own families who support our work and keep us grounded.

CONTENTS

C. LATENCY—Clinical papers and outreach

Overview

SERIES EDITORS' FOREWORD

This is the first volume in a series which Oliver Rathbone has entrusted us to co-edit. Initially, the series will focus on a spectrum of psychoanalytic leaders whose ideas have generated a tradition of thinking and working in particular ways.

By definition, such pioneers venture further into unknown or unclaimed territories—opening up new areas of theoretical inquiry and/or therapeutic work. As trailblazers, they often inspire others to expand their work and to build on their ideas through research, clinical developments, or practical applications. However, in the case of many psychoanalytic pioneers beginning with Freud, the diverse elaborations over the decades renders it virtually impossible for one reviewer to encompass the rich results of the respective leader's catalytic contribution to the field.

Thus, to do justice to its own conceptual framework and respective lines of development, each volume in the series will have two or three co-editors. Preferably, these will represent different "generations" and intercontinental locations to expedite a comprehensive compilation, by commissioning new papers from an international pool of both young and more senior experts in the field.

The proposed format of each volume in the series is similar to this one:

Historical frame

A section which provides the reader with a general overview of the tradition, its origins, historical milestones, and evolution of new developments. Training of professionals and theoretical elaboration of the school of thought by major figures will be highlighted.

Clinical applications
This section aims to illustrate the expansion of theoretical concepts and technique, and their methodical application to clinical work with babies, children, adolescents, adults, families, and/or groups.

Outreach and current applications outside the consulting room
This section reflects how the particular school of thought has informed the practice of allied professionals, and influenced contemporary thinking in other academic disciplines and social systems.

Personal reflections and accounts
This last section gives the reader an opportunity to experience the evolution of each tradition through the understanding of participants active in the process of its growth and the development of its ideas. It also contains pertinent historical accounts and personal recollections of the pioneers involved.

Having worked successfully to bring this current book to fruition, as series editors we will provide guidance to future co-editors to produce a comparable integrative and comprehensive body of work on the origins, evolution, and contemporary practice of diverse schools of thought in psychoanalysis, which in turn may serve as a further catalyst and reference resource for didactic purposes.

We hope you enjoy reading this first volume of the series, giving voice to the Anna Freudian school of thought and practice, characterized by its innovative and creative nature.

Norka Malberg and Joan Raphael-Leff
September 2011

ABOUT THE EDITORS AND CONTRIBUTORS

Steven Ablon, MD, adult and child psychoanalyst, is a training and supervising analyst at the Boston Psychoanalytic Society and Institute, and associate clinical professor of psychiatry at the Massachusetts General Hospital, and Harvard University Medical School. He has close links with the Anna Freud Centre, and has attended the colloquia at the AFC for the past 25 years. Dr Ablon has published widely in the psychoanalytic literature on subjects including the therapeutic action of play, dreams, technique, and affect. He has also published four books of poetry.

Debbie Bandler Bellman is a psychoanalyst (British Psychoanalytic Association), and a child and adolescent psychotherapist, having qualified from the Anna Freud Centre training in 1979. She was a training supervisor and seminar leader for the AFC, and is a training analyst for the Association of Child Psychotherapists. She currently works in private practice. She is a past editor of the *Journal of Child Psychotherapy*, and co-editor of *Transference and Countertransference: a Unifying Focus of Psychoanalysis*, published by Karnac (Arundale & Bellman, 2011).

Michela Biseo, BA (Hons), MSc, is a child and adolescent psychotherapist and parent–infant psychotherapist, trained at the Anna Freud Centre (graduated 2002). She has worked in multidisciplinary child and adolescent mental health teams in the NHS. Currently, she works as a parent–infant psychotherapist in PIP, the Parent Infant Project at the AFC. She also practises as a child psychotherapist at the AFC and in private practice. She teaches infant observation on the UCL/AFC masters course, and teaches on various AFC "Early Years" courses for professionals working with young children.

Mark Carter, MA, MSc, trained at the Anna Freud Centre, qualifying in 2005. He is currently joint locum team manager of a NHS mental health service for children and youth with neuro-developmental difficulties, and is also clinical lead for a referral service covering local mental health teams for children and adolescents in a London borough. For six years he taught "nursery observation" on the Anna Freud Centre/UCL MSc in Psychoanalytic Developmental Psychology. Professional experience includes psychoanalytic psychotherapy with children/adolescents with learning disability and/or social communication difficulties; and mental health work in secondary schools (particularly secondary pupil referral units).

Minna Daum has more than 20 years' experience as a systemic psychotherapist. Her particular area of interest lies in child maltreatment and the family justice system, and specifically in adult personality disorder and its impact on children's emotional development. In her 12 years at the Anna Freud Centre she has been responsible for work relating to children at severe risk (early intervention, court assessments, and work with children in out-of-home placements).

Hedde Maartje Evers, MA (Leiden University, the Netherlands), MA, MSc (AFC/UCL), is a psychologist and a child and adolescent psychotherapist. Having worked with children and their parents in various child and adolescent mental health settings for more than a decade, Hedde was one of the last trainees to complete the full Anna Freudian child analytic training in the summer of 2009. Her special interest is analytic work with young children and their parents, and she is currently completing her doctorate in psychoanalytic child and adolescent psychotherapy (on the experience of the therapist's pregnancy and its impact on psychoanalytic child psychotherapy practice). She works on a voluntary basis at a centre for refugees and migrant workers in Israel.

Audrey Gavshon qualified at the Hampstead Child-Therapy Course and Clinic in 1964; worked at the Kilburn (now Brent) Child Guidance Centre (1965–1967) and since then at the Anna Freud Centre where she was very involved in the clinical teaching of the child psychotherapy training, supervised child psychoanalytic cases, and led an AFC clinical group. For many years she ran clinical seminars for trainees and staff; treated children and adults (parent work) in the family support service, and was a member of the training committee and of the study group on "Developmental disturbance: qualitative research on aspects of child psycho-therapy". She also taught and supervised psychotherapists in Bologna. Her publications include: "The Analysis of an Atypical Boy" (*PSC* 42, 1987) and "The Analysis of a Latency Boy: the Developmental Impact of Separation, Divorce and Remarriage" (*PSC* 45, 1990).

Anat Gedulter-Trieman, BSW (Hons), MA (Hons), from Hebrew University in Jerusalem, trained in child psychotherapy at the Anna Freud Centre (1993–1998), where she later assumed the roles of the nursery consultant and supervisor of clinical trainees. For nearly three decades she has been working analytically with children, adolescents, and adults in various capacities. She also trained as an adult psychoanalyst and is now a member of the British Psycho-Analytical Society and the Association of Child and Adolescent Psychotherapy (ACP).

Viviane Green, BEd (Hons), MA, is an adult and child psychotherapist in private practice. She graduated from the Anna Freud Centre in 1989, and became head of the AFC clinical training from 1999 to 2009. She is now programme manager of psycho-dynamic counselling with children and adolescents at Birkbeck College, London. In addition she has developed child psychoanalytic training programmes in Utrecht for the Dutch Psychoanalytic Institute, and developed course modules and taught in Italy and Brazil. From 2006–2011 she was co-editor of the *Journal of Child Psychotherapy*. She is widely published and the editor of *Emotional Development in Psychoanalysis, Neuroscience and Attachment Theory—Creating Connections* (Brunner-Routledge, 2003).

Hillary Hamburger, MA, in clinical psychology: following training, and internship at a psychiatric hospital she served for many years as vice chair and then chair of the Johannesburg Psychoanalytic Psychotherapy Study Group. Anxious to find a meaningful way to continue participating in the wider struggle in the new South Africa, now no longer battling apartheid but rather the profoundly damaging consequences of that system, the Hamburgers converted a large industrial building on the borders of Alexandra township, which became Ububele, a psychotherapeutic training and resource centre. Hillary continues in private practice while acting as director of the Ububele Therapeutic Nursery School.

Tony Hamburger, MA, in clinical psychology, Witwaterstrand University, Johannesburg: after completing two internships (at TMI, a children's hospital, and at Tara, a large psychiatric hospital), he went into private practice as a psychoanalytic psychotherapist. He is a foundation member, past chair and treasurer of a professional psychoanalytic study group. He has been director of Ububele since 2000, designing and implementing the various programmes. He acts as facilitator in counselling courses and workshops for HIV/AIDS workers and trainer/supervisor at a professional and lay counsellor level.

Trevor Hartnup obtained an honours degree in French and a postgraduate diploma in social work before training at the (then) Hampstead Clinic where he qualified in 1975, and worked there part-time until 1980. Now retired from the NHS Child Mental Health Service, he works in private practice as a child, adolescent, and adult psychotherapist.

Angela Joyce is a training and supervising analyst of the British Psychoanalytical Society. She originally trained in teaching and social work before psychotherapy and then became an adult analyst in 1995. She completed the training in child analysis at the Anna Freud Centre in 2000. She has been a member of PIP, the Parent Infant Project since soon after its inception in 1997 and is also training lead for the child psychotherapy service at the Anna Freud Centre. She teaches widely and has written contributions to various books on development, child analysis, and parent infant psychotherapy. She has recently co-edited (with Lesley Caldwell) *Reading Winnicott* (New Library of Psychoanalysis Teaching Series, 2011).

Justine Kalas Reeves, MSW, DPsych, qualified as a child and adolescent psychotherapist at the Anna Freud Centre in 2003. Her most treasured and pleasurable learning and working experience while at the AFC was working as group leader in the toddler service. She works with children and adults in private practice in Washington, D.C., and is a candidate in adult psychoanalysis at the Psychoanalytic Institute of the Contemporary Freudian Society.

Ehud Koch, PhD, is a graduate of the Hampstead Clinic child-therapy course 1962–1966, and was a staff member of the Hampstead Child Clinic, 1966–1967. He is emeritus assistant professor of psychology, Department of Psychiatry, Case Western Reserve University, Cleveland, Ohio, 1967–1992. Since 1992 he has been in private practice in Boston, and has been an instructor in psychology, Psychiatry Department, Harvard University, from1992 to the present.

Sheila Levi, MA, MSc, MPhil, is a chartered clinical psychologist and child-adolescent psychotherapist. She trained and worked as a clinical psychologist at Bogazici University in Istanbul, Turkey. She developed the therapeutic programme for earthquake survivor children after the mass trauma in Adapazari, Turkey as part of her work in the Tel Aviv Trauma Centre. Empirically she studied the effects of circumcision on Turkish Muslim boys at Exeter University. She holds a MSc in Psychoanalytic Developmental Psychology from UCL/Anna Freud Centre. She began clinical training at the AFC and completed at the BAP. Currently, she teaches clinical training for the AFC and the BAP. Currently she teaches in the infant observation programme of the BAP, and works with children and adults in private practice, and within the NHS at Barnet, and at Enfield CAMHS specialist services for children and families with neurodevelopmental disorders.

Laurie Levinson, PhD, in clinical psychology from the City University of New York, trained at the Hampstead Child Therapy Course and Clinic, now the Anna Freud Centre (graduated in 1977). She is on the faculty of the Institute for Psychoanalytic Education affiliated with NYU Medical School, an active member of the Association for Child Psychoanalysis, and is in private practice.

Christiane Ludwig-Körner, MSc, PhD, is a clinical and educational psychologist, psychoanalyst (IPA, DPG), training analyst, and supervisor, with degrees in client centred psychotherapy, behaviour therapy, and gestalt therapy. She is a professor emeritus of the University of Applied Science, Potsdam, professor of clinical psychology and educational psychology at the International Psychoanalytic University, Berlin, and head of the Parent–Infant Centre, Potsdam. Over the past 35 years in clinical practice and academic work she has led training programmes for practitioners working with infants and parents, and for kindergarden teachers. She is the author of more than 50 single-author publications in the fields of clinical and educational psychology.

Norka T. Malberg, DPsych, is a child and adult psychoanalyst who qualified from the AFC as child and adolescent psychotherapist in 2005. She continued working at the AFC as clinician, seminar leader, and coordinator of collaborative outreach projects in schools and hospitals for three years. She taught seminars at the BAP on Anna Freud and the development of psychoanalytic research. Previously she had worked as a counselling psychologist in private practice in the USA and was assistant professor of psychology at Universidad Diego Portales in Santiago, Chile where she developed numerous clinical outreach projects. She also worked as clinical consultant to schools in Zurich, Switzerland from 1996–1998. Currently she is a faculty member of the continuing education section of the Western New England Psychoanalytic Institute in New Haven, Connecticut, where she teaches a course on Anna Freud; she is also clinical supervisor for the Child FIRST programme at the Clifford Beers Child Guidance Clinic in New Haven, CT. She continues her role as clinical consultant to the AFC in London.

Paddy Martin, MSc, qualified as a child and adolescent psychotherapist from the Anna Freud Centre in 2007, since when he has worked for the AFC court assessment service. He teaches a module on "intergenerational transmission of attachment" for the AFC Parent Infant Project.

For the last seven years has also worked for the North Middlesex Hospital paediatric liaison team, and teaches a series of seminars on psycho-somatic disorders for third year trainees at the British Association of Psychotherapy. He is a member of the *Journal of Child Psychotherapy*'s editorial committee.

Linda C. Mayes, MD, is a child and adult psychoanalyst. She is Arnold Gesell professor of child psychiatry, pediatrics, and psychology in the Yale Child Study Center, and a faculty member since 1985. She is special advisor to the dean in the Yale School of Medicine, where she established a laboratory for studying infant learning and attention, and a neuro-physiology laboratory for studies of startle response and related indices of emotional regulation in children and adolescents. Currently she oversees the developmental electrophysiology laboratory that includes dense array electro-encephalography to study brain activity in real time. She is an alumna and faculty member of the Western New England Psychoanalytic Institute. Since 2003 Linda has been chair of the directorial team of the Anna Freud Centre.

Federica Melandri, MSc, DPsych, graduated in clinical and community psychology at the University of Padua, Italy. She trained at the Anna Freud Centre as a child and adolescent psychotherapist, holding a joint training post with the West London Mental Health NHS Trust and the Anna Freud Centre (2001–2006). She achieved a doctoral degree in child and adolescent psychoanalytic psychotherapy at University College London. A member of the ACP and the Italian professional body of psychologists and psychotherapists, she currently works in private practice in Bologna, Italy.

Nick Midgley, DPsych, qualified as a child and adolescent psychotherapist at the Anna Freud Centre in 2002, and now works there as a clinician, a senior research fellow and as programme director for the MSc in Developmental Psychology and Clinical Practice. Nick's work is widely published in peer review journals and he was winner of the Anna Freud Foundation Essay Prize in 2007 for his paper about Anna Freud and the "Matchbox School" in Vienna in the 1920s. He was joint editor of *Child Psychotherapy and Research: New Directions, Emerging Findings* (Routledge, 2009) and is currently writing a book for the New Library of Psychoanalysis on the work of Anna Freud. In 2010 Nick received an Early Career Achievement Award from the British Psychoanalytic Council, recognizing his contribution to advancing psychoanalytic knowledge and practice.

Jack Novick, PhD, child, adolescent, and adult psychoanalyst, graduated from the Hampstead Clinic in 1969 and the British Psycho-Analytic Institute in 1971. He was on the faculty of the Hampstead Clinic from 1970 to 1977. He is a training and supervising analyst of the International Psychoanalytic Association and serves on numerous institute faculties. In addition to writing an array of articles published in peer-reviewed journals, the Novicks have authored four books: *Fearful Symmetry: the Development and Treatment of Sadomasochism* (1996), *Working with Parents Makes Therapy Work* (2005), *Good Goodbyes: Knowing how to end in Psychotherapy and Psychoanalysis* (2006), and *Emotional Muscle* (2010).

Kerry Kelly Novick is a child, adolescent, and adult psychoanalyst who graduated from the Hampstead Clinic in 1970 and was a staff member from 1970–1977. She did her adult training through the New York Freudian Society. She is a faculty member of the Michigan Psychoanalytic

Institute, the Michigan Psychoanalytic Council, the New York University Psychoanalytic Institute, the New York Freudian Society, the Chicago Center for Psychoanalysis, and the University of Michigan Medical School. With Jack she has worked with children and families for 40 years and joined other colleagues to found the Allen Creek Preschool, a non-profit psychoanalytic school in Ann Arbor, Michigan.

Ava Bry Penman trained at the Anna Freud Centre (1971 graduate), and is a lecturer in psychiatry at Harvard Medical School, and Cambridge Health Alliance (teaching and supervision). She is a member of the faculty, the Psychoanalytic Institute of New England, at Needham, Massachusetts. She undertakes supervision and is in private practice for children, adolescents, and adults in Brookline, Massachusetts.

Inge-Martine Pretorius, PhD and D Psych, qualified as a child and adolescent psychotherapist at the AFC in 2004. She is the manager of the parent–toddler service at the AFC. She is a clinical tutor for the MSc in Psychoanalytic Developmental Psychology at University College London and the AFC where she organizes and teaches the child development course. She works part-time in the NHS. She has published in the field of molecular genetics and psychoanalysis, and is co-editor, with Marie Zaphiriou Woods, of *Parents and Toddlers in Groups: a Psychoanalytic Developmental Approach* (Routledge, 2010).

Patricia Radford, a child and adolescent psychotherapist, graduated from the Hampstead Clinic training in 1964. She began her career as a teacher, and shortly after as a psychiatric social worker. She was part of the Anna Freud Centre clinical staff for more than 30 years. During her tenure, she taught courses and supervised clinical trainees. She was a seminar leader for the nursery observation module in the AFC/UCL MSc programme for many years. She worked as clinical consultant to the Robinsfield Primary School for more than ten years. She continues to run a parent discussion group and works in private practice.

Joan Raphael-Leff, PhD, psychoanalyst (fellow, British Psychoanalytical Society) and social psychologist, leads the UCL/Anna Freud Centre academic faculty for psychoanalytic research. Previously, she was head of University College London's MSc in Psychoanalytic Developmental Psychology, and professor of psychoanalysis at the Centre for Psychoanalytic Studies, University of Essex. For 35 years she has specialized in emotional issues of reproduction and early parenting, with more than 100 single-author peer-reviewed publications, and nine books, including: *Psychological Processes of Child-bearing*; *Pregnancy—the Inside Story*; *Parent–Infant Psychodynamics—Wild Things, Mirrors and Ghosts*; *Spilt Milk—Perinatal Loss and Breakdown*; *Ethics of Psycho-analysis*. Founder and first international chair of COWAP (IPA's Committee on Women and Psychoanalysis) in 1998, she provides training for practitioners working with teenage parents, and is consultant to perinatal and women's projects in many high and low income countries.

Helen Ritzema, BSc, DipHE (nursing studies: child), MSc, MACP, graduated from the Anna Freud Centre in 2007. She is currently employed within Cambridgeshire and Peterborough NHS Trust as a research child and adolescent psychotherapist, as part of the National IMPACT (Improving Mood with Psychoanalytic and Cognitive Therapies) study into adolescent depression. Prior to training to be a child and adolescent psychotherapist she was a paediatric nurse working on a cardiology ward at Guy's and St Thomas' NHS Trust.

Luis Rodríguez de la Sierra, MD, is a child and adolescent psychoanalyst, and training analyst, British Psychoanalytical Society. He qualified as a psychiatrist in Barcelona and London, where he also trained as a group therapist. He worked for many years in the NHS and at the Anna Freud Centre, and now works at the London Clinic of Psychoanalysis and in private practice. He lectures and teaches in the UK and abroad, and has published papers on child analysis and drug addiction.

Anne-Marie Sandler, now a retired child psychoanalyst, is slowly winding up her adult psychoanalytic practice. She grew up in Geneva, Switzerland and studied child psychology with Jean Piaget. She obtained a lic. es sc. in 1949, and came to London to study at the Hampstead Child Therapy Course and Clinic in 1950 (graduating in 1955). She served for many years as a member of the education committee and worked in the blind children's nursery, writing several papers on the vicissitudes of their development with Doris Wills, and others with her late husband, Joseph Sandler. She was the director of the Anna Freud Centre, formerly the Hampstead Clinic, from 1993–1996.

Natalia Stafler trained as a child and adolescent psychotherapist at the Anna Freud Centre, graduating in 2006, after which she worked as a toddler group leader for two years at the Anna Freud Centre, and managed the Primary Schools Project. In addition to private practice she worked as a child psychotherapist in TAMHS (Targeted Mental Health in Schools), a government funded project between the AFC and the Tavistock Clinic.

Mary Target, PhD, is a psychoanalyst and clinical psychologist. She has been professional director of the Anna Freud Centre since 2003. She is also professor of psychoanalysis at UCL, director of the MSc in Theoretical Psychoanalytic Studies, and academic and research organizer of the professional doctorate in child and adolescent psychoanalytic psychotherapy. Mary is a fellow of the British Psychoanalytical Society, and an associate clinical professor at Yale University, New Haven, CT. She is a member of the IPA research, and psychoanalysis and universities committees, and of the ad hoc working group on child-only psychoanalytic training. Within the British Psychoanalytical Society, she is chair of the universities liaison committee, hon. sec. of the curriculum committee, and a member of the communications and outreach committee. She serves on several editorial boards, including that of *The Psychoanalytic Study of the Child*. She has written widely and her research is in the areas of attachment and social understanding, psychoanalytic training, and psychotherapy outcomes.

Frances Thomson Salo, PhD, is a member of the British Psychoanalytical Society and a training analyst and past president of the Australian Psychoanalytical Society. She is an associate researcher for the Murdoch Children's Research Institute and has published in the infancy field. She is associate professor on the teaching faculty of the University of Melbourne graduate diploma/masters in infant and parent mental health, and consultant infant mental health clinician in the Centre for Women's Mental Health of the Royal Women's Hospital, Melbourne. She is international chair of COWAP, the IPA Committee of Women in Psychoanalysis, a member of the London editorial board of the *International Journal of Psychoanalysis* and of the Anna Freud Centre international advisory board.

Doris Venguer, MA, in clinical psycho-pedagogy, is a clinical psychologist and child psychotherapist. She graduated from the AFC in 1988, and has been in private practice since 1989. She worked at the Government Children's Hospital in Mexico City until moving with her family to Zurich in 1995. She has worked as a consultant for early childhood and provided parent guidance, diagnostic assessments, and non-intensive psychotherapy for children and adolescents in a school setting in Zurich since 1998.

Peter Wilson qualified from the Hampstead Child Therapy Course and Clinic in 1971. He worked in several child guidance clinics in London and in the Brent Consultation Centre. He became senior clinical tutor at the Institute of Psychiatry, and principal child psychotherapist in Camberwell, London. He then moved on to be the director of the Brandon Centre and later of YoungMinds, a national child mental health charity. He has written numerous chapters and papers and a book, entitled *Young Minds in Our Schools*. He is currently clinical adviser to The Place2Be, a national child mental health charity providing comprehensive school based counselling services.

Elisabeth Young-Bruehl is a psychoanalyst based in Toronto, where she is a member of the Toronto Psychoanalytic Society. She published *Anna Freud: A Biography* in 1988 (second edition, 2008) and *Hannah Arendt: For Love of the World* in 1982 (second edition 2004). Her other books include *The Anatomy of Prejudices* (1996) and the forthcoming *Childism: Confronting Prejudice Against Children* (2012). Currently, she is the general editor of *The Collected Writings of D. W. Winnicott*.

Marie Zaphiriou Woods graduated from the Anna Freud Centre in 1977. She trained as a psychoanalyst from 1990 to 1994 and is now a fellow of the British Psychoanalytical Society. She was the psychoanalytic consultant, and then manager of the Anna Freud Centre parent–toddler group service from 1999 to 2008. Marie teaches and supervises for a number of training schools, and is a training analyst for the British Association of Psychotherapists. With Inge-Martine Pretorius she co-edited *Parents and Toddlers in Groups: a Psychoanalytic Developmental Approach* (Routledge, 2010).

PREFACE

This book takes the reader through the developmental journey of a school of thought which inspired and continues to influence the work of child psychotherapists everywhere, even if sometimes they are unaware of or do not acknowledge the fact. The structure of this book is meant to introduce the reader to the birth, growth, and development of the Anna Freudian Tradition from a perspective of *developmental lines*, by addressing the early development of this tradition and the conflicts and innovations arising from the interaction between the internal and external world of the organization, and by reflecting the developmental crises in the life of this small, non-profit institution with its rich history of service to the community.

Anna Freud's vision, as depicted in the initial part of this book, was that of a centre of clinical practice and research excellence, a place of learning and growth for both children and grown-ups. In addition to the consulting room, the Hampstead Nursery and the toddler groups served as settings where grown-ups learned from children through detailed observation and playfulness, and where troubled children developed within developmentally driven environments.

The clinical training at Maresfield Gardens was one of the most complete and challenging learning experiences any professional could encounter. This book seeks to reflect the richness of the training and the *legacy* it has left in our psychoanalytic community by highlighting clinical papers written by alumni, and by commissioning professionals associated with the Anna Freud Centre to reflect on the impact of their relationship with the AFC on their personal and professional lives.

Clinical work has always been at the heart of the Anna Freud Centre and as such, it represents the main body of this book. These narratives, often shared and discussed during Wednesday meetings at the Clinic, illustrate therapeutic journeys embarked upon by young people and their therapists. They are examples of the skilled observational, technical, and theoretical insights acquired during the learning experience of students at the Anna Freud Centre.

At the present time, both analytic clinical work as well as clinical training have taken new developmental pathways. Specialized training courses around topics very near to Anna Freud's heart, such as children in foster care, work with borderline pathology, children and the courts, and parent–infant work, continue to be offered to multidisciplinary participants. Moreover, the possibility of an IPA sponsored training constitutes one of the current objectives of the directorial team. Recently, a newly developed child psychotherapy service headed by seasoned clinicians (some contributors to this book), was established in order to increase the number of intensive analytic cases seen at the Centre (the AFC website has information on how to donate funds to this effort).

As a second year trainee at the AFC, I attended a local conference and after eagerly presenting my work a colleague approached me and asked: "Is it true that at the Anna Freud Centre you are allowed to do psychotherapy on the front steps?" Well, perhaps not always on the front steps of the Centre, but since its inception, Anna Freud's vision was of a child psychoanalytic theory which could be transposed to other fields, and most importantly that could be applied to environments outside the consulting room. All through this book you will find examples of such work in schools, hospitals, and the legal system. You will also find work with hard to reach populations such as foster children and refugee families. So, yes! Anna Freudians do like the challenge of working outside the consulting room.

This book is filled with many voices, the voices of children and their families and their psychotherapists, and the voices of alumni whose own developmental paths were influenced by the experience of having trained at the Anna Freud Centre. Together, these voices help to weave the history of an institution, its legacy, and its growing pains. In doing so, they pay homage to the often unassuming and humble woman whose vision continues to live on in the work of her students, and the children and families who benefit from it. That, in the opinion of this editor, is the true legacy of Anna Freud. The stubborn conviction of her ideas and our wish to share them with others were the key motivations behind the development of this book.

Norka Malberg,
New Haven, CT, March 2011

PROLOGUE

This book honours a long-standing innovative tradition. It celebrates Anna Freud's contributions—her corpus of writing, empirical testing of psychoanalytic concepts, and their application in child psychotherapy and applied work far beyond the consulting room. Above all it focuses on her main achievement—the Hampstead Child Therapy Course and Clinic, and its evolution into the Anna Freud Centre.

This book is an attempt to render visible the principles underpinning work at Maresfield Gardens over the generations, guiding clinicians and scholars, both within and outside this school of thought. At this time of rapid change, we offer the book as a testimonial, hoping that psychoanalytic thinking will continue to inspire current and future managements, regardless of transformations in terms of the broad scope of Anna Freud Centre courses and interventions, and the interdisciplinary nature of research.

Fundamental principles of this tradition are outreach, training, and preventive as well as sustained therapeutic work. These involve the evaluation of clinical efficacy, scholarly attention to epistemic problems emphasizing close examination of psychoanalytic concepts (i.e monitoring clinical predictions rigorous note-taking, and systematic collation of data about the same phenomenon, followed by ongoing study group exploration); finally, a flexibility that allows for conceptual modifications arising in this interplay between theory, observations, clinical understanding, and technique, while retaining the basic tenets of psychoanalysis.

* * *

This book has several goals.

On one hand, it attempts to provide a clear and succinct summary of contributions of the Anna Freudian tradition to the field of child psychotherapy.

Some of these have now become common currency in clinical work of child psychotherapists across divergent theoretical groups: the reciprocal cross-fertilization of observation and psychoanalytic theory; the need to include the family in clinical work with children; the idea of transference as mitigated by the real active ongoing and necessarily dependent relationship of the child with his/her parents; the effect of the sex of the therapist; emphasis on the therapeutic alliance in children and adults alike, and latterly, the value of integrating a perspective of dynamic family reciprocity constitutive of the intrapsychic. Similarly, clinical concepts now adopted by child psychotherapists across theoretical schools include age-appropriate readiness; normal transitory delays; developmental deficits and the idea of disharmonious or uneven maturation across "developmental lines"; damaged self-representation; inadequate reflective capacity, and faulty ego structuralization in the case of abuse and trauma—and the need to modify technical procedures in these cases. Hence, timely identification of "toxic" pathogenic agents; distinction between "primitive" defences and more sophisticated ones; identification with the aggressor; altruistic surrender; interactive mechanisms. And, the need for "developmental guidance" and psycho-educational supplements for carers.

A second goal is to trace and acknowledge the expansion of psychoanalytic theory and therapeutic technique over the years.

We address this by including an introduction to each part of the book, written by a senior clinician who presents an overview of transitions, clinical application, and current developments. This is followed by detailed observations and intensive psychoanalytic case work, including lively verbatim material from each of the specified age-groups. The clinical chapters, from the younger generation of graduates across the world, illustrate the therapeutic process. In true Anna Freudian tradition, each part also includes an example of outreach application. The importance of work outside the consulting room is now accepted by child psychotherapists of all persuasions, and many psychoanalytically informed institutes around the world now run services in schools and doctors' surgeries, while graduates of child psychotherapy trainings work in children's centres, hospitals, court services, and prisons, and consult to a variety of professionals and practitioners who work with babies, children, and young people.

A final aim of our book is an invitation to revisit Anna Freud's work while considering the needs of today's children in different settings, with modifications to meet exceptional situations.

The book comprises four parts.

The initial part provides a framework for the reader to embark on the developmental journey of an institution, its people, its mission, and diverse range of applications. This includes an introduction to the Centre's current vision as well as historical, didactic, and biographical chapters focused on Anna Freud's legacies of theory, training, and praxis.

The second part delineates a series of "developmental phases" beginning with infancy and ending with late adolescence, providing examples of case work with each of these age groups, and applications elsewhere—thus highlighting how the Anna Freudian tradition has been both preserved and modified in clinical work and outreach in the context of ever-changing sociocultural realities.

The third part focuses on specialized work in the Anna Freudian tradition, including court assessment projects, work in paediatric psychology, toddler group outreach, and applications of such thinking to consultative work with groups of lay and professional workers, including psychologists, social workers, counsellors, midwives, education welfare officers, teachers, and nursery staff …

Finally, the fourth part of the book provides a series of brief personal commentaries from faculty members and alumni who trained at the Centre over the decades, reflecting their own experiences of training, particular technical challenges, and theoretical transitions from a practitioner's perspective.

* * *

As editors, our goal was clarity—of language, structure, and content. We believe the book is accessible to professionals and lay readers alike. It is truly an international product. Not only do the contributors originate and live in many different countries, but the editing too has been a trans-continental affair—we co-editors each resided at various times during the book's preparation in Europe, North and South America, Africa, Australasia, and the Middle East, operating across time zones, on email, Dropbox, Blackberry, Skype, and telephone, with one of us bleary-eyed and the other bushy-tailed; one snowbound, enveloped in sweaters and heaters, while the other sweltered under a swirling fan, through incapacitating and joyful personal life events, electronic glitches, and some major political crises. Nonetheless, the product is robust despite or perhaps due to this hybrid nature of its 36 month gestation, from inception at the 2008 Colloquium to its book-launch on November 4th, 2011.

Our book constitutes an introduction to the evolution of Anna Freud's thinking and application of her ideology in community projects during the war years and after. It provides fine-grained in-depth illustrations of the nature of clinical work as it has evolved in the consulting room, and applications outside it. Ultimately, it offers an overview of the psychoanalytic principles underpinning the Anna Freud Centre's age-old mission of improving the emotional well-being of children and young people.

In keeping with the Anna Freud tradition, the Centre continues to be multifaceted, teaching, treating and conducting natural observations and empirical studies, boosted by laboratory based experiments and outcome research projects with the specific aim of translating scientific findings into effective and innovative interventions for troubled children and families. And despite cessation of its training in child and adolescent psychoanalysis, the AFC remains committed to providing psychoanalytically informed academic and practical trainings, and a wide variety of evidence-based clinical services, including intensive child analysis and parent–infant therapy.

Psychoanalytic schools of thought have proliferated over the decades, enriched by some cross-fertilisation amongst them. Between these covers you will find the roots and branches of one extended family tree. We trust that by illuminating the Anna Freudian tradition in such great detail, our book will delight aficionados, and serve as a vibrant teaching and learning resource for students and practitioners alike.

Joan Raphael-Leff,
London, September 2011

PART I

ANNA FREUD: HER WORK AND LEGACY

Overview

CHAPTER ONE

The Anna Freud Centre today

Mary Target

It is an honour to write this brief introduction to such a welcome and timely book. I am highly aware of how much the Centre has changed, in some important ways almost out of recognition. This is especially true in relation to child psychotherapy and child psychoanalysis, and to a lesser extent in relation to the kinds of research and training which are carried on now, and their integration or otherwise with clinical activity.

Strong cohesion had, in the days of the Hampstead Child Therapy Course and Clinic, been created by an overriding commitment to psychoanalytic theory and treatment, by unquestioned loyalty to Miss Freud as the Centre's leader and founder, and by nearly all professional staff participating right across the Clinic's domains of treatment, research, and training, so that all staff knew each other and worked together continually. And, very importantly, by the presence of the Centre's young patients and their families, together with their therapists, the Centre's own symbolic "children": every cohort of trainees labouring away full-time for four to five years, with nearly all the training on site, Maresfield Gardens, a home for this international group of committed young people.

The atmosphere of the Hampstead Clinic and the early Anna Freud Centre are movingly revived each year at the AFC November Colloquium, where a group of alumni gather. For them I imagine Tuesday and Wednesday may perhaps always somewhere be tinged with the anxiety and excitement of presenting or hearing a new profile or paper!

That was how the Centre was when I arrived in 1988 to do some research on the outcome of child psychoanalysis. It was roughly the same place I read about in the copious material (800 files of assessments, weekly reports of the analytic process and of the painstaking parent work, research group minutes, and hundreds of Wednesday papers), which I felt privileged to absorb as I prepared my PhD. This was a retrospective study of child psychoanalytic outcomes at the Centre, enabled by *George Moran* and Peter Fonagy, which we continued after George's tragic death. George, who liked people to keep busy, also got me to sort out a lot of archive materials relating to the early history of the Centre, and it was this material which made very real to me what I had begun to understand from analytic publications and biographies. In the painstaking notes, minutes, observations, and correspondence, there were principles and priorities forming a backbone for the Centre's work.

* * *

I would like to introduce this book by naming what seemed to me some central enduring principles. However, first it is important to acknowledge the great gap in the Centre's earlier identity left by the closure of the four to five year full-time training in psychoanalytic psychotherapy for children.

Closure of the training:

In 2003 Anna Freud Centre's board reluctantly took the decision that heavily subsidizing the training was taking a large proportion of its income, raised with difficulty for other purposes, treatment, and research, and that as most trainees by then went on to work in the NHS, the NHS should meet its responsibility to fund the training. The incoming directorial team of myself, Linda Mayes, and Peter Fonagy set about first trying to negotiate with the NHS to provide secure funding on a new basis, then when that proved impossible, to establish a collaboration with the British Association of Psychotherapists to provide a joint training and clinical psychotherapy service. For different reasons, the intensive work on both initiatives was unsuccessful. We are currently very hopeful about the possibility of contributing to a new child psychoanalytic training in collaboration with the Institute of Psychoanalysis and other psychoanalytic child or adolescent centres in London. Ideally, although this is a distant goal, this could eventually lead to the fulfilment of one of Anna Freud's hopes, to have child analytic training (without requiring prior adult analytic training) recognized by the IPA as a route to membership, and the AFC could play a part in that. One of the Centre's many distinguished alumnae, Dr Jill Miller of Denver, has laid a vital foundation for this possibility through her successful work to create such a "child only" route to membership of the American Psychoanalytic Association.

Principles and applications of the Anna Freud Centre's work in the twentieth and twenty-first centuries

The Hampstead Clinic and Anna Freud Centre's dedication to the emotional well-being of children has several strong branches—theoretical, educational, therapeutic, research, all extending into social involvement and international collaboration. Let us look at some of these, past and present:

Theoretical tradition: In Anna Freud's day the Hampstead nurseries and Clinic were founded on a psychoanalytic model of normality and pathology, including theoretically based clinical assessments such as the developmental lines and profile which mapped each child's pattern of emotional growth. The uniqueness of these diagnostic methods lay in the development of systematic ways of observing and integrating the interaction of internal and external influences, framed by a strong metapsychological framework.

Education and training: was always at the heart of the Centre. During the war, training the staff of the War Nurseries began the creation of a whole generation of future child psychoanalysts. With the inception of the Hampstead Child Therapy Course a series of training and post-qualification activities developed in order to satisfy what Anna Freud felt were important professional development requirements. The clinical groups and the Wednesday meetings connect us to those activities even in such different times. The annual colloquium was and is a time for clinicians to discuss clinical work and explore common ground.

Therapeutic tradition: Child analytic thinking took many forms at the Hampstead Clinic: intensive and non-intensive psychotherapy with children and parents, and collaboration with allied professionals such as teachers and medical personnel in order to support children and their families. I would particularly like to mention the work of the social workers: all the hundreds of reports I read by Nicky Model and Barbara Grant impressed me by their penetrating delineation of what would now be thought of as systemic factors, and by their unsentimental but evident compassion. Research groups studied work with borderline, adopted, blind, or chronically ill children, and other special groups challenging and extending classical analytic principles. Preventive measures such as early intervention with toddler and nursery age children and their parents were also an important aspect of the clinical work at the Hampstead Clinic. All the clinical work went hand in hand with intensive study and discussion.

The research tradition was, as stated above, rooted in the understanding of specific disorders or conditions affecting development, and through conceptual research, especially the massive Hampstead Index (it must be admitted that "indexing" tends to be referred to as though an example of intergenerational trauma).

Social involvement and collaboration: There are numerous examples of this principle, through the decades, from work with war trauma; judicial and legislative consultation work to advocate the best interests of the child (Yale University); collaboration with child psychiatry services in very impoverished east London; work with paediatric patients on the wards of the Middlesex Hospital.

Today in the Anna Freud Centre many of these strong traditions continue, in twenty-first century incarnations:

The psychoanalytic model of normality and pathology is taught and adhered to as a broad framework, but it has become more interdisciplinary, incorporating contemporary thinking and evidence. For instance, the concept of mentalization posits a developmental line in the ego psychology tradition of Anna Freud, and I believe connects directly with the technique of developmental help, but is influenced by the work of Bion, the French psychosomatic school, Winnicott, Bowlby, as well as research in developmental and clinical psychology. It therefore offers bridges within and beyond psychoanalysis. The theoretical model of stages of early self-development, affect representation, experience of psychic reality, personality functioning and the family are underpinned by many theoretical and clinical psychoanalytic papers and an ongoing interdisciplinary discussion group (areas of exposition include: social cognition and attachment; personality disorder; aggression; violence; development of psychic reality; normal and neurotic development; relationship to other psychoanalytic theories and to research findings; mental experience as embodied, and new ideas on psychosexuality). Special clinically based groups in the Centre are developing their own models of parent–infant psychotherapy, work with toddlers and parents, work with personality disordered parents, and so on.

Theory based assessments include many measures developed for clinical and research work in areas such as parent–infant interaction, affect regulation, attention, coding of play and attachment narratives, etc.

The Anna Freud Centre now promotes a new, wider intellectual framework for psychoanalytic and related research, which includes developmental studies (identifying psychological and neural mechanisms underlying disturbance); therapeutic techniques specifically designed to address a developmental dysfunction, different age groups, and diagnostic problems; and a developmental neuroscience lab straddling psychodynamic developmental ideas, empirical psychology, and neuroscience.

Similarly, current programmes of education and training include popular short courses and workshops for clinicians and researchers in the field, covering a very wide range of areas. Some of the courses are delivered in association with UCL or to implement government priorities for professional training. Although far from psychoanalysis, they bring other professionals, young trainees, and older policy makers into the Centre, and connect us strongly with the world of child and family mental health today.

In addition, we run several high quality and popular University College London graduate programmes, developing the strong affiliation between our institutions started under the directorship of Mrs Anne-Marie Sandler. They include four master of science degree programmes (one taught 50% at Yale), a professional doctorate and a psychoanalytic PhD programme. The strong link to Yale Child Study Center is a vital and growing part of the Centre's identity and activity.

The annual Child Psychoanalytic Colloquium continues to be held at the Anna Freud Centre, now very ably organized by three child psychoanalysts who trained at the Centre, and the staff organize and present at many other international professional conferences.

The clinical orientation of the Anna Freud Centre is now more multidisciplinary, and multimodal. Treatments offered at the AFC still include both intensive psychoanalysis for children, and non-intensive therapy parent work, and therapeutic applications for specific disorders or populations (e.g., the parent–infant project, adolescents in crisis, maltreated fostered and adopted children, family relationship problems, and children undergoing dialysis). Developing and offering a range of evaluated treatments recognizes that children and families need a variety of treatments, and meets the challenge of the current policy agenda to widen access to psychological help for those most in need. Furthermore, integrative approaches may be important particularly for special clinical groups with complex problems such as families with severe adversity and/or very poor parenting. Studies show that common factors in the therapeutic process underlie the effectiveness of all talking therapies. A psychoanalytic model of the mind and of the therapeutic relationship can be extended through broader concepts such as "mentalization": all psychotherapies develop an interactional matrix in which the developing mind becomes a focus. In the area of prevention, the AFC has expanded outreach in the form of toddler groups in areas of great deprivation, school-based groups, work in prisons and hostels for homeless mothers and infants, and training of practitioners working with teenage parents and their children.

The AFC has burgeoned as a research centre studying a wide range of phenomena, including basic research on infant social-cognitive development; neuroscience of development and maltreatment; outcome research and systematic reviews (e.g., process-outcome of psychotherapies, evaluation of routine clinical effectiveness, Parent–Infant Project [PIP] Randomised Control Trial, and a very large study of the treatment of adolescent depression); and a range of studies of attachment: infancy, child, and post-adoptive placement. The Anna Freud Centre builds our wider scientific credibility and impact on policy by combining academic and clinical leadership with developmental psychopathology research.

Finally, in terms of contemporary social involvement and collaboration, most of the AFC's clinical projects now operate in the community, many in collaboration with other leading state and voluntary services (e.g., Great Ormond Street Hospital, the Marlborough Family Service, the Tavistock Clinic, Kids' Company, Islington CAMHS and Local Authority, the Brandon Centre). Our strong and growing academic links with Yale and UCL extend the clinical collaborations to research, training, and educational opportunities.

In sum, the Anna Freud Centre has lost a central plank of its original identity through no longer having the intensive psychoanalytic training, but it has gained in range and impact in other respects and across a much wider sphere. The original classical child psychoanalytic focus has broadened, and the developmental understanding of normality and pathology cuts across treatment models and reaches a much wider professional audience. Our research intersects with work on behavioural genetics and social/affective neuroscience, all the time focusing on aspects of parent-child relating, and its effects on the child's growing internal world. There has been great change, but also continuity, and the Centre remains a place where people come from all over the world to think about how to understand and help children and families. We continue to draw strength from thinking about their complex developmental problems in depth, respecting complexity and being ready to find new solutions—in theory and in practice—to improve and extend what can be offered.

CHAPTER TWO

Anna Freud: the teacher, the clinician, the person

Elisabeth Young-Bruehl

Very seldom in the history of psychoanalysis has a contributor appeared who could be and do everything to the highest level—and wear all the hats so beautifully. An adult and child clinician; a training analyst, supervisor, and mentor; both a theorist in and a historian of psychoanalysis as a science and a profession; an institution founder and builder, and an institution director; an expert extending "applied analysis" into other fields like paediatrics, social work, law; a model of integrity and ethical comportment, with virtues of the "classical" sort, acknowledged across all human endeavours and cultures—magnanimity, justice, moderation, courage. For most of her working life, Anna Freud was the spokesperson of psychoanalysis, its communicator—and probably the only one who could stand up and give a lucid hour-long lecture without a note.

In fact, Anna Freud was uniquely exceptional. For she was and did everything with the addition—both a magnificent advantage and a great challenge—of being her father's daughter, and the most obvious inheritor of his creation and his fame. In the history of fathers and daughters, which is a history replete with sexism, what she did and who she was, are hardly imaginable. Although the Greeks, with their renowned capacity for familial fantasy, were able to imagine a presiding male deity with a daughter worthy of his kingdom—a virgin daughter, renowned for her wisdom and her capacity to nourish wise (or wily) male mortal protégés like Odysseus. But even the Greeks could not imagine multi-talented Athena, woman warrior endowed with swift thoughts, as having a gift for understanding and helping children. Nor could they imagine Athena herself as a child—they had to picture her born full-grown, sprung out of the forehead of her father, Zeus!

I have always thought it curious that the consensus among analysts who marvelled at Anna Freud and wanted to honour her (in the *Gymnasium*-trained, European way) with a full complement of classical allusion, designated her an Antigone, a far less independent figure than Athena. In his desktop art collection, Freud had a treasured medallion given to him by his followers that presented on one side Oedipus and the Sphinx, and on the other Oedipus and Antigone. She was the strong-principled (the Greek name means "anti-bending" but also possibly "anti-child-producing") nursemaid daughter to her blind father Oedipus. In her father's manner, she was also the opponent of King Creon, who condemned her to death along with his son Haemon, her fiancé—for her attachment to nature's laws and defiance of his self-serving kingly decrees. Unlike Anna Freud, she accomplished nothing of her own; she was all defence.

Anna Freud herself helped foster this Anna-Antigone tradition by presenting herself as selflessly dedicated to *die Sache*, the psychoanalytic cause. She even wrote the first case study on selfless dedication. In her 1936 book *The Ego and the Mechanisms of Defence*, which she dedicated to her father on his birthday, her case study appears in a chapter on "Altruistic surrender" and other defences emergent in puberty. Unlike the Antigone fans who celebrated her, in that chapter Anna Freud showed a good deal of awareness that those who find themselves unable to be self-assertive and Oedipally triumphant will often sign over their ambitious wishes to male protégés and their erotic ones to girlfriends. They submerge themselves in a cause, and in every way possible avoid direct fulfilment of their wishes or gaining honours for themselves. From our present viewpoint, there is something self-constraining in being Antigone, and something collusive in an analyst who is willing to help celebrate Antigone's self-constraint.

We may wonder whether psychoanalysts did not want Freud to have a fully grown-up successor—except the few who coveted that role for themselves, and they sank under the weight of their own narcissism. The two of his original circle with great dedication to *die Sache*, along with great institution-building gifts and hospital research experience, Abraham and Ferenczi, died young. So, since 1939, psychoanalysis has had a positively Shakespearean kingly dynastic "succession crisis": with one father-daughter Lear-like play in it and a "play within that play" in which another—Melanie Klein—wanted to be the favoured daughter and ended up being just her very own version of a jealous sister.

Considering all the drama that swirled around her, particularly during the wartime "Controversial Discussions" in London, it is all the more remarkable that Anna Freud did and was, all that she did and was. When I wrote her biography in the mid-1980s, not long after her death, a few of her old associates from Vienna and Berlin were still alive to share their pre-war memories of her as well as their Hampstead memories. It was possible to construct a full, rounded portrait of her. The earliest generation of her students and collaborators in the Hampstead War Nurseries—many of them refugees from the Continent—were still alive to carry on her work at the Anna Freud Centre. Since then, since that brief moment between her death in 1982 and the outbreak of the complexities known as "The Freud Wars" in the late 1980s and on through the 1990s, with aftershocks up to the present, there has been no other good moment for a full-scale biography of the "life and works" sort developed—long before Freud—by the English descendents of Samuel Johnson.

So, it is all the more important to have the years since Anna Freud's death chronicled collectively by younger people who trained with her and took up her work when she was in her high old age and hoping that her programmes, her institutions, her ideas, would not suffer a "succession crisis". She was very fortunate in the people who came to study and work with her, often from far-flung places, as this volume attests. Full of life, and since renamed the Anna Freud Centre, her creation has survived her. But in her lifetime, when she was doing the succession planning for her own role, fate had not been kind to her. From 1948, when the brilliant *Kate Friedlander*, who contributed so much to the psychoanalytic study of adolescence and delinquency in the manner of Anna Freud's friend August Aichhorn, died before she could take up the role of director of the Hampstead Training Programme, to the time in the 1990s, when the brilliant *George Moran*, successor-designate to the directorship, died young of the motor neuron disease ALS, Anna Freud lost perfect multi-talented flame-keepers. And that last, tragic loss came just as the whole enterprise she and *Dorothy Burlingham* had created was beginning to enter into a period of crisis in external support and funding that changed it into an enterprise no single person could possibly have led. [Those whose names appear in the text in italics are followed in more depth in the Appendix.]

Since her death, directors at the Anna Freud Centre have had to divide her labour among themselves, in times when support of child psychoanalytic centres from public or private sources became even more tenuous. Under those conditions, no one of them—no one anywhere—could possibly have done all that she could do at the levels she attained. Her days had been filled with clinical work, with teaching, with case conferences (during which her summations and commentaries were the highlights), with meetings, and then, in the evenings and at the weekends, with reading dozens and dozens of reports on cases, on conferences, on group projects for exploring clinical phenomena or concepts, or for indexing and creating diagnostic profiles. (This at a time when paperless communications and electronic record-keeping were not even on the horizon.) She was running a laboratory, a scientific research project on a huge scale (with small budgets), a multifaceted clinic, two nurseries, and a training—perhaps the finest school in the world for students of psychoanalysis.

Looking back on her achievement, historically, it has a symphonic quality to it. In the first movement, culminating in *The Ego and the Mechanisms of Defence*, she laid the foundations for child analysis as she understood it, technically and theoretically, and tested her approach in her first small-scale institutions—a post-WWI *Hort* (a small school for displaced children), a school for children in analysis, a nursery—with her first group of collaborators (many of whom had small children of their own to learn from).

The coming of WWII took her into a period of work in group homes, residential nurseries, and a complex mixture of analytical work and child observation. The emphasis she had put earlier on Developmental Lines deepened, like themes being played in different keys.

A third movement began when she started the training programme at Hampstead after the war, and was able to start collating the work of many analysts and trainees and nursery workers, making a true research centre, and realizing that she had the situation for studying normal development. All of this came together in *Normality and Pathology in Childhood* (1964–5). Then, on the basis of that synthesis, she could clearly make distinctions between infantile neuroses—where her work had begun—and developmental disorders.

The culmination came over the next ten years: her clinical and observational research went largely down that developmental disorders path, with a big extension into the development of infants (in their relations with their caregivers). But she then changed mode and opened the path—the melody, the chorus—of her collaboration with Albert Solnit and Joseph Goldstein (supported, as always, by Dorothy Burlingham, the silent author) to produce the three volumes of *In the Best Interests of the Child*. I think it is no exaggeration to say that no other psychoanalytic book has had as profound an influence in the wider world on thinking about children and on policy towards children, as that hopeful finale, that "*An die Freude*".

In psychoanalysis, no realm of discovery is ever left behind; each developmental step of the science itself depends upon previous developments and draws what went before into itself. So it goes, too, with analytic explorers—and if they work for sixty years, as Anna Freud did, they certainly consolidate a lot of developmental steps! And her developmental story is particularly intense because psychoanalysis was her life, all day, every day; it was her *Lebensform*. This is a complicated legacy for a group of people to inherit and carry on, and it is a privilege to have a volume in which representatives of that varied group consider their individual and collective tasks and their—as Freud used to put it—*fons et origio*.

References

Freud, A. (1937). *The Ego and the Mechanisms of Defence*. London: Hogarth.

Freud, A. (1965d). Normality and pathology in childhood: assessments of development. In: *The Writings of Anna Freud, Vol. VI*. New York: International University Press.

Goldstein, J., Freud, A. & Solnit, A. J. (1984). *Beyond the Best Interests of the Child*. New York: Free Press.

Goldstein, J., Freud, A., Solnit, A. J. & Goldstein, S. (1986). *In the Best Interests of the Child*. New York: Free Press.

Historical Framework

CHAPTER THREE

Anna Freud and her collaborators in the early post-war period[1]

Christiane Ludwig-Körner

This chapter traces the origins of the Anna Freud Centre in London and some of the many women (and a few men) helped in those hard times of deprivation to build it up. [Those whose names appear in the text in italics are followed in more depth in the Appendix.]

When Anna Freud had to leave Vienna in 1938, she left many things behind which were dear to her. One of those was the Jackson Day Nursery created in February 1937. With the help of a generous donation from the American Edith Jackson, who gave her cases to Anna Freud for supervision, Anna Freud had just started to realize her life's dream: to create a psychoanalytic day nursery for less well-off children below the age of two. As a result of the growing anti-Semitism, the day nursery was not allowed to officially bear the name of Anna Freud. Thus, the project was purposefully brought into connection with the renowned Montessori Society, the more so as Anna Freud appreciated the work of Maria Montessori, and could use its premises. Staff members were the Montessori Nursery School teacher Hilde Fischer, her assistant Mizzi Milberger and the director of the nursery, Hertha Fuchs-Wertheim. Julia Deming, an American doctor, who also gave her child cases to Anna Freud for supervision, was in charge of the children's nutrition. The paediatrician Josephine Stross had attended psychoanalytical courses at the Vienna Institute. She was responsible for the preliminary examination and medical care.

It had been the wish of Edith Jackson and Anna Freud to gain more data from direct observation of early life, particularly of the second year which they considered especially important in leading from primary to secondary process function, as well as for the development of the

[1]Revised version of the article "Webereiter der Kinderanalyse. Die Arbiet in der "Jackson Kinderkrippe" und den "kriegskinderheimen", Luzifer-Amor, *Zeitschrift zur Geschichte der psychoanalyse*, 25, pp. 78–104, 2000.

superego, for drive control and cultivation of object relations. In the last annual report of the crèche, Anna Freud wrote:

> We know something about infants from developmental studies, from adults' retrospective reconstructions, and from child analysis with its microscopic view of the infant's inner life. What we need to see now are the actual experiences of the first years of life, from the outside, as they present themselves. Thorough knowledge of infancy is the goal (quoted by Young-Bruehl, 1988, p. 218).

In London, Anna Freud could resume this interrupted work in the "War Nurseries" she created.

The Hampstead Nurseries

When the bombing of London forced many families to take refuge in the Underground train station shafts, nurseries were urgently needed. In 1940, Anna Freud and *Dorothy Burlingham* started preparations to establish a children's home and by January 1941, the Children's Rest Centre was the first of three London War Nurseries to open in Hampstead, at 13 Wedderburn Road, NW3, supported by donations and furnished with the furniture of the former Jackson Nursery brought from Vienna. In February 1941 twenty-five children were cared for in this house. Most of them came from London's East End, which during the Blitz had been razed to the ground by the German bomb attack on London. Anna Freud needed many colleagues, because she upheld the idea of a care ratio of one adult to three/four children. However she could only offer a small salary. Nonetheless, many applied. The young German speaking women whom Anna Freud and Dorothy Burlingham employed had been driven out of their home country, and often had lost close relatives in the concentration camps. For them the work with Anna Freud and her circle offered a form of holding, and for some, temporarily, a substitute for family (personal interviews with *Hansi Kennedy*, 23.4.1997, Manna Friedman, 21.11.1996).

One of the first kindergarten teachers whom Anna Freud employed in the War Nurseries was Hedy Schwarz, who in Vienna had directed a Montessori Kindergarten. In the War Nurseries, she could take over a "completely installed Montessori Kindergarten" (Anna Freud, p. 367). It was from her that the then just seventeen-year-old *Hansi Kennedy* got to hear about the proposed opening of another house—the "Babies Rest Centre" at 5 Netherhall Gardens, very near the first house. *Hansi Kennedy* worked in the War Nurseries from 1941 until 1945 and took in all the knowledge which was offered to her in the regular team meetings and the training. About five workers in the Hampstead Nurseries, in parallel to their jobs, undertook additional courses at the university, completed their school exams or, respectively, started studies in psychology or social work.

It was from Hedy Schwarz that *James Robertson*, a Quaker and conscientious objector, and his young wife got to know that Anna Freud was looking for workers. *Joyce Robertson* had participated from the start, since the end of 1940, and her husband Jimmy joined early in 1941. Being a newly married English couple, they represented an exception among the mostly single, émigré Jewish women. Their opinion was important for Anna Freud since, coming from working class families, they could offer "translation help" not just on linguistic questions, but on cultural differences. In addition, James Robertson was one of the few men who worked in the war nurseries. His presence was important not just to extinguish incendiary bombs, but particularly to serve as model for identification in the place of the many absent fathers. Joyce and James Robertson contributed until the closing of the war nurseries.

Sophie and *Gertrud Dann* were part of the staff of the war nurseries from June 1941. Sophie Dann, a trained educator, children's nurse, and midwife, and her sister Gertrud, a trained nursery nurse and infant nurse, had to emigrate in 1939 from Augsburg to London. At first they earned their livings as maids until they both found lifelong work with Anna Freud. Sophie Dann was responsible for the care of infants, the mothers, and the milk kitchen, and later on also for the medical department; Gertrud Dann cared for the toddlers.

* * *

Every midday, when the children were sleeping, there were regular team meetings where observations on the children and newly occurring problems were discussed. Anna Freud strongly emphasized precise observation of the children, i.e. how they reacted to separations from their mothers and/or fathers; how they dealt with each other; their level of development, etc. All colleagues, be they educators, nurses, or students, were asked to note their observations on children on small cards. With that, Anna Freud followed her research interest on the one hand, and on the other, she met her obligation to deliver monthly reports to the financial "mother organization", the Foster Parents' Plan for War Children, Inc., in New York. Later, she used these records with Dorothy Burlingham (1942) in their books *Young Children in War-Time: A Year's Work in a Residential Nursery*, or respectively in *War and Children*.

Gertrud Dann remembers that in the beginning she was irritated, wondering what she was supposed to note, until Anna Freud told her: "Write down what is getting your attention as being 'particular'. Particular, because a child behaves differently than you expect or behaves differently than before" (Gertrud Dann, interview 21.11.1996). Anna Freud delivered theoretical explanations, but above all she transmitted her analytical attitude to those young colleagues and students, most of whom in the beginning understood nothing of psychoanalysis.

Thus Hannah Fischer, who had come to the Hampstead Nursery at the age of sixteen as the youngest student, remembers how Anna Freud talked about "pedagogic love".

> She meant a particular form of love, which we as educators should be ready to offer children; so that they feel accepted by, and safe with us; a type of love, which does not demand love in return—as is natural for parents—but which just belongs to children, and which sees in the children of one's own group representatives of the totality of all children. Unlike the love of parents, which belongs to a measurable number, meaning to their own children, pedagogic love of the entrusted child is inexhaustible, transferable from one child to another, from one group to another (Laible, 1982, p. 17).

Looking for further suitable colleagues, Anna Freud asked the certified psychologist and social worker *Dr Ilse Hellman*, a former assistant of Charlotte Bühler from Vienna, if she would be ready to take over the direction of the house at 5 Netherhall Gardens and care for the toddlers.

From March 1941 until the home closed in September 1945, she headed the children's home ("Babies' Rest Centre") in which up to fifty children were cared for. Her first visit to the War Nurseries already impressed Ilse Hellman, as she was used to another way of handling children. She remembers that she visited at mealtime, and even the one-and-a-half- or two-year-old children sat together at a big table, and were allowed to eat with relish with their hands, selecting what they wanted from a small buffet so they composed their meals themselves. This was a study on eating habits of children which had started already in the Jackson Nursery in Vienna with the help of the American Julia Deming.

This very different way of dealing with infants and small children irritated Gertrud Dann, who had previously headed her own kindergarten in Augsburg. She remembers one of her first working days:

> … and I realized that someone watched me and that this someone did not like what I was doing. I thought that I just cannot do anything different. I fed that baby as any other baby and this someone then came up to me and said: "I am Anna Freud." I did not ask "What actually did I do wrong?", but I was absolutely sure that something was wrong. Much later in a meeting people talked about children's nutrition, and then it came up. It is totally wrong to hold children … to educate them that they should not touch the food. The children should be allowed to "smack into" the spinach, into the millet gruel, that this does not matter, and one should not hold the babies in the way we had learned in baby-care—the baby holds the thumb and then one can [spoon] feed. Sophie said: "But the spinach and the fresh overalls …" Then Anna Freud said: "Does not matter. The fresh overalls—you can replace and wear another one, but the babies need to *know* what they eat." And the "Junior Toddlers" did eat really terribly. With the hands. [But] it did not take long, and then they learned quite fast to eat with a spoon. Yet then without drill. Then they, the children, learned voluntarily. And when they wanted, one would help them. Yet very soon they wanted to eat alone. And it was very interesting—that's what Miss Burlingham wanted to try—if a child, about one and a half years old, was able to decide for himself what the right food would be for the child. Thus, there were ten or twelve Junior Toddlers, sitting in a circle, though in a way that each of them saw the back of the other one. Each had a small table, on that table was a board with, I think, about ten small bowls. In each bowl was something different. A piece of meat, a piece of chocolate, a piece of cake, a salad leaf, totally different and in the middle there was an adult, who each time, when meat had been eaten, could add another piece into the bowl. We did this—I don't know—[for] perhaps three weeks. And then it was already absolutely clear that those dumplings had eaten the chocolate, the cake, the cookies, the others the meat, the piece of apple. That was quite interesting, but not yet necessarily proven. And then came the flying bombs, and one had to bring the children in the middle of the meals down into the cellar, and one had so much annoyed the children, and they were so furious that the meal was interrupted. There was no sense in starting this again. And Miss Burlingham sat always apart and was recording which child took meat or cheese. It was a very interesting experiment (interview: 14.7.1996).

Already then, Anna Freud was of the opinion that children had preferences and feelings, and that an early separation of mother and child could have pathogenic effects. She made efforts to include the parents as much as possible in this work. Mothers of newborns were encouraged to live in the house and to work there. In part, they were housekeepers which enabled them to breastfeed their babies. In the same way siblings were accommodated together to foster their relationship. In all homes the house was open night and day for visits of family members. After one year, the War Nurseries were restructured so that four to five children would each have a caregiver meeting their individual wishes and providing affection that is, "family groups" were introduced. Already then, the fundamental importance of the mother-child relationship and attachment was recognized by Anna Freud and taken into consideration in her practical work. James and Joyce Robertson later used their experiences from the War Nurseries when they started working with John Bowlby at the Tavistock Clinic on his research on attachment. (The Robertsons' film *A Two Year Old Goes to Hospital,* showing the effects of even brief separation, was instrumental in getting hospitals to allow parents to stay with their sick child.) Reciprocally, Anna Freud too was inspired by these colleagues. In practical ways she unequivocally made it clear that mother and child belonged together—an attitude which was always vehemently supported by Joyce Robertson.

Training

Already in November 1941, Anna Freud and Dorothy Burlingham decided to offer an informal training programme for the approximately twenty young women who worked in the Hampstead Nurseries. In training these colleagues, Anna Freud harked back to the times in Vienna in the Twenties, when she had held her famous seminar "On the technique of child psychoanalysis". Together with Siegfried Bernfeld and Willi Hoffer, she had created a psychoanalytical working group, the "Children's seminar" (*Kinderseminar*), which met regularly in the Berggasse. This group was composed of people with an interest in working with children, including August Aichhorn, Dorothy Burlingham, Berta Bornstein, Hedwig Hoffer, Muriel Gardiner, Edith Jackson, and others. There was, however, at that time in Vienna no well-established child psychoanalysis. But with this work, Anna Freud linked up to the courses of the Youth Welfare Office of the municipality of Vienna. "In a two year training course, where pedagogues and social workers participated alongside the candidates for therapy training, she had taught under the guidance of Willi Hoffer and together with August Aichhorn, Siegfried Bernfeld, and Editha Sterba a course on psychoanalytic pedagogical knowledge" (Laible, 1978, pp. 43f.).

With her current offer of training, Anna Freud succeeded in winning over many women who were working in the Hampstead War Nurseries on a voluntary base in return for board and lodging, with a bit of pocket money. The candidates lived in shared accommodation in three flats in London, as well as in a renovated warehouse and in a farmhouse in Lindesell, Essex (Anna Freud, Bd. III, p. 871). The demand for this training was so high that waiting lists of candidates were created and many had to be turned down. Except for the heads of department, who were teaching at the same time, and a few paid helpers, the care staff of the Hampstead Nurseries consisted entirely of training candidates. During financial shortages in 1942, staff had to work unpaid for four to six weeks (Anna Freud, Bd. III, pp. 871f.). The theoretical teaching was directly linked to the practical work in the nurseries, along the lines Anna Freud and Dorothy Burlingham had already practised in the Jackson Nursery. It included the working stations: babies from ten days until three months, babies from three to twelve months, milk kitchen, toddlers from one to two years, kindergarten (two to five years), children's school (five to nine years). In addition there were the transient periods in the sickroom and in the air-raid shelter.

By the time of the closure of the Hampstead Nurseries, sixty-six candidates were trained: twenty-eight of them had received a training of at least two years, some of more than four years (Anna Freud, Bd. III, p. 873). Many of the colleagues who acquired psychoanalytical fundamentals in Anna Freud's training courses wanted to gain more competence, as they felt they often reached the limits of their capacities when dealing with traumatized children—and this marked the beginning of a child analytical training.

The countryside

After the bomb attacks increased, it had to be calculated which would be the greater danger for the children—potential physical damage by bombs or a psychic one, if, as a protection of their bodily integrity, they would be evacuated to the countryside and thus separated from their attachment figure. When in summer 1941 a third house was available in Lindesell, Essex, with the name "New Barn", the older children were brought there as it was assumed that they would be better able to manage the separation. A short distance from this home (four minutes' walk over the fields) another little house could then be rented, "The Farmhouse". Both houses were considered as a unit (Die Schriften der Anna Freud, Band II, 1939–1945, Kriegskinder, pp. XVI–XVII). "New Barn" was directed by *Alice Goldberger*, a social worker and crèche nurse from Berlin. Due to petrol rationing, Anna Freud and Dorothy Burlingham could only visit the homes in the countryside one Sunday a month, whereas they were present in the London War Nurseries on a daily basis (interview with Gertrud Dann, 14.7.1996).

From the time these homes were set up Martha Herzberg contributed as well; during the entire period of their existence she headed the household of the War Nurseries without payment. Julia Weiss, initially Sigmund Freud's secretary, was responsible for the book-keeping and the correspondence of Anna Freud, who had an intensive exchange of letters with mothers and soldier fathers of the homed children. She was employed as assistant to the director of the War Nurseries. The paediatrician Josephine Stross, who had already worked in the Jackson Nursery, took over the medical care of the children. From 1942 on, *Dr Anneliese Schnurmann*, a sociologist, also worked on a voluntary base in the War Nurseries in London until their closing in 1945. During the time when the bomb attacks increased and the children had been evacuated to the countryside, Anneliese Schnurmann helped out in the London office. She typed and took care of the payment of the salaries. Many years later, when interviewed as a senior child psychoanalyst, she commented with a grin that "if nothing would have become [out] of me, I would have been a good secretary" (interview with Anneliese Schnurmann, 24.11.1996).

With the end of the war, the purpose of the Hampstead War Nurseries was fulfilled and by September 1945 the children's homes were dissolved. James Robertson had the particular task of reintegrating the children in their families or finding adoptive or foster families and homes for those children who could not return to their families. Out of a total of 191 children who had been cared for in Anna Freud's War Nurseries, 101 later returned to their parents. Ten of those children had lived for over five years in the nursery. Twenty-three children continued to be cared for as day children within the context of the Foster Parents' Plan (Anna Freud, pp. 840f., 865, 869).

Care for children rescued from the concentration camps

When in 1945 children who survived the concentration camps were brought to find a new home in England, appropriate caregivers were looked for under whose charge those children could learn to deal with their traumatic experiences. Acknowledged through their work in the War Nurseries, Anna Freud's colleagues seemed to be the right choice for such work. *Oscar Friedmann* and Alice Goldberger were charged with the task of setting up an appropriate team, since more than 1000 children were anticipated. They had a group of thirty-five colleagues and prepared to receive the children, who were expected to arrive in England first in May, then in July, and finally in August 1945. Many of those children and young people were so undernourished and sick that they could not begin the journey from the death camps to England right away. Those who came to England had no adult relatives on the continent who could care for them.

Alice Goldberger and Oscar Friedmann recognized how important it was for the small children to be integrated as soon as possible in stable small groups or to find appropriate parents for adoption. Among them were six three- to four-year-old orphans, who as babies and infants had been cared for in a group in Theresienstadt. Small for their age, the intense attachment among them was remarkable. When separated, they would fight and support each other against the adults who wanted to care for them (Moskovitz, 1983). Lady Clarke, the wife of the Member of Parliament for East Grinstead, Sussex, made available for them one of her houses, "Bulldogs Bank" in West Hoathly, Sussex for one year under the condition that Sophie and Gertrud Dann were the caregivers for this group of small children. Sophie Dann got to know Lady Clarke at a presentation given by Anna Freud; henceforth, she looked after the two sisters and became their "guardian angel" (Gertrud Dann, 20.11.1996). The Foster Parents' Plan for War Children, Inc., New York, which had supported the Hampstead Nurseries from 1940–1945, now took over the financial support of the Bulldogs Bank children.

On October 15, 1945, after several years in Theresienstadt, another month of waiting in Prague, and two months in the reception camp at Windermere, Westmorland, they were finally brought to the country house "Bulldogs Bank" where Sophie and Gertrud Dann spent a year caring for this group of small children. (On these children, Anna Freud reported in detail together with Sophie Dann in her article "Gemeinschaftsleben im frühen Kindesalter", 1951.)

For the four- to nine-year-old children, Sir Benjamin Drage offered his wonderful manor house "Weir Courteney" in Lingfield, Surrey. He and his family withdrew into the smaller part of the house in order to give the children enough space. Alice Goldberger took over this group, supported by Sofie Wutsch, who had come with Ms Herzberg from Austria, working until now in the War Nurseries as cook. Eight months later, another eleven children, who had survived the Nazi regime in Germany by being hidden, were integrated into this group. Thus a total of twenty-four children aged between three and fifteen were cared for. From 1946 on, *Manna Friedman* joined the staff as an additional colleague. Together with Alice Goldberger, she spent three years caring for this group of children, into which a year later the last of the "Bulldogs

Bank Kinder" who was not adopted, became integrated. This children's home was not directly subordinated to Anna Freud. Yet through the relationship between Alice Goldberger and other colleagues of Anna Freud, there was a close exchange.

In an interview about her work there, *Manna Friedman* says:

> I think these were my happiest years. This was something very special. First, it was in the countryside in a wonderful old house with a beautiful garden—a paradise for children. And we had those children, which needed to be rehabilitated and whom one could make so happy, because they were used to nothing. (...) and it was the most wonderful work, because they were just filling you up with gratitude and they were also therapeutic for me. I know, when I arrived there ... I arrived there with my violin and looked through the window and saw these six-year-old children with shorn hair, who danced, and there I stood outside and started crying. It was a fantastic work ... And there were many helpers, many. People almost sought to work there as volunteers. And sure, we got a salary. It was not very much, but we got money. (...) Hence, it was a fabulous healing through this work and through this spirit with these children. You see, all this time, I was here in England and worked with the children, with the survivors. And this was for me naturally like a therapy, since I knew that my siblings were no more there (12.7.1996).

Anna Freud and Dorothy Burlingham visited this children's home regularly. "And then, we arranged sometimes little children's concerts, and that was always a great day, when Anna Freud came" (interview with Manna Friedman, 12.7.1996).

Child Guidance Clinics

In October 1944 *Kate Friedlander* received from Sussex County Council the mandate to organize an Education Counselling Service (Haager, 1986, p. 67). As a psychoanalyst, she experienced it as a challenge to apply her psychoanalytical knowledge differently than in individual treatment, and hence to develop modified methods of treatment (Friedlander, 1946, 1947). Lydia Jacobs, a psychiatric social worker, who had been trained in psychoanalysis and whom Kate Friedlander knew from the working group around Anna Freud, was one of the first colleagues in the Child Guidance Clinic. All those working there were supposed to have psychoanalytical knowledge, so colleagues who were scheduled for it trained themselves in weekly discussion groups over a period of more than a year. In January 1946 the first two Child Guidance Clinics were opened in Horsham and Chichester—the third being added in February 1947 in Worthing. Each Child Guidance Clinic consisted of a team: one psychiatrist, one child psychologist or child therapist, one psychiatric social worker, and one secretary. Anneliese Schnurmann and Hansi Kennedy were among the first colleagues of the Child Guidance Clinics in Chichester.

Employment in the Child Guidance Clinics allowed them to gain good clinical experience, since not all who attended the Hampstead Training Courses could work there. Moreover, the training candidates needed patients. These were referred partly by the Child Guidance Clinics, and also by Dr Augusta Bonnard and Dr Liselotte Frankl. Both of them also taught in Anna Freud's training programme and offered three more internships in the East London Child

Guidance Clinic (Kennedy, 1995, p. 350). Liselotte Frankl, a medical doctor and psychologist, joined after the early death of Kate Friedlander in 1949. She became the psychiatrist responsible for advanced training and was later also employed at the Hampstead Child Therapy Clinic.

Hampstead Child Therapy Clinic

With the help of the financial support of the Field Foundation in New York, it became possible in 1951 to buy the house at 21 Maresfield Gardens which was just a stone's throw away from the former Hampstead children's homes. When its renovation was finished, the Hampstead Child Therapy Clinic was opened here in February 1952, directed by Anna Freud. In the facilities of this house there were already six treatment rooms, one playroom, offices, a small library, and a classroom for the training candidates. Four years later, a second house was bought in the same street with the support of the New Land Foundation and inaugurated in May 1956 in commemoration of Freud's 100th anniversary. And in 1967, with donations of the Foundation for Research in Psychoanalysis in California it became possible to purchase a third building (Kennedy, 1982, p. 131), number 12 Maresfield Gardens, where a kindergarten was established in the lower floors with the furniture from the Jackson Nursery. The extensive work of the Anna Freud Centre—as the Hampstead Child Therapy Training Course and Clinic was renamed in commemoration of Anna Freud (in 1984, two years after her death)—took place particularly within these three houses with the three interlinked fields: training, therapy, and research.

In 1954, Dorothy Burlingham finally realized her long-cherished wish to open a kindergarten for blind children. On the premises of 21 Maresfield Gardens a small additional building was constructed, designed and executed by Ernst Freud, to be adequate for the needs of blind people. Later, an additional house, number 14 Maresfield Gardens was bought, so that in 1968 after renovation, it was possible to create appropriate working conditions for the continuously expanding areas of interest and the respective increase of staff.

Attached to it was a counselling service for the parents of blind babies. The colleagues undertook home visits to observe the children in their own domestic environment. In addition, a counselling service for mothers, the Well-Baby Clinic, was established—with the aim of advising young mothers in their handling of their babies, be it on medical issues, psychological or educational questions like sleeping or eating habits, weaning, sanitary education, etc. The responsibility for this lay with Josephine Stross, the directing child physician of the clinic. In the mornings, a Play Group was offered for children with their mothers. Thus, those who had previously attended the Well-Baby Clinic could be further accommodated with their children. In 1957, out of this arrangement developed the Nursery School group, which was directed by Manna Friedman until her retirement in 1978:

> When I got employed at the kindergarten, Anna Freud asked me: "Did you ever think about studying this child psychoanalysis?" There I said: "No." "Why not?" And there, I told her: "Because I prefer working with the ego of a child, instead of with the unconscious." And she did accept that. No, I was never particularly interested in it. I wanted to know much about it and learn. But much more on a theoretical level than to apply it therapeutically with children (interview with Manna Friedman, 12.7.1996).

Initially, this Nursery School was also created to offer possibilities for training candidates and personnel to observe the normal course of development. In the first ten years it "offered a half-day programme for children of a largely middle class clientele" (Kennedy, 1982, p. 133); thus, there were among them also children of analysts. Manna Friedman, who had worked in large children's groups in an Israeli kibbutz, remembered how she was initially irritated by the psychoanalytical kindergarten work with this small group of children of middle or upper class people (interview with Manna Friedman, 19.3.2000). Then from 1966 on, the kindergarten focused on "children from underprivileged and disadvantaged families", who grew up under spatially and economically confined living conditions (Kennedy, 1982, p. 134).

Manna Friedman recollects many "pearls of thought" from Anna Freud. Often, she would have said that it was important to save children from the experience of being denied "the pleasure of being good":

> For Anna Freud there existed one main rule in the kindergarten: everything is allowed that makes fun and what does not lead to damaging oneself or others. Did children do something which was not allowed, then they had to sit down on a bank with the comment: "I leave you sitting here [so] that you can think about it." Anna Freud proposed for this the name "thinking bank" yet this was abandoned since it seemed not useful to link thinking with punishment.

During her daily work training candidates were often present:

> They observed what and how I was working with the children. And how, for example, I was dealing with a child in a certain situation; did not interpret it, what you would perhaps be doing in a therapeutic session, but just being pedagogical (interview, 19.3.2000).

Manna Friedman in turn learned much from the fact that regular reporting had to be done on the children. Those reports were then discussed in depth by Anna Freud with the training candidates. "That was in fact my training on the analytical level. There, I have learned a lot. Furthermore, I participated in a Montessori-course, because in the beginning I did not open that nursery alone" (interview, 19.3.2000).

> In the beginning, it wasn't easy for me, in a clinic, where everybody was psychoanalytically trained and I was the only one there in educational work. But this thinking, this empathizing deep into the behaviour of the child, I was … to learn, what it actually means, if a child is aggressive, in order not to say: "So! that one doesn't do!" I anyway did not work like that. I always said I did not work in this nursery in a different way than I had worked in the kindergarten in Israel with fifty children … The pedagogical part, that's what I am good at. And naturally I like to mother people and children, hence this work with these children offered me a lot of satisfaction. But sure, I have learned, why I do something, how I do it (interview with Manna Friedman, 12.7.1996).

For instance, she remembers a very "greedy" four-year-old girl, whose behaviour caused difficulties. When she told Anna Freud in supervision about it, the latter asked her, how she would feel if she imagined that this girl was two years old. She advised treating that girl on an intellectual level as a four-year-old and her "greedy part" as that of a two-year-old girl. Laughing, Manna told me that this girl had now become a very successful businesswoman.

Anna Freud also thought that education included a certain amount of discipline. Some thought that Anna Freud remained deep down in her heart more a pedagogue than a psychoanalyst. Also within the psychoanalytical training she was the "teacher", for whom it was obvious to read the reports of all training candidates regularly and in a disciplined way. There were weekly reports and reviews every two months. In meetings she decided above all whether a child needed psychoanalysis or not.

Manna Friedman remembered observing the process:

> It was also she who assigned the children who needed psychotherapy to the psychoanalysts. With a good intuition she knew the strengths and the weaknesses of the training candidates. Thus, Anneliese Schnurmann got the "artistic" children, and in turn, Alice Goldberger had a particular talent to deal with children which were not very intellectual (interview with Manna Friedman, 19.3.2000).

Commenting about the Nursery, Manna Friedman added:

> After ten years (from 1966 on), we changed the whole programme, and we took also children from underprivileged families and children who did not really have difficulties, yet whose parents had problems with accommodation or unemployment. Thus, the kindergarten was then open from in the morning, like it is also now, until the afternoon at four, for that we had much more the type of child (…) with whom I always had worked. So, this way I liked it certainly more, even though it was hard work, but wonderful. I always preferred to identify with this group of children [than] with those who had it all. There, I thought it was luxury for me. There, I once told Anna Freud: "This is actually not real work for me, this is—here, I am a luxury good!" And she replied: "No, this is very important, these children, they need someone, who will also tell them sometimes, No!" But [they] were fabulous children and they all handled their lives well (12.7.1996).

On another occasion (26.11.1996) she commented:

> These children, some of them were educated too liberal[ly], hence there was never a "no", very little limits put. And the children found that difficult. And it was me who had to set the limits. There had to be, as she [Anna Freud] said, built up a benign superego, so that they got a feeling that it would be much nicer to behave decently, than always have their own will. Thus this was really a difficult time, to arrive there …. And all in all, it was wonderful work. And this I did for twenty-one years. And always continued learning, and also the students, who came to us for observing, could learn always something more.

Conclusion

The experience which Anna Freud and her colleagues had gained in the War Nurseries and countryside children's homes, the Hampstead Child Therapy Clinic and the Child Guidance

Clinics were incorporated into the concepts of child psychoanalysis: in the notion of the relevance of building up attachments, the effect of separations, the influence of substitute mothers, group education, the consequence of traumas and their treatment, and more. Furthermore, this understanding also gave the initial impetus to development of parent–infant therapy and therapy for very young children, as well as formulations in the field of early developmental help and in day care providers.

References

Bolland, J. & Sandler, J. (1965). *Die Hampstead Methode*. Munich: Kindler, 1977.

Essenhigh, C. (1995). Interviews with Hansi Kennedy and Clifford Yorke. *Child Psychotherapy*, *21*(3): 347–374.

Frankl, L. (1964). Die Hampstead Child-Therapy Clinic. In: P. Federn & H. Meng (Eds.), *Psychoanalyse und Alltag* (pp. 189–204). Bern: Hans Huber.

Freud, A. (1957). The contribution of direct child observation to psychoanalysis. In: *The Writings of Anna Freud, Vol. V* (pp. 95–101). New York: International Universities Press. German edition: Direkte Kinderbeobachtungen und Psychoanalyse. In: *Die Schriften der Anna Freud, Bd. 6*. Frankfurt/M.: Fischer Verlag, 1987 (pp. 1701–1706).

Freud A. (1969). Research at the Hampstead Child Therapy Clinic and other papers. In: *The Writings of Anna Freud, Vol. V.* New York: International Universities Press. German edition: Forschungsprojekte der "Hampstead Child-Therapy Clinic" (1957–1960). In: *Die Schriften der Anna Freud, Bd. 6*. Frankfurt/M.: Fischer Verlag, 1987 (pp. 1627–1631).

Freud, A. (1980). *Gemeinschaftsleben im frühen Kindesalter* (pp. 1162–1204). Köln/Opladen: Westdeutscher Verlag, Jahrbuch der Psychoanalyse 1961/1962. Wiederabgedruckt in: A. Freud, D. Burlingham (1971) Heimatlose Kinder. Frankfurt/M.: Fischer Verlag, 1971 (pp. 165–217).

Freud, A. & Burlingham, D. (1942). *Young Children in War-Time: a Year's Work in a Residential Nursery*. London: George Allen & Unwin. German edition: *Kriegskinder: Jahresbericht des Kriegskinderheims Hampstead Nurseries*. London: Imago, 1949.

Freud, A. & Burlingham, D. (1943). *Infants without Families: the Case for and against Residential Nurseries*. London: George Allen & Unwin. German edition: Anstaltskinder. Berichte aus den Kriegskinderheimen "Hampstead Nurseries" 1943–1945. In: *Die Schriften der Anna Freud, Bd. 3*, 1980.

Freud, A. & Dann, S. (1951). An experiment in group upbringing. *Psychoanalytic Study of the Child*, *6*: 127–168. German edition: *Jahrbuch der Psychoanalyse*, *2*: 201–224.

Freud, W. E. (1983). Funeral tribute. In: Anna Freud 1895–1982 [special issue]. *Bulletin of the Hampstead Clinic*, *6*(1): 5–8.

Friedlander, K. (1946). Some notes on the organization of a child guidance service. *New Era in Home and School*, *7*: 170–174.

Friedlander, K. (1947). Psychoanalytic orientation in child guidance work in Great Britain. *Psychoanalytic Study of the Child*, *2*: 343–357.

Furman, E. (1995). Memories of a qualified student. *Child Psychotherapy*, *21*(3): 309–312.

Geissmann, C. & Geissmann, P. (1998). *A History of Child Psychoanalysis*. London: Routledge.

Gilbert, M. (1996). *The Boys: Triumph over Adversity*. London: Weidenfeld & Nicolson.

Haager, J. (1986). Kate Friedländer (1902–1949). *Leben und Werk*. Cologne: Diss. Universität Köln.

Harmat, P. (1988). *Freud, Ferenczi und die ungarische Psychoanalyse*. Tübingen, Germany: Edition Diskord.

Laible, E. (1978). Anna Freud und die Entwicklung der Psychoanalyse. *Jahrbuch der Psychoanalyse, 10*(2): 41–62.

Laible, E. (1982). Anna Freud—von der Arbeit ihres Lebens 1895–1982. *Studien zur Kinderpsychoanalyse, 2*: 13–30.

Ludowyk, G. E. (1963). The analysis of a young concentration camp victim. *Psychoanalytic Study of the Child, 18*: 484–510.

Moskovitz, S. (1983). *Love Despite Hate: Child Survivors of the Holocaust and Their Adult Lives.* New York: Schocken.

Mühlleitner, E. (1992). *Biographisches Lexikon der Psychoanalyse.* Tübingen, Germany: Edition Diskord.

Wolffheim, N. (1958). Kinder aus Konzentrationslagern. *Praxis der Kinderpsychologie und Kinderpsychiatrie, 7*: 302–312.

Young-Bruehl, E. (2008). *Anna Freud: A Biography* (2nd edition). New Haven, CT: Yale University Press.

CHAPTER FOUR

From the Hampstead War Nurseries to the Anna Freud Centre

Inge-Martine Pretorius

The Anna Freud tradition developed and was sustained through the child psychoanalytic training. This chapter traces the origins of the tradition that gave rise to a remarkably thorough way of understanding, describing, and assessing a child's development.

The Hampstead War Nurseries

The Anna Freud Centre—formerly known as the Hampstead Child Therapy Course and Clinic (HCTCC), is a direct descendant of the Hampstead War Nurseries (1941–1945). Directed by Anna Freud and *Dorothy Burlingham*, the three nurseries provided wartime homes for children whose family life had been temporarily or permanently disrupted by the war conditions (*Burlingham* & A. Freud, 1942; A. Freud & *Burlingham*, 1944).

The Children's Rest Centre in Hampstead was the first nursery to open in January 1941. It received ten children, some accompanied by their mothers, seeking refuge from the East End of London, which had been reduced to rubble in the first Blitz. In the summer of 1941, two additional buildings were equipped and opened. The Babies' Rest Centre in Hampstead was a large residential nursery for babies and young children, caring for up to fifty children. The country house, called New Barn, was an evacuation residence for thirty children aged between three and six years (*Burlingham* & A. Freud, 1942; Hellman, 1983). When the three buildings were all working at capacity in 1941, staff cared for 120 children who were between ten days old and six years old.

Although the nurseries aimed primarily at repairing physical and psychological damage already caused by the war and preventing further damage, they also provided a tremendous opportunity for research and teaching (*Burlingham* & A. Freud, 1942). The children presented the possibility for longitudinal studies of child development. To this end, Anna Freud trained her staff to become observers and to keep detailed records. This method of recording observations, which Anna Freud had pioneered in her "experimental" Jackson Nursery in Vienna in 1938, developed into an important research tool in psychoanalytic child observation (Hellman, 1983). All staff members meticulously recorded their observations of children's behaviour on index cards and these observations were discussed.

Most importantly, attached to the nursery, was a theoretical and practical training course for children's nurses and teachers. Nursery staff used their rest hours to attend a series of courses prepared by more senior members of staff, many of whom had pre-war teaching experience. For instance, Dr Josefine Stross taught anatomy, first aid, nutrition, and children's diseases, while Hedwig Hoffer (wife of Willi Hoffer) and *Dorothy Burlingham* taught Freud's writings. Anna Freud thought highly of *Dr Kate Friedlander,* who taught the "fundamental concepts of psychoanalysis". Nursery staff rotated between departments to learn to handle babies, toddlers, nursery, and ill children (Young-Bruehl, 2008). (Those whose names appear in the text in italics are followed in more depth in the Appendix.)

When the Hampstead War Nurseries closed in 1945, a number of nursery workers undertook further training as psychologists or as psychiatric social workers in order to qualify for work in the increasing number of child guidance clinics being established in Great Britain after the war. However, many felt insufficiently prepared for the child psychotherapy they were expected to do and sought a comprehensive training that would include a personal psychoanalysis. They urged a number of senior psychoanalysts to establish a formal child psychotherapy training course (Sandler, 1965).

The Controversial Discussions in the British Psychoanalytical Society (BPaS) (1943–1944) that threatened to label Anna Freud and her work as "extreme" provided an additional impetus for the creation of an Anna Freudian training programme (Young-Bruehl, 2008). The BPaS resolution of June 1946 allowed for the three theoretical groups (Freudians, Kleinians, and Independents) to have equal representation in the Adult Psychoanalytic Training and on committees of the society (King & Steiner, 1991).

With the help of Kate Friedlander, Anna Freud founded the Hampstead Child Therapy Course (HCTC) in 1947. This four-year full-time course in child psychoanalysis aimed to train "child experts". Eight students enrolled to form the first cohort, seven of whom were former Hampstead War Nursery workers. Lectures, seminars, and (five sessions per week) personal analyses were provided by a group of psychoanalysts who were members of the BPaS. Lectures and seminars were given in the teachers' homes. Treatment cases were provided by Kate Friedlander who was in charge of the West Sussex Child Guidance Service and by Dr Augusta Bonnard, director of the East London Child Guidance Clinic (Sandler, Novick & Yorke, not dated, in archive.)

Anna Freud introduced a memorandum of her Hampstead training scheme in psychoanalytic child psychotherapy to the Training Committee and the board of the BPaS. The Training Committee secretary John Bowlby and Sylvia Payne were moderately supportive, while Donald Winnicott worried that this training programme might lower the standards of psychoanalysis in England (Young-Bruehl, 2008). Anna Freud became weary of the ongoing debate, writing to Kate Friedlander in September 1947, "The Training Committee is, so far, more disagreeable than ever. If I were not the only representative from our side in it, I would look for the first opportunity to withdraw" (as quoted in Young-Bruehl, 2008, p. 331).

An "Institute for the psychoanalytic study of the child"

As student numbers and the scope of the course grew, there was an urgent need for a clinic in which students could offer psychoanalytic treatment to children and which would form the centre for the research projects arising from clinical cases. The generosity of the Field Foundation in New York enabled Anna Freud to purchase a house at 12 Maresfield Gardens in November 1951 for £6253 7s 1d (A. Freud, 1952, April 26). Anna Freud and her brother Ernst Freud chose furniture, equipment, and curtains costing £840 2s 5d (A. Freud, 1952, April 26). The enthusiasm was great:

> The new clinic became a matter of interest, excitement and speculation to all members of the Training Course and students and staff helped in painting woodwork and making toys. The waiting room is gay and arresting in its own right, with bright blue paint, a dresser on which toys are arranged, light wood tables and blue canvas chairs, a stand for books and magazines and a counter where children buy orange and lemon squash and parents can get coffee or tea, while they wait during examinations or sessions. Opposite the waiting room is the library [later called the Common Room], the centre of the student life in the clinic. Looking over the garden, with large windows, light polished wood floors and furniture, with the books on the shelves which line the walls giving the only highlight of colour, this is a pleasant room of reading, talking and the writing of reports. Each Wednesday, the library is transformed as staff, students and occasional visitors crowd in to take part in the weekly discussion of cases, chosen for presentation on account of some special point of interest. On the two floors above the ground floor, there are seven treatment rooms, and in the basement, the nursery and the refectory where staff and students have lunch and tea (History of the Hampstead Clinic, 1954, pp. 1–2).

Anna Freud was pleased with her new Clinic: "It is a most pleasant place. It looks so gay and charming that one regrets not being a problem child oneself" (as quoted in Young-Bruehl, 2008, p. 340). The Hampstead Child Therapy Course and Clinic (HCTCC) opened to patients in February 1952. The clinic staff included Anna Freud (honorary director), Drs Augusta Bonnard, Willi Hoffer, and Josefine Stross (honorary consultants), Dr Liselotte Frankl (psychiatrist in charge), and Mrs Bianca Gordon (psychiatric social worker and child therapist). By April 1952, the Clinic had received fifty-three referrals and ten cases were in treatment (nine were in five times weekly psychoanalysis).

The areas chosen for investigation were:

1. The interrelation between the neurotic or other mental disorders of mother and child (simultaneous analysis of parent and child).
2. The comparison of analytic findings with the observed facts of early development of children, by analysis children who were brought up in the Hampstead War Nurseries.
3. The analytic investigation of children deprived of their parents' care from an early age, such as institutionalized and concentration camp children (A. Freud, 1952, April 26).

The Clinic reflected Anna Freud's two principles of studying children: to combine research with service, and to complement psychoanalytic treatment with the study of normal development. It differed from the traditional child guidance clinics in that its orientation was entirely psychoanalytic, and the bulk of treatment offered was full psychoanalysis.

A strong sense of enquiry, flexibility, and individual approach characterized the early years of work: "There are no hard and fast rules of procedures and form filling is kept to a minimum. The method of examination of every case referred is decided according to the particular circumstances" (History of the Hampstead Clinic, 1954, p. 4). Anna Freud explained the reason for embarking on simultaneous analyses of mother (and occasionally, father) and child: "There was a conviction growing in many persons, that every neurosis or disturbance in the child is due to a disturbance in the mother. Well, that is right *if* it is true. And we were interested to see if it *is* true" (Anna Freud's emphasis) (A. Freud, 1965).

With the expansion of the work at the Clinic, a house at 21 Maresfield Gardens was acquired. It was opened on May 6, 1956, on the occasion of the Freud centenary commemoration. This house made fourteen treatment rooms and other facilities available. In 1967, 14 Maresfield Gardens was acquired and opened on March 23, 1968.

By 1965, the Clinic had expanded considerably. Anna Freud said,

> Although we are called Hampstead clinic, we are not only a clinic. I would like to think of it as an "Institute for the psychoanalytic study of the child". We have many departments and treat a great number of children. But we try to divide our time fairly evenly between training, preventative work, therapeutic work and what we call "clinical research"—not research in the academic sense (A. Freud, 1965a, p. 2).

Therapeutic work and clinical research groups

By 1965, between seventy and eighty children were coming daily, five times a week for psychoanalysis. There were three simultaneous analyses of parent and child. Attached to the therapeutic service was the diagnostic service which was elaborating the developmental profile (which became the Provisional Diagnostic Profile). Very detailed records were kept of clinical and diagnostic work that formed the basis for psychoanalytic research, in which both staff and students participated. The large number of research groups met under the direction of one senior person to explore a particular interest. These included the diagnosis research group, development of blind children, simultaneous analysis of mother and child, borderline research group, borderline psychotic research group, the index, concept research group, and clinical concept group (Sandler, 1965).

Preventive and educational services

The Clinic's aim of combining training, service, and research was reflected in the preventive and educational services. The Well-Baby Clinic, a medico-psychological service, aimed to relieve early tensions arising between mother and infant, in areas of sleeping, feeding, weaning, and toilet training, as well as the repercussions of these bodily experiences on the infant's developing mind. The play group for toddlers (under three years) and their mothers met once a week to support the young child's transition from home to community life and nursery. The nursery group for blind children aimed at helping mothers understand the needs of their unsighted children at the various stages of development. The nursery school was attended by a small group of children aged three to five years, some of whom received psychoanalytic treatment at the Clinic. The educational services also included discussion groups for nursery school teachers, paediatric consultants, and lectures to professional organizations (Sandler, 1965).

The child therapy course

Since the beginning of the child psychoanalytic training course, a new group of two to eight students enrolled every year or every alternate year. The course changed over the years, but the essential requirements remained the same: a personal analysis (five sessions per week) starting prior to entry and continuing throughout the training, supervised child analytic cases, weekly child cases and parent-work, and attendance at case conferences, lectures, and seminars (theoretical and clinical). Weekly reports (short summaries of the week's treatment) were required from students and staff. In addition, longer reports involving theoretical formulations were prepared for each analytic case once a term (Sandler, Novick & Yorke, n. d.).

In 1993, an MSc course in Psychoanalytic Developmental Psychology was established together with University College London. This one-year full-time course became the pre-clinical year for the child psychoanalytic training.

In the 1990s the course was changed from full-time to part-time to enable students to take up the NHS training posts (Midgley, 1997). The training conformed to the regulations of the British Association of Child Psychotherapists and students were eligible for membership upon qualification. In collaboration with UCL, an optional professional doctorate was added to the curriculum in 1996 affording students the possibility of carrying out independent research to obtain a doctorate in psychoanalytic developmental psychology (DPsych). With the 2001 intake, the requirement for personal analysis decreased from five to a minimum of four sessions per week (which was in line with the child psychotherapy trainings at the Tavistock Clinic and the British Association of Psychotherapists).

The child psychoanalytic training was the heart of the Anna Freud tradition which was gaining and international reputation. According to Yorke, the Clinic was "a psychoanalytic centre offering the most comprehensive child-therapy training, services and research facilities to be found anywhere in the world" (1983, p. 16).

Becoming a "child expert"

Students came from many countries besides Great Britain, including Australia, Canada, Germany, Hungary, India, Italy, Israel, New Zealand, South Africa, Sweden, Switzerland, the Netherlands, and the USA. The tremendous diversity of educational and professional backgrounds among the students was a source of enrichment, but also of potential friction. Some students struggled with a disconcerting jarring in their sense of being an accomplished adult:

> Prior to coming to the Clinic these people typically have attained some degree of success—on occasion even status—either as staff or faculty members. ... Yet when they become students at

> the Clinic, these same people—after first having given up their jobs, often their friends, homes and country, and perhaps even more often, while in the process of giving up their life savings and going into debt—must in effect become full-time beginners in a field in which the distance separating the beginner from the proficient is measured often … in terms of decades (Lopez & Campbell, 1972, p. 3).

The course was rigorous and challenging:

> All feel that the clinic's training programme in child-psychoanalysis is by far the most thorough, carefully planned and indeed the most profound educational experience that they have ever had. All also feel that the programme is at the same time, by far the most stressful educational experience they have ever had (Lopez & Campbell, 1972, p. 1).
>
> By means, almost of literal immersion, the course provides the students with a degree of concentration, opportunity for reflection and with it, internalisation which, it seems to us, is probably impossible for a part-time course to provide. *We do not believe any of the students think there exists a better way to study psychoanalysis* (Lopez & Campbell, 1972, p. 3).

L'amour de travail

Anna Freud, who represented "the most respected—indeed revered—person in psychoanalysis today" (Lopez & Campbell, 1972, p. 6) and a special link to Freud, inspired and guided the staff and students. One student wrote, "She brought a sense of joyous commitment and a search for freedom to so much of what she did" (Heinicke, 1983, p. 81). Others emphasized her enthusiasm: "She could induce 'l'amour de travail'" (Luissier, 1983, p. 87). All were inspired by her masterly capacity to teach and her clarity of thought which was reflected in her dictum, "If the thought is clear, the words will be clear" (Vas Dias, 1983, p. 91). It was her capacity to see the world from the child's perspective that made her a brilliant clinician. Her nephew Ernst Freud wrote, "She had a rare gift of being able to identify and empathise intuitively with us children and an endearing habit of seeing the world through the child's eyes herself" (W. E. Freud, 1983, p. 7).

Playfulness

Playfulness is at the heart of the Anna Freud tradition. This is first evidenced in the War Nurseries in a "letter" written by *Ilse Hellman, Sophie* and *Gertrude Dann* to Anna Freud and Dorothy Burlingham, in December 1942. Using a reprint of an "annual report of a residential War Nursery", the writers have blocked out sections of text and added some in German and Yiddish to form a highly amusing and moving thank-you letter (Hellman, Dann & Dann, 1942). Playfulness emerged particularly at birthdays and anniversaries. Nicky Model and *Clifford Yorke* gave a memorable rendition of *Albert and the Lion* at various celebrations, including at Anna Freud's 80th birthday celebration. Peter Wilson's piano "Improvisation on the Index" was so popular that Anna Freud commented, "Mr Wilson, you're wasting your time being a child psychotherapist!" (personal communication). Marianne Parsons revived the playfulness with "The Anna Freud Roadshow" at the Graduates Weekend in 1993. The nimble

"Annettes" performed the inimitable "There's no business like shrink business". The show also included "Epistemorphilia" or "Let's fall in with research" set to the tune of *Let's Fall in Love* (Parsons, 1993).

Conclusion

With the appointment of new directors in 2003, the Centre's mission turned to innovative services and the training drew to a close. New applicants to the child psychoanalytic training were turned away from 2004. With the qualification of the last two students in July 2009, the training closed. Just over 170 students had become "child experts" at Anna Freud's "Institute for the psychoanalytic study of the child".

References

Burlingham, D. & Freud, A. (1942). *Young Children in War-Time: a Year's Work in a Residential War Nursery*. London: George Allen & Unwin.

Freud, A. (1952, April 26). Letter to Maxwell Hahn of the Field Foundation. Anna Freud Centre Archives, London.

Freud, A. (October, 1965). Hampstead Child-Therapy Clinic: an informal seminar presented to the National Institute of Child Health and Human Development, Bethesda, MD. Anna Freud Centre Archives, London.

Freud, A. & Burlingham, D. (1944). Infants without families: the case for and against residential nurseries. In: *The Writings of Anna Freud Vol. III. Infants without Families: Reports on the Hampstead Nurseries: 1939–1945* (pp. 541–664). New York: International Universities Press, 1973.

Freud, W. E. (1983). Funeral tribute. In: *Anna Freud* 1895–1982 [special issue]. *Bulletin of the Hampstead Clinic, 6*(1): 5–8.

Heinicke, C. (1983). Personal tribute. In: *Anna Freud* 1895–1982 [special issue]. *Bulletin of the Hampstead Clinic, 6*(1): 81.

Hellman, I. (1983). Work in the Hampstead War Nurseries. *International Journal of Psychoanalysis, 64*: 435–439.

Hellman, I., Dann, S. & Dann, G. (1942). *Annual Report of a Residential War Nursery: a thank-you letter.* [Unpublished manuscript.] Anna Freud Centre Archives, London.

History of the Hampstead Clinic (1954). [Unpublished manuscript.] Anna Freud Centre Archives, London.

King, P. & Steiner, R. (Eds.) (1991). *The Freud-Klein Controversies 1941–45.* London: Routledge.

Lopez, T. & Campbell, D. L. (1972). *Some Difficulties in the Path of Being a Hampstead Student.* [Unpublished manuscript.] Anna Freud Centre Archives, London.

Luissier, A. (1983). Personal tribute. In: *Anna Freud* 1895–1982 [special issue]. *Bulletin of the Hampstead Clinic, 6*(1): 87.

Midgley, N. (Ed.) (1997, Autumn). *Anna Freud Centre Newsletter.* Anna Freud Centre Archives, London.

Parsons, M. (1993). *The Anna Freud Roadshow.* [Unpublished manuscript.] Anna Freud Centre Archives, London.

Sandler, J. (1965). The Hampstead Child-Therapy Clinic. In: *Aspects of Family Mental Health in Europe* (Public Health Paper No. 28) (pp. 109–123). Geneva: World Health Organization.

Sandler, J., Novick, J. & Yorke, C. (not dated). *The Hampstead Child-Therapy Course and Clinic.* [Unpublished manuscript.] Anna Freud Centre Archives, London.

Vas Dias, S. (1983). Personal tribute. In: *Anna Freud* 1895–1982 [special issue]. *Bulletin of the Hampstead Clinic*, *6*(1): 91–92.

Yorke, C. (1983). Memorial tribute. In: *Anna Freud* 1895–1982 [special issue]. *Bulletin of the Hampstead Clinic*, *6*(1): 15–18.

Young-Bruehl, E. (2008). *Anna Freud: A biography* (2nd edition). New Haven, CT: Yale University Press.

CHAPTER FIVE

The Diagnostic Profile: an invaluable clinical tool

Trevor Hartnup

Key diagnostic concepts and their evolution

Anna Freud's procedures for the assessment of children and adolescents were in use at the Hampstead Clinic (later the Anna Freud Centre) from the 1960s into this century. They developed from her study of the role of the ego in psychic functioning previously elaborated in *The Ego and the Mechanisms of Defence* (A. Freud, 1966c). Her diagnostic concepts derive from close observation in clinical and nursery settings examined in a research-minded way through the psychoanalytic perspective of Freudian structural theory. They were intended to be applied by child experts not simply for the purpose of diagnosis with a view to treatment, but also to provide assistance to parents and professionals in their decision making in the best interests of children's development. With this in mind, she approached the task of assessing normality as well as pathology.

Her approach to this differed from the diagnostic categories prevalent in the Fifties and Sixties and still predominant today in the NHS. Rather than categorize symptoms on the basis of observable behaviour, she concentrated upon understanding what lay behind them, through study of the development of the child or adolescent who was either troubled or troublesome to others and the environment in which they grew up.

The assessment was structured by the Diagnostic Profile and the concept of Developmental Lines. The task was to create a profile of child development in psychoanalytic terms. In other words, the Profile and Developmental Lines were ways of expressing the assessment material in a way that would describe the inner world of the child and the ongoing processes of development, in terms of the interactions between the drives, the ego, the superego and the external environment.

It was apparent to her that many apparent symptoms in childhood arise from stresses inherent in development itself. Indeed, the absence of such normal indicators of stress might itself be a cause for concern. For her the most important indicator of pathology in childhood was the failure to progress developmentally.

Introduction to the Diagnostic Profile and Developmental Lines

Anna Freud designed these two main frameworks for the assessment of development, which child psychotherapists who trained at the Centre learned to apply, and carried with them into their professional practice.

The emotional and psychological development of the child is studied within the framework of Freud's structural model of the mind, namely the developmental phases of drive, ego and superego development, and the interactions between them, permutations of which produce the vast array of personalities and behaviours to be seen in children and adults.

The distinguishing feature of Anna Freud's work is the emergence of the ego as the main focus of study. The ego is regarded as the agency which determines the outcome of the biological givens of sexual and aggressive drives and the demands of the superego and the external world. The outcome of the ego's work is seen in the workings of the child's mind, in his behaviour and relationships as he develops.

The Diagnostic Profile

Anna Freud wanted to ensure that developmental factors received due weight in the diagnostic process. The interview with the parents elicited as full a history of the child and family as could be obtained. The child was seen, usually twice, for unstructured sessions of talk and play, and also by the psychologist for an assessment of intellectual functioning and personality testing. These interviews were written up in detail and the task of the diagnostician was to assemble the information within the format of the Profile and to compose an account of key aspects of the child's development according to this framework. This was a difficult task not because of the rigidity of the framework, but rather because of the many points of articulation on the Profile. My own starting point amid a sea of possibilities was to identify apparent contradictions in the material and work out how they might properly be reconciled in a provisional account of the child's psychic functioning.

The Profile underwent a number of revisions, but here is one late version which appears in full in Edgcumbe (2000), where the headings are explained in detail. These are much condensed here:

Reason for referral

Description of the child: Significant where the child behaved differently in different settings.
Family background and personal history: The manner in which the parents recounted the history and what they chose to include gives clues to the nature of their relationship to the child.
Possibly significant environmental influences: Positive and negative impact upon the child's development including organic factors.

Assessment of development: Drive development; progress through the drive phases (oral, anal, phallic, genital) but also the balance between the child's emotional investment in his objects on the one hand and the self on the other. (Edgcumbe illustrates this with a clinical example.)
Ego and superego development: An important consideration here is whether there are organic defects that impede the ego in its developmental tasks. The effectiveness and age-adequacy of defences are considered as well as their quality (e.g., rigidity/flexibility). Identifications are considered in this section as well as the child's affects and attitude towards them. The quality and age-adequacy of the superego is considered. Is it harsh or corruptible for example? Does it reward as well as punish? Does it function independently of outside support?
Genetic assessments—regression and fixation points: (This refers to the origins of psychological characteristics, not to what is carried in the genes.) The personal history, parents' descriptions, and observations by the diagnostician may indicate developmental tasks that have caused difficulty for the child from which the child may retreat by regression. Permanent regressions may distort or delay development.
Dynamic and structural assessment—conflicts: These require work by the ego. The earliest conflicts are external: e.g., between the child and his parents over the fulfilment of his wishes. Internalized conflicts take place within the psychic structure where the ego is faced with the demands of his impulses and the strictures of his superego with the threat of guilt. Conflict between opposing drives takes place between love and hate, passivity and activity or masculinity and femininity.
Assessment of some general characteristics: The outlook for development depends not only on the disturbance, but the range and quality of ego capacities to deal with disturbance: e.g., frustration tolerance, sublimation potential, the overall attitude towards anxiety, and the balance between progressive and regressive forces in the personality.
Diagnosis:

1. Disturbances of behaviour represent variations of normality.
2. Symptoms are of a transitory nature.
3. Conflicts of a neurotic-type permanent drive regression, with risk of infantile neuroses and character disorders.
4. Drive regression accompanied by ego and superego regression leading to borderline, delinquent, or psychotic disturbances.
5. Evidence of destructive processes at work (of organic, toxic, psychic, known or unknown origin) which have effected or are on the point of effecting a disruption of mental growth.

The Developmental Lines

Whilst the Diagnostic Profile aims to provide a cross section of overall functioning, the Developmental Lines represent a vertical framework of aspects of development over time, so that the dynamic process of development can be better understood when applied to a particular child. Such a framework might enable the clinician, or other professional, to identify whether developmental assistance is required and what form it might best take. Significantly, the concept of Developmental Lines appears in the chapter headed Assessment of Normality in Childhood.

It is intended to offer a response to parents' questions concerning child development and to their wishes to protect their child from future problems. It has to be said that Anna Freud was conservative in her estimation of the ability of professionals to predict the children's future personality. The thoroughness of the Profile and Developmental Lines indicates that caution. She notes that specific types of parenting do not lead to specific types of children. Such a view would leave out of account the variable development of the human personality and its complexity in each individual, and the fact that the impact of unpredictable life events upon children's development, for good and ill, depends upon their *timing* in relation to the child's levels of development in particular areas.

In this brief account it is possible only to outline aspects of the Developmental Lines:

1. *From Dependency to Emotional Self Reliance and Adult Object Relationships.*

This line follows the drive development as expressed in its source, aim, and object. The drives are the psychological representatives of the biological urges that manifest themselves in the behaviour of infants from the very beginnings of psychological and emotional development. The source of the oral drive is the mouth, the original oral aim is to suck, and the object is the feeding mother.

According to Anna Freud the original "relationship" is one of biological unity with the mother. Mother and infant include the other in their narcissism. (Since her day the psychoanalytic concept of "primary narcissism" in infants has been convincingly challenged by research.) The *part-object stage* followed based on the fluctuating urgency of the child's bodily need for the "object" whom the infant cannot yet see as a person in their own right. This is followed by the stage of *object constancy* enabling the child to maintain a positive inner image of the object irrespective of satisfaction or dissatisfactions. The *anal-sadistic phase* is characterized by ambivalence and the completely *object-centred phase* by possessiveness of the parent of the opposite sex and rivalry with the same sex parent. During *latency* the biological sexual drive diminishes (becomes latent), and the child's libidinal investment transfers to adults other than parents and to peers. *Pre-adolescence* sees a return to part object and ambivalent attitudes. *Adolescence* struggles to diminish the tie to the infantile object, to leave behind the pre-genital drives reawakened in pre-adolescence and establish genital relationships with objects of the opposite sex outside the family.

Anna Freud's elaboration of normal phases of psychological and emotional development shows why common reactions to events such as significant separations from the maternal object are as varied as they are, because the reaction to separation derives from the stage of development governing the psychological reality of each individual child. Working from the developmental phases, it is possible to say at what stage (but not what precise age) separations become non-traumatic. Anna Freud gives extensive examples of this. She says, for example: "It is only after object constancy … has been reached that the external absence of the object is substituted for, at least in part, by the presence of an internal object that remains stable; on the strength of this achievement temporary separations can be lengthened, commensurate with advances in object constancy."

This argument is followed through with the enumeration of several Developmental Lines, their phases, and the observable disturbances and achievements associated with them. In a summary such as this it is not possible to elaborate, but further examples of developmental lines indicate the developing capacities of the child's ego working within its own psychic reality to transform and manage conflicting parallel and simultaneous demands deriving from the drives, the superego, and the external world, in ways that carry the stamp of the particular child.

The line *From Suckling to Rational Eating* includes the establishment of feeding in face of fluctuations in the infant's appetite and intestinal upsets; weaning from liquids to solids; the transition to self-feeding; table manners, pleasurable sucking, food fads and beginnings of disgust in the anal phase; eating as independent of the relationship to the maternal object; irrational fears based on sexual theories (fear of getting fat, etc.); increase in rational eating.

The following also appeared in her original exposition:

From Wetting and Soiling to Bladder and Bowel Control
From Irresponsibility to Responsibility in Body Management
From Egocentricity to Companionship
From the Body to the Toy and from Play to Work.

These Lines share as their outcome the freeing of the drive activity from the relationship with the parental objects, and the child's assumption of responsibility. However, the quality of the relationship to the parents is essential to the achievement of this end. Disruptions impact upon the child according to the psychic reality of its developmental phase: separations before the child has achieved phase adequacy will tend to lead to difficulties expressed in terms of eating, toileting, or physical accidents. Childhood illness that requires the mother to resume responsibilities for care of the child's body may lead the child to regress in a co-operative way or fight to maintain its most recent achievements along developmental lines.

There were many developmental lines to be elaborated. Anna Freud herself added *From Physical to Mental Pathways of Discharge*, and *From Irresponsibility to Guilt*. Her colleagues elaborated developmental lines for anxiety and for insight, amongst others.

Regression and discrepancies of attainment

Anna Freud cautions that normal psychological development does not follow the same relentlessly forward course as normal physical development. Regression along developmental lines is a normal part of psychological development. Like advances, regressions may occur at different rates along different developmental lines. The recognition of these possibilities enables us to understand apparently contradictory manifestations in children and adolescents, and distinguish normal from pathological development. Regression may be induced by tiredness, or illness, other physical discomfort, anxiety, or distress, and it is invariably the latest acquisition of competence that is lost first. For her, the main indicator of pathology in children was when development ceased to advance or became distorted.

Anna Freud describes the combination of endowment and environment that may lead to discrepancies of attainment along the Developmental Lines. She emphasizes that these discrepancies are not pathological as such but represent the many variations of normality that may be encountered. She illustrates the usefulness of these Lines to the question: "When is a child ready for nursery school?" For example, the achievement of "object constancy" makes separation less upsetting and indicates readiness to engage with others, though the length of separations still has to be borne in mind. Similarly eating and use of the toilet depend upon developmental achievements.

Progress along developmental lines could be thought of as threads being woven progressively into what will become the tapestry of the adult personality. However, they are more like the development of the individual's own ego capacity to weave these emotionally invested psychological threads from sensory information into a meaningful form that represents the individual style or personality.

The potential application of developmental lines covers the whole field of provision of mentally healthy environments for children. Anna Freud co-operated with Solnit and Goldstein to produce three books on the implications of the Developmental Lines for courts and law-makers charged with determining the best interests of children. The chapter that contrasts the child's sense of time with the legal time frame for adoption is particularly telling. This leads me to a brief comment on the direct relevance of Anna Freud's diagnostic approach to the tasks facing child mental health services today.

Diagnosis in NHS services for children and adolescents

Since health services are now blessed with more treatments than can be paid for, the idea of value for money has led the UK necessarily towards reliance upon outcome research based upon the Diagnostic and Statistical Manual categories. In front line services where social policy meets patient need, the implementation of "what works for whom" inexorably drifts towards "what works for what", i.e., away from the person towards the symptoms. All illness impacts upon the personal relationships of the patient, but it is arguable that, in mental ill health, the patient's relationships with self and others are the main area of dysfunction, and affect most areas of life, including engagement in treatment.

In present day practice, psychotherapists often regard assessment as a brief therapeutic intervention in its own right or as the beginning of treatment. Anna Freud herself carefully distinguished the process of assessment from the intervention that might result from its findings. From that point of view, the clinician's diagnostic assessments of the patient's ego strengths and weaknesses, and the appropriate application of that understanding, have a place at the core of the treatment endeavour, whatever the intervention. It is at best wasteful, and at worst harmful, to apply the right treatment to the right symptoms in the wrong patient.

References

Edgcumbe, R. (2002). *Anna Freud: a View of Development, Disturbance and Therapeutic Techniques.* London: Routledge.

Freud, A. (1965). *Normality and Pathology in Childhood.* New York: Penguin University.

Goldstein, J., Freud, A. & Solnit, A. J. (1980). *Beyond the Best Interests of the Child.* London: Burnett.

Goldstein, J., Freud, A., Solnit, A. J. & Goldstein, S. (1986). *In the Best Interests of the Child.* New York: Free Press.

Contemporary Issues

CHAPTER SIX

Anna Freud's influence on contemporary thinking about the child

Anne-Marie Sandler

In this short chapter I hope to show how the ideas and discoveries of Anna Freud have had a considerable influence throughout England, Europe, and the USA, not only in the field of child analysis, but quite markedly in fostering new educational, social, and legal practices in regard to children and adolescents. However, as these new understandings became accepted and absorbed in the day-to-day mores, they also became disconnected from their original source. I believe this to be true in regard to the important changes which have occurred in the last decades in the quality of care in nursery schools, in the awareness of children's emotional needs in hospital, and in the new thinking on fostering and adoption issues as well as in many legal decisions concerned with the well-being and best interests of the child. Anna Freud played a central role in these changes but her initial input has long been forgotten.

Anna Freud's first paper "Four Lectures on Child Analysis" was published in 1927, followed a year later by "The Theory of Child Analysis" (1928). These papers were written for a psychoanalytic audience. However, as a clear indication of her lifelong desire to share her understanding of the psychological needs of children with parents, teachers, health visitors, social workers, and paediatricians, her third and fourth publications were addressed to the wider public and were named "Four Lectures on Psycho-Analysis for Teachers and Parents" (1930) and "Psychoanalysis and the Upbringing of the Young Child" (1934). In regard to Anna Freud's work, it is very important to remember that during her entire career she was engaged in studying both the normal as well as the pathological development of children and adolescents.

After 1945, with the closure of the War Nurseries, Anna Freud organized some training in child analysis in response to the needs of former war nursery staff, many of whom had moved on to work in child guidance clinics. Gradually, the idea of creating a specialized centre of child psychoanalytic learning took shape, in large part encouraged by Anna Freud's reaction to the controversial discussions, which had taken place at the British Psychoanalytical Society.

Thanks to Anna Freud's remarkable organizational skills and the purchase of a house in Maresfield Gardens in 1952, the Hampstead Child Therapy Course and Clinic, a charitable institution, officially opened its doors. It offered a full-time four-year course in child and adolescent psychoanalysis for child psychotherapists and a place where students would be expected to treat intensive and non-intensive psychoanalytic cases, often seen at reduced fees, and to work with the parents, especially with the mothers. They would also be asked to join and participate in research groups, studying various aspects of child and adolescent development and disorders. This new institution attracted a number of young people, who aspired to become experts in child and adolescent psychoanalysis, with a solid grounding in theory, and experienced in a variety of child and adolescent problems, informed by a clear understanding of development.

Anna Freud's enthusiasm in her work was infectious. All students at the Clinic were asked to write brief weekly reports on all their patients in therapy, many of them being seen five times a week. These reports were not easy to write, as they needed to be short and to precis the main movements of the material, if possible illustrated by an example. They were collected on Fridays so that Anna Freud could read them over the weekend. Anna Freud's capacity to recall all these short reports and to follow up the vicissitudes of the treatments of all the children and adolescents seen at the Clinic was astonishing.

A number of students were British but many others came from the USA and a variety of European countries and when they finally returned home, these dedicated and highly trained men and women took with them their analytic knowledge and their specific understanding of child development, gained from their working years at the Clinic. Thus in the USA, for example, in many centres, particularly New York, Yale, Ann Arbor, Cleveland, Seattle, Chapel Hill, and Boston, the influence of Anna Freud is still widespread. In Europe, her work is known in Greece and in some parts of Italy and Germany and, of course, in London, although the major influence of Winnicott's and Melanie Klein's publications have tended to overshadow Anna Freud's influence. It is certainly sadly true that in some parts of Europe and the USA and in large areas of Latin America, her work is only rarely mentioned.

Defences

In the sphere of psychoanalysis proper, there is no doubt that Anna Freud's book, *The Ego and the Mechanisms of Defence*, published in English in 1936, established her as an important psychoanalytical contributor. Although faithful to her father's discoveries, the ideas in the book were original and creative in their own right. It is difficult to realize nowadays, when the idea of mechanisms of defence are included in everyone's psychoanalytic references, how courageous it was to write a book concerned with the ego when all the rage was to explore the vicissitudes of the id. Anna Freud was warned in no hidden way by a number of senior colleagues in Vienna that the ideas contained in her book, although interesting, would be open to considerable criticism. Yet Anna Freud felt strongly that the need to study the ego's response to the urges of the unconscious drives was of great importance for psychoanalysis. Her book became a classic, read by most psychoanalysts to this day.

Anna Freud's interest in developmental issues was already visible in this, her first book, as she attempted to differentiate between primitive defences and later ones, which required a more mature ego. Denial, projection, and introjection, for example, were thought to be more primitive than sublimation or reaction formation. In view of later development in psychoanalysis, it is also worth noting that Anna Freud described in her book two specific defence mechanisms, the identification with the aggressor and a form of altruistic surrender, which have the common feature of involving an interaction between the child and someone else in his world. These two defences describe what would now be called projective identification.

Anna Freud also underlines in her book the importance of not only interpreting the transference of early instinctual wishes and phantasies, but also to be aware of the "transference of defence". She pointed out how in this form of transference, analytic attention has to be focused on the ego, on its specific defensive strategy, rather than on the instinctual drives and the wishes associated with them.

Inner world

From 1945 onwards, Anna Freud wrote, among many others, a series of papers which examine and extend the understanding of the inner world of the child and the adolescent. She wrote for example on infantile feeding, on aggression, on certain types and stages of social maladjustment, on the role of body illness in the mental life of children, on the emotional and social development of young children, on pre-adolescence and on adolescence, to quote but a few. These more obvious analytic publications were again interspersed with papers specially written for the general public, for parents, health visitors, and teachers, as for example her publications "On Nursery School Education: its Uses and Dangers"(1949a) and "Entrance into Nursery School: the Psychological Pre-Requisites"(1960a). They were followed a few years later by work on "Psychoanalytic Knowledge and its Application to Children's Services" (1964), "Residential versus Foster Care" (1966), "Expert Knowledge for the Average Mother" (1949b), and "On the Interaction Between Paediatrics and Child Psychology" (1975). Here again we witness her lifelong commitment to psychoanalysis and to the dissemination of her understanding to everyone who has contact with children. Her aim was to foster a better understanding of the complexities of human development and of the various levels of maturity of the child in his or her interaction with the demands of the wider world.

Anna Freud was convinced that children developed best in stable relations within an intact family and that the role of the mother was crucial in establishing healthy bonding. But as the result of her experience in the War Nurseries, she had also become an expert in residential upbringing of young children. Even though Anna Freud was not in favour of residential upbringing, she knew that many children, because of death, illness, divorce, or other reasons had no choice but to be sent away, and she found it important to share her psychoanalytic knowledge and indicate measures which could be used to minimize the damage to the children's attachment, personality, and cognitive as well as emotional development. Two of her papers, the one on "Answering Teachers' Questions" (1952) and the other entitled "Answering Paediatricians Questions" (1961) illustrate this desire to inform.

Observation

Anna Freud discovered early in her career that detailed observation of young children was of great importance in deepening understanding of the child's development. She believed that it gave the informed analytic observer, working with children, a chance to add to the knowledge gained from the reconstructed image of children obtained during the course of the analysis of adults. She believed that observation of the child not only would confirm her father's psychoanalytic framework but would also lead to further refinement of some earlier hypothesis. Anna Freud did not expect her observational work to affect major revisions of theories, but she felt convinced that they would give the student of psychoanalysis a precious basis on which the psychoanalytic theory and its application would flourish.

When the Jackson Nurseries, a place which cared for children aged one to three years, opened in Vienna in 1937, one of the first things that Anna Freud did was to ask all the helpers to write down in detail any behaviour of the children which they had noticed and had interested them. She provided for each worker pencil and paper, which became part of the working uniform of the staff. The same method of observation was used in the War Nurseries, where the age of the children ranged from babyhood to nursery years, and were an integral part of the Hampstead Clinic curriculum.

Observations concerning any and every aspect of infant and child behaviour were assembled carefully at the end of each day and discussed. They then were filed thematically and referred to later when certain specific topics were taken up or when papers were written. Anna Freud gathered, for example, at that time, numerous and detailed observations of the reactions of the various children in her care to separation from their mothers or their carers. The impact of what was observed helped her to understand much more fully the vicissitudes of the children's efforts to cope with the challenge posed to them by the new situation. Thanks to the detailed material that had been assembled, she could describe how each child, not only displayed obvious distress and longing, but how each of them found regressive or progressive solutions to cope with this overwhelming situation. A detailed picture of each child emerged, revealing which mechanisms of defence they used, which phantasies could be deducted from their play, and how new relationships to the staff were slowly constructed or avoided. She also observed the crucial role of the body as well as the mind in the attempts of these small children to reorganize their inner and outer world. The various observations also describe the practical measures taken to minimize the damage to the children and the ways the children reacted.

This example about separation and loss is but one area of interest. Over time, Anna Freud had gathered a treasure of detailed observations on a large variety of children and adolescents of all ages and these observations were used later in her descriptions of feeding or toilet training problems, of the development of aggression and anxiety, of learning and behavioural problems of all kinds, and of a further variety of disorders. They facilitated the formulation of extremely detailed descriptions of the many intertwining constitutional, maturational, and environmental factors which contribute to a child's development. To acquire a solid understanding of the enormous complexity of normal and pathological development, Anna Freud felt that consideration of the strength of the drive, the role of the ego and superego, and the centrality of object relations as well as the influence of the outside world had to be carefully considered if one wished to get a clear picture of the child or adolescent's internal life.

Anna Freud stressed the importance of differentiating between the mind of the child, that by definition will show some signs of immaturity, and the mind of the adult and its particular importance when determining the readiness of the child for various events, such as the start of nursery or primary school, the reactions to going on holiday or the need to be hospitalized, to quote but a few examples.

Attachments

Anna Freud never relinquished her father's drive theory and his statement that the object is the thing, which allows the instinct to achieve its aim. Freud added that the object is not originally connected with it, but becomes assigned to it only because of being particularly fitted to making satisfaction possible. Although for a long time, Anna Freud thought that the first six months of life were mostly biological, it did not mean that she was not deeply interested in the central role for the child of the parents, particularly of the mother. She stated categorically that object relations is a basic topic in child psychoanalysis. She gradually conceded that vital psychological events occur from the very beginning of life. She wrote in a report on the War Nurseries that "the attachment of the small child to his mother seems to be to a large degree independent of her personal qualities and certainly of her educational ability."

As a result of her observations, she believed that "the figure of the mother is for a certain time the sole important representative of the whole outer world." She described how out of the initial "stomach love" of the baby, there develops "a real attachment to the mother, which is personal, exclusive, violent, is accompanied by jealousy and disappointment, can turn into hate and is capable of sacrifice". The relationship to mother gradually extends to father and to the siblings. She observed and described how the growing child internalizes bit by bit the wishes, the prohibitions, and the characteristics of his parents, these most important objects, into his own internal world and how this shapes the child's developing ego and superego, the development of his personality, his emotional life, and cognitive capacities.

In her therapeutic work at the Hampstead Clinic, Anna Freud always involved the parents. She felt it important to help the parents to feel recognized and possibly helped with their own problems. She was also very aware of the effort for parents to bring their child to treatment and the need to acknowledge the specific difficulties which can occur at certain periods in the therapy. At the same time, she was very clear about the necessity of maintaining confidentiality in the case of latency and adolescent patients. Yet she was convinced that to consolidate progress and changes, the parents needed to be given some information and support to help them sustain their child's efforts and changes. The work with parents was more intensive with pre-latency children or with children with specific deficits.

Developmental lines

In 1965, Anna Freud produced her second book, *Normality and Pathology in Childhood: Assessments of Development*, in which she described her theoretical thinking concerning the central role of development in the understanding of childhood and adolescent pathology. She introduced the concept of lines of development and described the use of diagnostic profiles. The Developmental Lines were based on the belief that the careful study of surface phenomena allowed the analytically trained child therapist to grasp the functioning of the child's inner life. It showed how the interactions and interdependence between maturational (internal) and environmental (external) determinants can be observed and how each interference can be seen to leave its mark on the individual's personality. The Developmental Lines provide the analysts with a series of predictable, interlocking, overlapping, unfolding lines, which are characteristic for each child's development.

The Developmental Lines enabled the psychoanalytic diagnostician to look at a specific child and, with the Diagnostic Profile, another instrument devised by Anna Freud, to try to assess the normal and the pathological components in that child's mental and physical life. Briefly, the Profile was an organized set of headings which, apart from some factual data, was essentially a set of metapsychologically framed assessments. As Anna Freud put it:

> In the analyst's mind, the whole bulk of material collected during the diagnostic procedure organizes itself into what may be called a comprehensive profile of the child, i.e., a picture that contains dynamic, genetic, economic, structural and adaptive data. This can be seen as the analyst's synthetic effort when dealing with disparate findings, or, conversely, as showing his diagnostic thinking broken up analytically into its component parts (1965, pp. 139–140).

Anna Freud did not believe that classical psychoanalytic treatment was the appropriate solution for all children's psychological difficulties. She was of the view that it should be offered only to children or adolescents whose developmental thrust had developed reasonably normally during their first years but who had failed to find a suitable solution to their Oedipal conflicts and their development had become blocked or reversed. With some young children, she believed that work with parents, weekly visits to a well-run toddler group, or attending the Clinic's nursery school would be sufficient to get the child back to the lines of normal development. But with many further children who showed deficits and distortions in their development, developmental help proved to be a necessary part of child analysis. It consisted mainly in an effort by the child therapist to verbalize affects and clarify thinking, to facilitate play, to help control impulses, and to offer the child a *new* "object" in his life, a person with a new approach to his problems, a new model for identification.

Finally, it is with the publication of *Normality and Pathology* that Anna Freud's distinctive dual interest both in normality and in pathology became clear. She was well aware of the complexity of assessing disturbances and, as a child psychoanalyst, she saw her role as twofold. On the one hand, she aimed at being a skilful, fully informed, and sensitive child analyst, able to help children and adolescents in the consulting room. On the other hand, she saw herself as an educator, a researcher, whose role was to inform parents, teachers, paediatricians, and all the professionals whose work brought them in touch with families, of the latest insights of psychoanalytically informed understanding. In this way, her widespread influence was evident, with many of her ideas becoming household concepts, although not always ascribed their origin.

References

Freud, A. (1927). Four lectures on child analysis. In: *The Writings of Anna Freud, Vol. I* (pp. 3–50). New York: International Universities Press.

Freud, A. (1928). The theory of child analysis. In: *The Writings of Anna Freud, Vol. I* (pp. 162–175). New York: International Universities Press.

Freud, A. (1930). Four lectures on psycho-analysis for teachers and parents. In: *The Writings of Anna Freud, Vol. I* (pp. 73–121). New York: International Universities Press.

Freud, A. (1934). Psychoanalysis and the upbringing of the young child. In: *The Writings of Anna Freud, Vol. I* (pp. 176–188). New York: International Universities Press.

Freud, A. (1936). *The Ego and the Mechanisms of Defence.* London: Hogarth.

Freud, A. (1949). Nursery school education: its uses and dangers. In: *The Writings of Anna Freud, Vol. IV* (pp. 545–559). New York: International Universities Press.

Freud, A. (1949b). Expert knowledge for the average mother. In: *The Writings of Anna Freud, Vol. IV* (pp. 528–544). New York: International Universities Press.

Freud, A. (1960a). Entrance into nursery school: the psychological pre-requisites. In: *The Writings of Anna Freud, Vol. V* (pp. 315–335). New York: International Universities Press.

Freud, A. (1961). Answering pediatricians' questions. In: *The Writings of Anna Freud, Vol. V* (pp. 379–406). New York: International Universities Press.

Freud, A. (1964). Psychoanalytic knowledge and its application to children's services. In: *The Writings of Anna Freud, Vol. V* (pp. 460–472). New York: International Universities Press.

Freud, A. (1965). *Normality and Pathology in Childhood: Assessments of Development.* Madison, CT: International Universities Press.

Freud, A. (1966e). Residential versus foster care. In: *The Writings of Anna Freud, Vol. VII* (pp. 223–239). New York: International Universities Press.

Freud, A. (1975). On the interaction between paediatrics and child psychology. In: *The Writings of Anna Freud, Vol. IV.* New York: International Universities Press.

CHAPTER SEVEN

The clinical training: 1947–2009—commemorating a tradition

Viviane Green

From the inception of the Anne Freud Centre, until 2003, when the trustees and new directorial team took the decision to close it, the training in child psychoanalysis had been at the heart of the organization. In 2009 the last two remaining trainees qualified. In this chapter I will focus mainly on the last twenty years of the training and in so doing hope to convey something about its special ethos, and some qualitative aspects of the Anna Freudian way of understanding and thinking about children and adolescents.

The origins

The establishment of an independent training, in what came to be thought of as the Anna Freudian tradition, arose from a fraught period when it became increasingly apparent that there would be no seamless accommodation within the British Psychoanalytical Society. The Controversial Discussions, coupled with a disheartening period of presenting a training scheme to the training committee and the board of the British Psychoanalytical Society, culminated in Anna Freud's resolve to offer her training independently. In doing so Anna Freud held onto a metapsychology which emphasized a primarily psychosexual organization as distinct from Klein's view of psychic life constellating around paranoid schizoid and depressive positions. In Anna Freud's view there were no constitutional givens such as envy, nor did she adhere to early unconscious fantasy. Finally, theoretical and technical emphasis was given to the defences. The move to establishing a separate training led simultaneously to fostering a spirit of independence but perhaps also a degree of isolation or marginalization from the mainstream.

The early years of the training

The clinical training, formally established in 1947 by Anna Freud with help from *Kate Friedlander*, was originally known as the Hampstead Child Therapy Course. In 1951 the Centre opened its own clinic which was to provide training cases. (Those whose names appear in the text in italics are followed in more depth in the Appendix.)

The training offered a profoundly intensive, rigorous, and thorough psychoanalytic understanding of children and adolescents. Intake of trainees varied but depending on demand tended to be every two years. From the outset the training was international, attracting trainees from the countries of Europe, North and South America, Canada, India, Israel, Australasia, and South Africa. The majority of trainees were well established in a wide variety of previous professions and an almost universal experience was having to relinquish a prior professional identity and accepting an inevitable "regression" in becoming a beginner in the new world of child psychoanalysis.

Trainees, visitors, and families and their children were left in no doubt that they were entering a world focused on childhood. The physical setting itself, in particular the waiting room, with its (erstwhile shabby chic and latterly modernized) furnishings, many toys, children's books, and welcoming receptionists who could offer juice and biscuits declared that this was a place for children. Unlike the neo-brutalist post-war architecture of some NHS buildings or the later practical but rather featureless purpose-built premises, the houses in Maresfield Gardens, each with its attractive garden, suggested a (rather well-to-do) "home". In writing this a poignant memory returned of the Anna Freud Nursery (closed in the late 1990s) housed in the basement of no. 12 and giving out onto a garden well equipped with swings and slides. Until its closure trainees could gaze from the common room windows and continue their informal observations of young lives. Something of the "family" atmosphere also characterized the training itself. The number of trainees never exceeded nineteen and was more usually significantly smaller. Year groups ranged from two to six trainees but were more usually about four. A loyal and long-standing core staff group taught and supervised several generations of trainees.

From the outset there was a sense within the organization that clinical cases treated by both trainees and practising staff were highly invested in, and the subject of, ongoing psychoanalytic curiosity and concern. Anna Freud, having read all the "weeklies", reputedly knew the details of every case. Following her death in 1982, with the aim of providing stability, *Hansi Kennedy* and *Clifford Yorke* became the Centre's new co-directors. Until her retirement in 1993, Hansi Kennedy held the clinical cases in mind in a remarkable fashion characterized by her humane, humorous, clear-sighted, and sturdy understanding of how children, particularly young ones, functioned. On one memorable occasion I managed to persuade her out of retirement to address a group of visiting Dutch child psychotherapists on her work with under-fives. When the precise interpretations to a young child were not very meaningful she spontaneously offered, "After all, all they hear are friendly noises." In this she captured the ways in which an ongoing spirit of inquiry allowed moves away from entrenchment within classical theory—marking the trend into what became consolidated into a developmental approach where the qualitative aspects of the therapeutic relationship are increasingly emphasized (Hurry, 1998; *Edgcumbe*, 2002; Green, 2003). Following the Wednesday Scientific Meetings, *Hansi Kennedy*, taking up Anna Freud's mantle, gave highly succinct summaries following case presentations replete with further questions with which the audience could engage. Fortunately there was a period when these Wednesday Scientific Meetings were minuted and published in the *Bulletin of the Anna Freud Centre.*

This sense of being "watched over" meant that, at best, trainees felt known, held, and supported by their seminar leaders, supervisors, and the overseeing body, the training committee. At worst this sense could give way to feeling over-scrutinized. Whatever the vicissitudes of an individual's training experience, almost all would subsequently voice their view of a sense of real solidity which would strike them in their post-qualification years.

The training's hallmark was rooted in its earliest beginnings where psychoanalytic understanding, observation of different age groups, and clinical research dynamically informed each other. Many of the principles which guided the training had been established earlier during the War Nursery years (1941–1945). During those early years nursery staff gained broad hands-on experience with normally developing and sick children, and in conjunction with this attended a range of taught courses offered by more experienced professionals. Presciently, Anna Freud also stressed the importance of a child's early attachments. The importance of continuity of care was emphasized in a context where many children had been deprived of this, having been separated from their parents. Her insights, that attachments to main caregivers needed to be preserved, and long separations (e.g., during periods of hospitalization) were to be avoided, have had a direct impact on social policy. Already one can see the importance Anna Freud attributed to the psychosocial realities of a child's life which were later to be incorporated into the first section of her provisional Diagnostic Profile.

Anna Freud's emphasis on the value of hands-on experience, matched with close observation of children, led to her singular contributions which were intrinsically married to her father's developmental psychosexual theories. Freud's understanding of children at different stages of development was drawn largely from retrospective reconstructions on the couch, from young adults and older patients, whereas Anna Freud's understanding rested on live observations of children. This was reflected in her Developmental Lines, where Anna Freud drew a finely grained picture of stages related to psychic preoccupations rooted in the early relationship to the main caregiver. Throughout its duration, the training continued to emphasize the value of observations and proved invaluable in helping trainees develop their internal working models of what constituted normal development and what presaged a more problematic trajectory. Undertaking a two-year mother-infant observation was a requirement of the Association of Child Psychotherapists (ACP). In addition, Anna Freud Centre trainees also conducted weekly observations in a toddler group and nursery, thus offering an intimate understanding of dyadic and peer-group relations in the early years.

Probably all trainees in the last twenty (-plus) years would have been taught or supervised by one or more of the following: *Hansi Kennedy, Clifford Yorke, Anne Hurry, Rose Edgcumbe,* Anne-Marie Sandler, Maria Berger, Pat Radford, Marie Zaphiriou Woods, Audrey Gavshon, and Pauline Cohen, all of whom had known Anna Freud. This is not an exhaustive list but suggests something of the continuity within the "tradition".

The last years of the training

Over the years there were several important changes to course requirements and the broader context in which the training took place. The training was accredited by the Association of Child Psychotherapists, a professional body recognized by the government Department of Health. As such, training requirements met those standards and they in turn reflected the needs and demands of the National Health Service Child and Adolescent Mental Health Teams (CAMHS). The ACP is a small professional body with a membership of just under 800 members at any one time. It was therefore a remarkable achievement (in the 1990s), spearheaded by senior members, to negotiate with the NHS and establish funded training posts. Trainees could undertake their training in CAMHS teams. In many meetings held between the profession and the NHS it is reiterated that while funding child psychotherapist trainees is an expensive proposition on a per capita basis, the very low rate of attrition followed by many years of service make us a good investment! Certainly the advent of these posts changed the training landscape. The Anna Freud training was very successful in securing a number of these posts for its trainees but inevitably demand outstripped supply. Trainees without a funded post gained their clinical experience in an honorary capacity as interns in NHS or in voluntary sector organizations (sometimes paid), with a number of cases obtained through the Anna Freud Centre.

The training has always been arduous in terms of its demands on the trainee but originally trainees also worked, often in the NHS. At some point the training became full time and took place entirely within the Centre. Generous scholarships covering training school fees, supervision, and analysis were available to UK trainees. Self-funded trainees either had to have personal means of support or undertook the training incurring substantial debts. The more recent training posts meant that the training had to be restructured. Attendance at the training school now took place on one day a week when papers or diagnostic assessments were presented. Seminars, as before, took place on two evenings a week. There is no doubt that the training posts proved an excellent training environment for the trainees who would then work in the UK context. Invaluable experience was gained from being part of a multidisciplinary team. However, with the contracted hours of training at the Centre there was less opportunity for trainees to have informal common room exchanges and hear about each other's cases. There was a different sense of "belonging" to the institution. However, some work such as running toddler groups was available for trainees and that reinforced a more "professional" side to being a trainee.

In order to capture some of the changes I will contrast one or two aspects of the training experience of the final 2004 cohort who qualified in 2009 with the cohort who qualified nineteen years earlier in 1990. Those of us who qualified in 1990 (and earlier) saw three cases: an under five, latency, and adolescent, at the frequency of five times a week. The 1990 cohort (and those of the decade-plus earlier) would, in addition to their intensive cases, have treated around three non-intensive cases. Additional requirements included parent work, social histories, and diagnostic assessments, all with the majority of cases provided by the Clinic. Indexing, where a completed clinical case was indexed with clinical examples drawn from sessions to illustrate core psychoanalytic concepts, was also a requirement and within the tradition of the concept groups originally set up by *Professor Joseph Sandler.* Somewhere along the line indexing was dropped as a requirement but in the meantime other requirements had multiplied in line with changing practices in the National Health Service.

The 2009 trainees, in addition to the requirements listed above, would have treated six non-intensive cases. Many trainees would also have undertaken a number of additional family assessments as members of a multidisciplinary team. They also had experience of consulting to allied professionals. The frequency of treatment requirement was dropped to four times a week for two cases. In exceptional circumstances, where a particular CAMHS service had real difficulties in providing cases at this frequency the training committee agreed to two cases at three times a week. While this represented an at times regretted change, nonetheless this was still more than the usual three cases at three times a week frequency undertaken by those from other trainings.

The written work requirements of the Anna Freud training were well over and above the ACP minimum requirements. Individual sessions, weeklies, monthlies, six monthlies, and closing reports were the ongoing Sisyphean tasks. As caseloads increased weekly reports became monthly. These, in conjunction with the social histories and diagnostics meant that trainees not only had to record the transference/countertransference experience of being with a child but also to link and integrate the experiences to psychoanalytic understanding and concepts.

This systematic approach was important in offering a "map" within which the trainee could learn to navigate their way through developmental and unconscious waters. Those wishing to make a strong case for a greater pluralism might criticize the approach as one leading to rigidity. However, one likes to think that this "orientation" was not at the cost of exercising independence of thought; rigidity was not inherent in the system but only in the way it might be applied.

Trainees wrote two clinical papers, one on an intensive case. (Some of these are presented in this book.) The clinical accounts, presented at the Wednesday Scientific Meetings, reflected the training's emphasis on the therapist using all their creativity and analytic understanding to get in touch with their patients through play. Latterly trainees presented very complex, developmentally delayed, traumatized cases which often featured abuse, severe breaks in continuity of care, and parental mental health problems.

Until its demise in 1995 the *Bulletin of the Anna Freud Centre*, edited by Barbara Sullivan (now available on PEP-WEB), regularly published trainees' clinical papers as well as mother-infant, toddler, and nursery observation papers, and hence stands as a record of the rigorous nature of clinical work. These initial experiences of appearing in print were encouraging for trainees who had an interest in publishing further. The *Bulletin* also testified to the several outside influences trainees were privileged to have heard such as the lectures given by Professor Mark Solms in the early years of neuropsychoanalysis.

In 1993, the pre-clinical year of the training became incorporated into an academic master of science degree programme in psychoanalytic developmental psychology conferred by University College London. It could be undertaken on either a one-year full-time or two-year part-time basis, the latter making this a more realistic proposition for many would-be trainees. In addition to psychoanalytic theory, the MSc offered lectures on attachment theory and child developmentalist research, as well as observation of an infant in the family, and nursery or toddler group observations, so that future trainees began with a broader frame of reference.

They were also research-literate having trained in methodology and completed their own research assignments.

Then in 1999/2000, following the groundwork done by Professor Peter Fonagy, the training, in conjunction with UCL, offered the possibility of undertaking a professional doctorate in psychoanalytic psychotherapy with children and adolescents (DPsych). The Anna Freud Centre trainees were the first to undertake this clinical doctorate, followed by the Tavistock child psychotherapy training (through the University of East London). (In 2006 a second MSc was established at the AFC in Psychodynamic Developmental Neuroscience in collaboration with UCL and Yale University Child Study Center.)

In an "evidence based" culture the clarion call from both outside and within the profession, to produce not only research-aware but research-active child psychotherapists, grew ever louder. The absence of evidence within the field became untenable and had to be redressed. It became critical for clinicians to be able to engage publicly with testing questions as to the robustness of their treatment modality and also to be able to produce research on a range of topics including therapeutic outcome, treatment efficacy, and heuristic questions. A number of students signed up for the doctorate and to date four have completed and a further three will be submitting in the near future.

In alumnae such as Dr Jill Hodges and Dr Miriam Steele, the Centre already had a long history of clinicians undertaking research, and in some cases those who remained primarily as committed researchers also training as clinicians. Currently, the Centre has a number of AFC trained clinicians such as Tessa Baradon (PIP manager), who combine delivering a clinical service with research. In the course of the doctorate getting underway and a greater number of trainees beginning to engage with research questions, there were some significant debates within the Centre, and subsequent publications reflected these discussions about the limits and possibilities of different underlying epistemologies and quantitative versus qualitative research methods. It is widely recognized within the profession that the Anna Freud Centre, particularly under the present directorial team, continues to be in the forefront of research activity and that those who have emerged from the training are making a significant contribution.

Tradition and revision

In this final section I would like to highlight further some features of the particular cultural milieu at the Centre which gave the training its particular stamp.

The Anna Freud Centre had a history of clinical and conceptual research groups arising out of which were a number of significant publications. One of these was Anna Freud's and *Dorothy Burlingham's* seminal work on the development of blind children. Others included simultaneous analysis of mother and child, a research group on borderline personality, the Index, and interest groups on adoption and bisexuality. This culture meant that there was a fund of understanding held in the minds of seminar leaders and supervisors who had participated in these study groups. If one had the luck to be supervised by someone who had taken part in a group relevant to one's case, the expertise offered was invaluable, as one could both work with the clinical material at hand, and in supervision begin to understand how issues were also germane to a particular group. This history also fostered a cast of mind where it was possible to go on questioning received wisdom, and to generate one's own questions. The work of the borderline group was a good example of how understanding of anxieties and defences built on Anna Freud's work on the ego and defences could help conceptualize the nature of overwhelming and disintegratory anxiety in these children. Clinical technique altered in the process. Exploring this "deficit" in borderline children led to revisions of working in a way that would not escalate the child's anxiety to dysregulatory levels, with a view to fostering and strengthening developmental processes. (An example of the enduring understanding is evident in B. Smith's (2000) published treatment case of a borderline child.)

The provisional diagnostic profile

As much has been written elsewhere about the provisional Diagnostic Profile (PDR) (A. Freud, 1962; Edgcumbe, 2002; Green, 2003) a few points will suffice: the regular diagnostic meetings, chaired by Dr Clifford Yorke in the 1980s and later by Dr Duncan McLean, constituted a crucial part of the training experience for all generations. The PDP invited the diagnostician to engage in a very detailed assessment of the child or adolescent taking into account external and internal factors resulting in a psychoanalytic formulation of the difficulty.

The challenge was to move from the immediate experience of being with the child in the interviews to a second order understanding reflecting on different aspects of their psychic organization through the developmental perspective inscribed in the different sections of the Profile. While the developmental "story" was different for each child the underlying assumption was that the child's inner emotional landscape was fashioned through a dynamic interplay between forces from within the child and impacted upon from without. The PDR took as a given that development was a weave of many threads in a series of intricate interdependencies between maturational sequences, experiences afforded or withheld by the environment, and developmental steps reflecting the growing internal psychodynamic organization.

It is worth mentioning that while "constitutional" factors were taken into account this metapsychological view did not ascribe an "innate" strength to affects such as aggression, envy, or destructiveness, but (where these might be marked features in a child's presentation) tended to understand them as a failure in the early relationship.

One section of the Profile focused on the ego, anxiety, and defences—areas where Anna Freud made her original contributions. The nature and degree of the child's anxieties and the relative strength or fragility of the child's ego in coping with distressing experiences were given careful consideration, and this included areas of resilience.

At the heart of emotional development lay the relationship between the child and his/her primary caregivers: the manner in which they were inscribed in the child's internal world sculpting his/her conscious and unconscious, affective, and fantasy life. In the course of learning how to put together the psychic jigsaw, trainees imbibed and applied a range of psychoanalytic concepts. They had to learn to work within a format that was never intended to be an exhaustive box-ticking exercise but an invitation to try to define the salient areas to consider with a particular child. Complex issues such as the relative contributions of internal and external factors, what was deficit, what was conflict; and how did these dynamically interact, were factors to be teased out in the discussion of each child.

These many strands woven into the child's inner psychic organization were also to be thought about when making a recommendation. Trainees would have to take a view on the nature and underlying causes of the presenting problem, the child's internal object world, and his/her capacity to make relationships, and other overarching considerations such as whether the child's development was moving forwards, backwards, or was stuck. Discussion also focused not only on questions of intensity of treatment but questions around the timing and nature of treatment, i.e., should parent work start first, should there be a family intervention? In some cases, it was a useful learning experience for trainees to know that some cases needed additional referral to other agencies such as social services or that individual treatment was not indicated whereas a referral to specialist setting such as a boarding school might be.

The experience of the Wednesday Meetings and other opportunities to hear about other clinicians' cases on a regular basis was an important part of the training. Regrettably, in the last years of the training there were few opportunities to hear staff presenting at these meetings.

This concentrated and systematic way of understanding a child offered a framework which could later be modified and applied in different contexts, e.g., undertaking court assessments. The Profile proved a useful tool and was tailored by Moses and Egle Laufer for assessing adolescents at the Brent Adolescent Centre. In the early part of the decade a group led by Dr McLean produced a revised version. Other members of the group were Jenny Davids, Angela Joyce, and this writer. The challenge, as we struggled to make room for sometimes jostling frameworks, was to incorporate considerations drawn from contemporary developmental and attachment research (such as meeting the child's need in its safety seeking and its "theory of mind") without jettisoning the profile's psychosexual metapsychology. This drew the disapprobation of some who felt that a fundamental aspect of Anna Freud's (and her father's) legacy had been tampered with, but at the same time it says a great deal about the flexibility inherent in the tradition that it was not preserved in aspic and that "modernization" could occur.

Communicating with the child

There was also something in the training's DNA that imparted a sense of the importance of play as a therapeutic medium and simply as the expressive medium through which children expressed their internal preoccupations. A good example of engagement with a hard to reach atypical child can be found in Audrey Gavshon's paper presented at a Colloquium on the same topic, where she described the ways in which communication could lie outside words when they let their "fingers do the talking". Play can be serious, hard work but there is a way in which supervisions, teaching, and the trainees' own capacities to play meant that playfulness and a lightness of touch were encouraged in the technique.

At the AFC there are still ongoing weekly clinical groups. During the period when the training existed these were attended by both staff and trainees. In the collegial atmosphere there was continuing focus on questions of technique as well as psychoanalytic understanding. Discussions revealed the different shades of opinion or rather emphasis held within the culture which encompassed classical, Winnicottian and Intersubjectivist stances as well as more specific interests in attachment theory or neuroscience.

A developmental perspective within child psychoanalysis

A common thread can be found in the publications of those trained within the tradition that can best be summed up as a "developmental perspective". *Anne Hurry*'s work (1998) laid the groundwork when she spelt out her understanding of the ways in which the therapist acted as an integrated transference object and a new development object. *Rose Edgcumbe* (2000) meticulously traced the ways in which in Anna Freud's thinking the different stages of the child's psychic growth were embedded in his psychic fantasies and expressed in symptoms. The broadening frames of reference were captured in this author's book (Green, 2003) which sought to integrate approaches from psychoanalysis, attachment theory, and neuroscience. Again, in the clinical accounts attention is paid to the ways in which the child's level of development shapes its internal worlds and the therapist's responses and understanding. More recently, the careful consideration paid to a specific phase is captured in a publication on toddlers by Marie Zaphiriou Woods and Inge Pretorius.

An ending and new beginnings

The Anna Freud's Centre current organizational mission is described on its website (http://www.annafreud.org). Several of the founder's original aims have been recast and revitalized into a contemporary context with a continued emphasis on research and clinical projects. Nonetheless, the decision to close the clinical training started by Anna Freud and to reset the direction of the Anna Freud Centre provoked an outcry from several quarters including the ACP, the professional body which prided itself on its pluralism. This decision had an ongoing undulating effect within the organization itself. The final training committee comprised of myself as the head of training, Duncan McLean, Mary Target, Marie Zaphiriou, Tessa Baradon, and Janine Sternberg as an external member, was keenly aware that trainees (and indeed staff) were experiencing the effects of a rapidly changing organization. These effects were felt in myriad ways and thus extra care was taken to protect the training's quality and standard. It was helpful that the final cohort were all in training posts but there was also inevitable sadness for all involved.

Subsequent to the decision, the directors (with the backing of the trustees) undertook to see if a training funded by the NHS could be resuscitated by joining forces with the British Association of Psychotherapists as a sister voluntary sector organization. A good deal of time and effort by the directors and the head of training was devoted to a protracted series of negotiations with both the National Health Service and the British Association of Psychotherapists. Regrettably, although this move initially had the full backing of the ACP, after a number of key decisions by the NHS and then by the BAP, such a partnership proved impossible. It is probably also true that the Anna Freud Centre itself, in its long overdue need to set a course for the next stage of its life, had made some strategic miscalculations. We might have been in a stronger negotiating position with the NHS had the training still been running. The BAP ultimately did not wish to join forces, preferring to maintain its own training's integrity. Currently discussions are underway with the Institute of Psychoanalysis to see whether and how an Anna Freudian tradition can continue within its child training.

At the risk of being accused of being "tribal", it is this writer's view that in its demise something very precious was lost and this is a view echoed by many others. The training shaped generations of us with a sense that what was really important was simply being in a room with a child and learning to trust and work with one's own creativity to get in touch with what mattered to the child. Following this, although one had to learn the "trade" so to speak, clinical understanding was fostered in an atmosphere of apprenticeship which encouraged you to use your own psychoanalytic mind. Hedde Maartje Evers captures her experience (training 2003–2009) thus:

> I came to the Anna Freud Centre as a young psychologist from the Netherlands keen to begin the most thorough and in depth child analytic training I had been able to find. Little did I know then how rich, fulfilling and intensive my training at the Anna Freud Centre would really turn out to be. The training was all encompassing, and my seven years at the Anna Freud Centre were certainly amongst the busiest and the most formative years of my life. I feel very privileged to have been able to train at the Anna Freud Centre and to have been taught, supervised and "brought up" psychoanalytically by such dedicated and excellent child clinicians.

It is a striking testimony to the "visionary" aspects of its founder that the training produced international alumnae who had very varied careers in the public, private, and voluntary sectors and several of whom pioneered specialist services. Many still attend the annual Colloquium at the Anna Freud Centre. They are a group too, whose work is reflected in their publications covering a broad range of clinical work and research. Most of all they have impacted on the lives of many individual children worldwide.

References

Edgcumbe, R. (1995). The history of Anna Freud's thinking on developmental influences. *Bulletin of the Anna Freud Centre, 18*(1).

Edgcumbe, R. (2000). *Anna Freud: A View of Development, Disturbance and Therapeutic Techniques.* London: Routledge.

Freud, A. (1965). *Normality and Pathology in Childhood.* London: Hogarth.

Freud, A. (1965). The concept of Developmental Lines. In: *Normality and Pathology in Childhood* (pp. 62–92). London: Hogarth.

Freud, A. (1972). A psychoanalytic view of developmental psychopathology. In: *The Writings of Anna Freud, Vol. VIII.* New York: International Universities Press.

Gavshon, A. (1988). Playing: its role in child analysis. *Journal of Child Psychotherapy, 15*(1): 47–62.

Green, V. (1995). Developmental considerations and diagnostic assessments. *Bulletin of the Anna Freud Centre, 18*(3).

Green, V. (Ed.) (2003). *Emotional Development in Psychoanalysis, Attachment Theory and Neuroscience.* London: Routledge.

Green, V. (2009). Intensive psychotherapy. In: A. Horne & M. Lanyado (Eds.), *Handbook of Child and Adolescent Psychoanalytic Psychotherapy* (2nd edition). London: Routledge

Hurry, A. (Ed.) (1998). *Psychoanalysis and Development Therapy.* London: Karnac.

King, P. & Steiner, R. (1991). *The Freud-Klein Controversies 1941–1945*. London: Tavistock.

Midgley, N. (2009). Research. In: M. Lanyado & A. Horne (Eds.), *The Handbook of Child and Adolescent Psychotherapy: Psychoanalytic Approaches*. London: Routledge.

Miller, M. J. & Neely, C. (2008). *The Psychoanalytic Work of Hansi Kennedy: from the War Nurseries to the Anna Freud Centre (1940–1993)*. London: Karnac.

Sandler, J., Holder, A., Dare, C. & Dreher, A. U. (1997). *Freud's Models of the Mind: an Introduction*. London: Karnac.

Smith, B. (2000). From the "drunken boat" to the "Chinese junk": the treatment of an 8-year-old boy with severe ego impairment. In: T. Lubbe (Ed.), *The Borderline Psychotic Child*. London: Routledge.

Tyson, P. & Tyson, R. (1990). *Psychoanalytic Theories of Development*. New Haven, CT: Yale University Press.

Zaphiriou Woods, M. & Pretorius, I. M. (Eds.) (2010). *Parents and Toddlers in Groups: a Psychoanalytic Developmental Approach*. London: Routledge.

PART II

CLINICAL WORK AND APPLICATIONS OF ANNA FREUD'S DEVELOPMENTAL TRADITION

A. INFANCY

Observations, interventions, and applications

Overview

CHAPTER EIGHT

Overview of theoretical and clinical applications, and current developments

Frances Thomson Salo

Infancy

The range of psychodynamic interventions in infancy has changed enormously since Anna Freud's day but I think she would have been interested in the explosion of knowledge about infants and pleased about therapeutic developments.

Infant capacities

With new research technology, knowledge about the capacities of babies is increasingly augmented by studies in neonatal temperament and attachment, and from neuroscience. A different kind of knowledge is gained from psychoanalytic infant observation which offers a fine-grained way of coming to know the baby in his or her family over one or two years.

All these provide evidence for our intuitive understanding that in the baby's developing sense of self from birth, active agency, differentiation and recognition of self and other, and a capacity for empathy, are important.

The world of the baby is interactive from the start. Newborns actively process information and can imitate their parents' facial gestures even in the first hour. Imitation has been described as a two-way bridge that bears psychological traffic from birth and helps the differentiation of self and other (Meltzoff, 2005). Babies want above all to be enthusiastically enjoyed by their parents, to matter to them, to be in their mind. They can show their pleasure by smiling in the first week. A mirroring system for matching expressive states between people is active in the brain probably from birth and provides a neurobiological basis for empathy and intersubjectivity, the capacity to understand the feelings of other people and share subjective experiences. From the second month onwards babies are capable of complex relational feelings. When they feel that they have successfully captured another person's attention and approval, they have a sense of pride; they can feel shame if they cannot entrance their parents or feel misunderstood or disliked.

In a two-parent family a baby's father usually becomes quickly important, offering an exciting experience of difference. His being a third person in a close relationship with the baby's mother enables the baby to explore feelings about being both included in that relationship and sometimes feeling excluded. By about two months most babies gain considerable pleasure from their siblings and by the following month they will, when interacting with one person, reach out with vocalization and gesture to include a third person in their interactions. Differentiation continues to develop and five-month-old babies have been shown to discriminate between boy and girl toddlers. They have a capacity in their first year to differentiate between good and bad and to prefer the helpful other to an unhelpful one (Bloom, 2010).

The process of separation occurs within the envelope of attachment, that deep emotional bond formed between babies and the adults who look after them. While the attachment relationship is universal, the way that parents and babies express it differs in different societies. Securely attached babies explore their world with pleasure and can find comfort from their carers when they need this. When things go well and their anxieties are sensitively responded to, a secure attachment relationship is imbued with good self-esteem. Parents who were themselves insecurely attached to their own parents are likely to have babies who find it difficult to explore and be comforted. Parents who have unresolved traumatic events in their own attachment history are significantly more likely to have babies whose attachment relationships are disorganized, making it difficult in turn for them to find security and comfort.

The role of parents in promoting mentalization and repairing emotional rupture in relationships is seen as one of overriding importance. It is now established that a baby's comprehension of language allows her/him to understand words that are frequently repeated and to begin to enunciate them by six months. Confirming Freud's hunch, evidence from the field of neuroscience has contributed to the view of early relational experiences as a template through which subsequent experiences are filtered and shape brain structure. There is increasing evidence of the effect that a mother's anxiety and mood disturbances have on her unborn baby, and new knowledge of risk factors for parenting such as unresolved bereavement and trauma. Recent research has indicated that a mother's negative attitude to her infant in the first month is significantly more likely to predispose him/her to insecure attachment forty years later (Broussard & Cassidy, 2010). How to intervene becomes ever more important.

* * *

Clinical applications and current developments

The Parent–Infant Project of the Anna Freud Centre is located within the tradition of psychoanalytic parent–infant psychotherapy developed by Selma Fraiberg (1980). It is clearly described by a number of PIP psychotherapists in the book *Practice of Psychoanalytic Parent Infant Psychotherapy: Claiming the Baby*, by Tessa Baradon and her colleagues (2005). The therapist functions as a "container" for those parental projections that are directed towards the infant and through interpretation s/he tries to shape the parents' representations so that the effect of the projections on the infant is lessened. The Parent–Infant Project has offered both short and long term therapy to parent–infant dyads and has also developed a number of group models, while incorporating some elements of Anna Freud's idea of "developmental guidance" as well as a Watch, Wait and Wonder stance (Cohen et al., 1999).

Clinical and research evidence suggest that rather than viewing only the mother (or parents) as the patient, both the parent–infant relationship and the infant should be recognized as needing therapeutic intervention. There is general acceptance that an intervention can target different entry points such as a parent's behaviour or their representations, or the infant's, and this will affect all parts of the parent–infant system. While the infant is present in sessions, to support parental function and avoid undermining this, the PIP staff have focused their therapeutic interventions more on the parents, aiming for a therapeutic position that is poised equally between parents and infant. Change in parental interaction or representations could be viewed as regaining or beginning to develop an internal good object through the availability of a new object, the therapist. Videoing parent–infant interaction to discuss with the parents has been found to be very helpful in modulating troublesome projections. Striking results can be achieved relatively quickly in this work, changes in disorganized attachment patterns taking longer to consolidate.

New clinical methods and target populations commingle. There has for some time been a greater awareness of the need for specificity in matching interventions with different kinds of patient difficulties. Recognition of the crucial importance of early intervention has impelled many innovative and creative approaches worldwide, including work with traumatized and refugee populations. Thus the Anna Freud Centre PIP has been extended to include work with mothers in drop-in hostels and in prisons and the PIP staff has increasingly publicized this work in articles and conference presentations, culminating in a second book, *Relational Trauma* (Baradon, 2010). This approach has spread worldwide as it became more widely known through the annual PIP International Study Day held in conjunction with the Colloquium in which invited participants from around the world work with PIP staff using video and DVD clips to gain a closer understanding of the dynamics behind differing techniques of the work.

The approach became further known as Anna Freud Centre graduates began working in countries overseas, with local variations, mainly in the USA but also Australia and South Africa. Engaging with the infant in the presence of the parents to understand the meaning of the infant's experience re-presents the infant to the parent (Thomson Salo, 2007). This is thought to increase reflective thinking in both parent and infant. The PIP therapists, also drawing on the contributions from neuroscience, have included speaking *to* the infant as an element in their work. With very premature infants, the high rate of anxiety and trauma experienced by their parents has prompted clinicians to develop therapeutic interventions that are appropriate to the different stages of the parent and infant journey through the neonatal intensive care unit. Other developments involve offering a group experience for parents and infants who have experienced family violence in the first year, to mitigate the effect on the infant's development. Related developments are the exploration of effective interventions that mothers with serious mental illness would find acceptable, and for adolescent mothers if they experience difficulty in seeing their baby as a person (Jones, 2007).

PIP staff have also responded to requests to help develop services and trainings in a number of countries such as USA and South Africa, for example, to meet basic infant mental health needs in health facilities in areas with overstretched resources (see chapter 20). The therapeutic interventions described are being clinically refined at the same time as they are being researched empirically in order to become clearer about the effective therapeutic factors (Fonagy, 2010).

The three papers that follow in this part describe a psychoanalytic infant observation, clinical intervention, and developmental guidance with mothers and infants, illustrating the urgent need to intervene as early as possible with troubled families. Nick Midgley's chapter conveys the fine-grained observation of an infant over his first two years as he painfully struggles with a situation that Midgley characterizes as maternal ambivalence that is close to being unmanageable. Midgley clearly illustrates the gains for knowledge in carrying out an infant observation and the growth of the therapist's capacity to become more containing in therapeutic encounters. Despite the intrusion that the infant experiences there is an absence of expectable anger until the emergence of later ADHD-type symptoms. The paper also raises a question about the self-selected nature of observed families and whether in very difficult observations more could be done for the mother and infant apart from the containing presence of the observer.

Michela Biseo's chapter shows how the therapist's sensitive interventions combined with necessary technical modifications enable parents and infants to evolve the possibility of a different way of relating. In the first mother-infant dyad she describes, working with an interpreter unexpectedly allowed the infant the possibility of a benign male figure to whom to relate. In the second dyad, she explains how working with video with a traumatized mother, who actually did some of the filming of her infant herself, empowered the mother to transform a traumatic experience in which she had felt victimized to one in which she felt she had some agency. This contributed to her being able to see her infant son in a more joyful and desiring way.

Sheila Levi describes some innovative work with a psychologically traumatized immigrant mother and her physically damaged and silent baby, and the technical modifications this necessitated in offering mother-infant psychotherapy in their home setting, and in her native tongue. She illustrates the need to recognize the mother's own unresolved traumatic experience before the incapacitating maternal ambivalence towards the infant and authority figures can be overcome.

The work described by Midgley, Biseo, and Levi exemplifies the best in the Anna Freudian tradition of understanding the meaning in the carer-infant communications, and finding flexible ways to intervene more effectively with troubled families, as well as honouring Anna Freud's commitment to make this available to those most in need.

References

Baradon, T. (Ed.) (2010). *Relational Trauma in Infancy: Psychoanalytic, Attachment and Neuropsychological Contributions to Parent–Infant Psychotherapy*. Hove, UK: Routledge.

Baradon, T., Broughton, C., Gibbs, I., James, J., Joyce, A. & Woodhead, J. (Eds.) (2005). *Practice of Psychoanalytic Parent Infant Psychotherapy: Claiming the Baby*. London: Routledge.

Bloom, P. (2010). *How Pleasure Works: The New Science of Why We Like What We Like*. New York: W. W. Norton.

Broussard, E. R. & Cassidy, J. (2010). Maternal perception of newborns predicts attachment organization in middle adulthood. *Attachment & Human Development, 12*: 159–172.

Cohen, N., Muir, E., Parker, C., Brown, M., Lojkasek, M., Muir, R. & Barwick, M. (1999). Watch, Wait and Wonder: testing the effectiveness of a new approach to mother-infant psychotherapy. *Infant Mental Health Journal, 20*: 429–451.

Fonagy, P. (2010). The changing shape of clinical practice: driven by science or by pragmatics? *Psychoanalytic Psychotherapy, 24*: 22–43.

Fraiberg, S. (Ed.) (1980). *Clinical Studies in Infant Mental Health: The First Year of Life* New York: Basic.

Jones, A. (2007). Levels of change in parent–infant psychotherapy. *Journal of Child Psychotherapy, 32*(3): 295–311.

Meltzoff, A. N. (2005). Imitation and other minds: the "like me" hypothesis. In: S. Hurley & N. Chater (Eds.), *Perspectives on Imitation: from Neuroscience to Social Science*. Cambridge, MA: MIT Press.

Thomson Salo, F. (2007). Recognising the infant as subject in infant-parent psychotherapy. *International Journal of Psychoanalysis, 88*: 961–979.

Observation

CHAPTER NINE

Aggression in relation to emotional development: an observation of an infant and his family in the first two years of life

Nick Midgley

> The mother ... hates her infant from the word go. I believe Freud thought it possible that a mother may in certain circumstances have only love for her baby boy; but we may doubt this. We know about a mother's love and we appreciate its reality and power. Let me give some of the reasons why a mother hates her baby, even a boy ...
> ... The baby is a danger to her body in pregnancy and in birth.
> The baby is an interference with her private life, a challenge to her preoccupation.
> To a greater or lesser degree a mother feels her own mother demands a baby, so that her baby is produced to placate her mother ...
> He is ruthless, treats her as scum, an unpaid servant, a slave.
> She has to love him, excretions and all ...
> He tries to hurt her, periodically bites her, all in love.
> He shows disillusionment about her.
> His excited love is cupboard love, so that having got what he wants he throws her away like orange peel ...
> At first he does not know at all what she does or what she sacrifices for him. Especially he cannot allow her to hate.
> He is suspicious, refuses her good food, and makes her doubt herself, but eats well with his aunt.
> After an awful morning with him she goes out, and he smiles at a stranger, who says "Isn't he sweet?."
> If she fails him at the start she knows he will pay her out forever.
> He excites her but frustrates her—she mustn't eat him or trade in sex with him
>
> —(D. W. Winnicott, "Hate in the Countertransference", 1949, pp. 73–74).

Introduction

Psychoanalysis has a long history of attempting to understand the place of aggression in early infant development. Freud himself struggled about whether to regard aggression as an aspect of the sexual instinct (1905), or the self-preservative instinct (1914), or as deriving from a distinct death drive (1920). Others have continued to grapple with a psychoanalytic conception of early infantile aggression, ranging from Abraham's introduction of the oral- and anal-sadistic stages of libidinal development (1924), through to Klein's work on the primacy of destructive phantasies in early emotional development (1957), and the work of Independent analysts such as Balint and Fairbairn on aggression as not innate but a result of frustration (Rayner, 1991).

And yet, as Anna Freud pointed out at the end of the 27th International Psychoanalytic Congress on the theme of aggression, in 1971, all of these debates somehow failed to remove many of the doubts and uncertainties about the status of aggression, including "the part played by aggression in normal infantile development" (1977, p. 152). In the same speech Anna Freud went on to suggest that one productive way forward might be through the use of mother-infant observations, because these "provide important data as to the links between aggressive development and the incidence of maternal care or maternal deprivation" (1977, p. 169).

Of course mother-infant observations are never theoretically "objective", and to that extent cannot be used to settle theoretical disagreements over the status of aggression. Nevertheless, observations at least oblige us to find empirical support for the hypotheses we have, and do so in a unique setting to assess the links between "aggressive development and the incidence of maternal care". Moreover, since Anna Freud made her comments, there have been a number of contributions to the psychoanalytic study of aggression which manage to avoid the split between "nature" and "nurture" that seems to have been such a stumbling block for earlier psychoanalytic thinking (e.g., Cohen, 1993; Fonagy & Target, 1993; Perelberg, 1995; Harris, 1998; and Mitchell, 1998).

Most contemporary psychoanalytic contributions to this topic, to a greater or lesser degree, pay tribute to the pioneering work of D.W. Winnicott, whose thinking about aggression and emotional development spans the whole of his career (1939, 1947, 1950, 1960c, 1963a, 1963b, 1964; Philips, 1988), and whose important 1950 paper on "Aggression in Relation to Emotional Development" is the source of this paper's title. There have also been valuable observational studies of the subject, such as Henri Parens's monumental work, *The Role of Aggression in Early Infancy* (1979), which I have benefitted from greatly.

It therefore seems a good moment to try to explore once again the issue of aggression in relation to emotional development, integrating psychoanalytic thinking with observations I conducted over a two-year period of the relationship between a baby, whom I will call Wayne, and his mother, Cathy.

Family background

Wayne is the third child of a family living on a rough council estate in south London. It is a close-knit community, in which Wayne's mother, Cathy, lives on the same estate where she was born and grew up. She herself was the youngest of six children, with a ten-year gap between herself and her nearest sibling—a brother said to have gone "strange" when Cathy was born, who is now extremely violent. All of Cathy's siblings and their families live on the same council estate, as does her mother, known by everyone as Nan, a pillar of the local community who was once invited by the queen to have tea at Buckingham Palace. Wayne was her nineteenth grandchild at the time the observation began; several more were born before it ended.

Cathy, who is in her mid-twenties, was described to me by the health visitor who helped set up the observation as a "rough diamond". Cathy enjoys such a reputation, and looks suitably rough with her short black hair, a nose stud, and tattoos along her arm. Her favourite hobby is watching horror movies, sitting up late at night with videos of *The Exorcist* or *The Boston Strangler*. But there is also a creative side to Cathy, whose paintings (albeit of monsters) illustrate the walls of the bathroom, and whose descriptions of her life and family—such as the death of her father when she was just nineteen, or the day she got married—are often poignant, heartfelt, and almost lyrical. Cathy enjoyed telling stories of how she was a tomboy at school, more interested in soccer than skirts, and frequently getting into fights. She was expelled from school for setting fire to a girl's hair with a Bunsen burner, and was thought by most people to be a "lesbo".

Cathy's husband, Andy, whom she met when she was sixteen, was her first boyfriend, and the first man, she said, to just accept her as she was. In contrast to Cathy's background, Andy is an only child from north London, and was effectively "adopted" into Cathy's extended family when they were married. Andy works as a postman, and in his few comments about his own family background implied that he did not get on very well with his family. Andy is rather soft-spoken and gentle, but I was told that Andy and Cathy argue frequently, Cathy accusing Andy of being "a lazy sod" who just sits around smoking dope. At times Cathy has been quite violent towards him, and I was told that sometimes he quite literally had to sit on her just to calm her down, she got so out of control.

Visiting Wayne's home for the observations was never a quiet event. In addition to Wayne and his mother, the two elder siblings, Martin (aged two when Wayne was born) and Gabriella (aged four) were frequently at home, as were Andy (often playing sick to get off work), Nan, and Cathy's best friend Donna, whose daughter was the same age as Gabriella. Huddled together in a small living room, where the television or the stereo (or both) were almost constantly playing at a loud level, it was sometimes difficult to focus on Wayne and his development, and this may well have been his experience too—lost amongst a wealth of stimuli and activity.

Observations

The first year

Wayne was a fairly robust baby, 8 lb. 10 oz. at birth, with a big round face, a large chin, and a good head of dark hair. Although the birth had been smooth, there were some complications afterwards and there had been a possibility that the baby was anaemic. This appears to have been handled badly by the doctors, who lost the results of Wayne's first blood test and failed to tell his parents what was going on. Andy shouted at the doctor and Cathy had a fight with the anaesthetist, but in the end everything had been fine. Over the coming months I was to learn that fighting with authority figures—teachers, health visitors, doctors—was a regular feature of this family's life. But for now there was relief that Wayne was safe and well, and he appeared to be sleeping well and drinking healthily from the bottle. Cathy had chosen not to breastfeed, explaining that she had smoked all through the pregnancy, and had been told that this "affected the milk".

Wayne was asleep during my first visit, the day after he had come out of hospital, tucked up so that I could not see him, but I saw him awake for the first time a week later, when he was ten days old:

> When I arrived Cathy was changing Wayne on the bed in the bedroom. She was trying to get his nappy on, and his legs were thrashing about. He wasn't crying but he was on the verge—making little snorting noises and squeals. Cathy talked to him all through changing and washing him—"Keep still you little toad," "You don't like getting dressed, do you?" She was trying to stop him from crying, and dealt with him firmly but sensitively. All through it Wayne had his eyes closed, until he was almost dressed. When she started putting oil on his face he opened his eyes, and became calmer. Andy joked about putting Wayne in the oven—baked Wayne for dinner. Cathy moved up close to Wayne's face and tried to get his attention, but he gazed around him without stopping at her face. Cathy commented that she knows he can't see properly yet, but that he recognizes her voice, and Andy's (first visit, 27.9.96).

Certainly Wayne's thrashing about could be understood as a mild example of "unpleasure-related destructiveness" (Parens, 1979) in response to the experience of having his nappy changed, the exposure of his skin to the air, the removal of the comfort of the contact with his soft clothes. That Wayne was able to deal with these unpleasurable stimuli without too powerful a "rage reaction" was no doubt related to the quality of maternal care. Both in the firm sensitivity of her holding, and the imaginative identification with her infant's experience, Cathy was able to modify Wayne's experience of unpleasure. She attributed intentionality to Wayne even if she thought he was physically incapable of seeing her, and imagined already that her voice—and her husband's—had a particular meaning for her child.

On the other hand, even at this stage there were suggestions of another aspect of the relationship. Cathy's sense that her milk could damage Wayne might suggest that she saw her love for her infant as deeply destructive; or perhaps the decision not to breastfeed was an attempt to escape from the neediness that this would imply? Likewise, Andy's comment about cooking Wayne in the oven and eating him is in some ways no more than a variant of the common adult comment about babies—"So good I could eat you up!"—but it has a graphically aggressive quality that I was to see on many occasions to come. (Before Christmas Cathy elaborated on the fantasy, describing how they would put Wayne in the oven as the Christmas turkey, that his brother and sister would eat an arm each, Cathy would have his leg, and they would leave his head to boil.)

Indeed, only a few weeks after the previous observation the interaction between mother and child was quite different. Wayne was now one month old. When I arrived, Cathy was clearly exasperated, screaming at Martin to tidy up his room while Gabriella was in tears. "There's not a fucking moment's peace in this house!" despaired Cathy, as the door bell rang and her Nan arrived. The observation continues:

> There was a fair deal of chat going on, with Cathy trying to control the behaviour of the kids and getting very short-tempered. A smell was coming from Martin, and Cathy called him a "smelly little shit" and almost hit him, then counted to ten, as if she'd learnt this as a temper control exercise. She started to feed Wayne with the bottle, saying "Get it in your mouth, you little turd," then explaining to me that this was the third time he'd had milk this morning ... Wayne drank from the bottle quite passively, not sucking very vigorously. His eyes were open, but looking away from Cathy, across the room to where Nan and Gabriella were sitting. "He doesn't seem that hungry," said Nan. "Yeah, I'm just feeding him to shut him up," replied Cathy, and took the bottle from his mouth.

It is painful to imagine how Wayne must have experienced this aggressive handling by his mother, one which is not responsive to his need but might be described as an "impingement". It is as if the act of nurturance (feeding) has been perverted into an aggressive attack, and Wayne responds not with aggression or upset, but by breaking off the visual eye contact that is such a crucial aspect of the mother-infant bond.

As for Cathy, there may have been numerous reasons why she could not control her aggression on this day, but I am particularly interested in the comment from Nan ("He doesn't seem that hungry"), which Cathy seemed to experience as a harsh superego telling her that she was a "bad" mother. Parens points out, in his discussion of the infant's early rage-reactions to painful stimuli, that in many cases where the infant was exposed to extreme frustration or hostility, one could often discover that the "mother's unconscious hate attached to past objects was displaced onto her child" (1979, p. 8). Such seems to be the case here. Nan was after all a kind of "supermum", who (as she often reminded people) had brought up six children in the difficult post-war years, run a crèche for the entire local community, and still took in several of her nephews, nieces, and grandchildren when their own parents could not cope. Cathy both depended on her mother and resented her intrusions.

At the end of November, when Wayne was two and a half months old, I observed a typical interaction in which the tension between Cathy and her own mother became apparent. Cathy had asked Andy to hold the baby while she attended to her other child's needs:

> Nan said that [Cathy] was "spoiling" Wayne, always having someone to hold him. Cathy said that he just started crying if she put him down, but to prove her point lay Wayne down in the seat of the comfy chair. "Go on then, prove me wrong," said Cathy, and sure enough Wayne, after wriggling for a moment, settled down into sleep.

In this observation one can see how Nan's voice, which Cathy may experience as critical or even persecutory, becomes externalized onto Wayne, whose "good" behaviour—settling down to sleep—is experienced by her as a deliberate attempt to make her look stupid in front of her own mother. I am reminded of Rozika Parker's (1997) description of "maternal persecutory anxiety", which she describes as involving "a mother's phantasised experience of herself as punished and tormented by her infant—no matter the difference in power between them, no matter that such phantasies may mostly be due to her own projections".

By January, when Wayne was four and a half months, the situation had become worse. Significantly, this period coincided with Nan having a hip operation, which made it impossible for her to climb the stairs to Cathy's flat. Cathy not only lost her mother's support at this time, but her mother's incapacity may well have increased her own feelings of anger and guilt. After she had been an almost constant presence in the first three months of the observation, I was not to see Nan again, although the children continued to visit her home regularly on the other side of the estate.

On this particular January morning Cathy was looking rugged and tired when I arrived, and Wayne himself had started teething, which added to the difficulties:

> Now it is time to dress Wayne, and Cathy is clearly not expecting it to be easy. She begins with the woolly hat, saying: "You're going to scream when I do this," but as she puts it on he doesn't seem to be getting upset. Then she takes his coat, and pushes his arms through the sleeves, quite roughly. He looks up at her, staying quite calm. He begins to kick his legs about, and Cathy tells me that this is it, the sign that he's about to start crying, but he doesn't. She wheels the pram into the doorway, then picks Wayne up in one hand by grabbing his coat by the scruff, like a cat with a kitten in her mouth. "Shopping bag!" she says, as she lifts him up and puts him in the pram …
>
> "This is the bit where he screams," she says, as she gets the blanket and lays it on top of him, but still he doesn't cry. She seems to feel he is not crying just to prove her wrong, and says that the other two do that as well, to "show her up". She shoves the blanket down in the pram, as if trying to make him cry. "You like it rough, don't you?" she says to him.
>
> Finally Cathy puts the hood up on the pram, and comes and looks at him. "Look at you," she says, "always smiling—not like your mum and dad who grumble all the time." She pauses for a moment, then starts telling me about a programme on TV the night before about a mother who twice left her children out to get rid of them. She says women like that should be "castrated", and complains that social services shouldn't have allowed this mother to have more kids. She says that the first time it happened the woman did it because she was depressed, and Cathy can understand that—she tells me that she was depressed after Martin was born, but that she'd been fine after Gabriella and Wayne were born.

This was a particularly painful observation. I could sense the conflict as Cathy struggled with her anger and frustration, taking it out on her child in her rough handling, while simultaneously trying to provoke his anger in order to externalize the feelings. When this failed—with Wayne once again responding not by becoming upset but by being relatively passive and inexpressive—Cathy was caught between feeling persecuted (he isn't crying to show her up) and acknowledging her own anger (it is she who is grumbling, and he who is smiling). It seems as if Cathy hovers between what Rozsika Parker (1997) calls "manageable ambivalence" and "unmanageable ambivalence"—the former a source of creative insight, the latter of intolerable levels of guilt.

The story of the "bad" mother who abandons her children and the failure of social services appears to act as a displacement of Cathy's own feelings of hatred, as well as strong superego condemnation of these feelings. Perhaps the wish for social services to have stopped the "bad mother" having more children suggests a wish for a benign parental figure who will intervene and protect her (and her children). In this context, the absence of Cathy's own father and her sense of Andy as ineffectual are perhaps relevant. Cathy is caught between severe condemnation of the bad mother (she should be "castrated") and sympathetic identification (Cathy too was depressed after Martin's birth), although she adds quickly that after Wayne's birth she was "fine".

Three weeks later, however, Cathy admitted openly for the first time that she was not "fine". She told me that she had been to see the doctor who had prescribed anti-depressants, which "knock her out" at night-time but leave her feeling dopey all day. She explained that her temper had been awful recently, and she had felt very close to being violent. Cathy told me that she never hits the children, but instead goes and locks herself in her room until she calms down. She went on to say that her mood was not due to the kids but to Andy, who never helps at home, and she feels as if she might kill him. She added that at the time of Wayne's birth she did not have post-natal depression, but she felt as if she did now.

With Wayne that day the interactions were more calm, but behind the subdued atmosphere there was a sense that Cathy felt overwhelmed by Wayne's "demanding" behaviour, which she seemed to experience as almost literally devouring:

> Cathy sits behind Wayne, explaining to me that this is because she is smoking a cigarette. Wayne senses her presence, and tries to turn his head to see her. "What is it?" says Cathy, putting down her cigarette, and coming over to stand above him. Wayne looks up and his arms and legs wave back and forth. "Why can't you ever stay in that chair?" says Cathy, as she picks him up and puts his face against hers. Cathy gives him a kiss on the cheek, then several more. He turns his face and mouths her. "You can't eat me," says Cathy, pulling him away from her face, and carrying him back to her chair, where she sits down with him lying back on her lap, his head resting against her chest.

In many ways this period was a turning point in the observation, and one way of discussing this is in terms of my own countertransference regarding the place I was given as an observer. In the first few months of the observation (until the Christmas break) I could not understand why this family had agreed to let me come and observe their infant, and often felt like a sack of potatoes stuck in the corner of the room. Nobody asked my name, or where I came from, or what I was doing. I wrote in my notes at the time:

> What is confusing is that I am allowed to go along, without creating a ripple, without any inquisitiveness on their part—just letting me sit in like it is neither here nor there ... They are almost amused at how boring it must be, and that nothing is happening ... And indeed I don't feel anything for the baby, no affection, no desire to pick it up and play with it, no sense of its character. ... I feel as if nothing is happening—which is of course ridiculous, when I think about it. So are they letting me feel the place that Wayne has—to fit in, not be a bother, not make a noise, not stir up any emotions? That it might be dangerous if Wayne made them feel anything too strongly?

By the spring term my feeling had changed completely. As Cathy struggled with her own aggression and the conflict between her own needs and those of her baby, I felt a desire in the countertransference to protect this family and look after them. The lack of questions about my own "real" life—where I lived, whether I was married or had children, what my study involved—might suggest a massive denial of curiosity, or perhaps a wish for an object who was interested, concerned, but had no demands of his own. I was "Mike", the "man from del Monte", as Cathy once put it in a rambling free association as she played with Wayne.

Wayne's needs, however, *were* the cause of great conflict, as Cathy oscillated between a fantasy of running away from her children and protestations of love. According to Winnicott, the infant's ability to integrate his own loving and aggressive feelings during the first two years of life depends to a great extent on how he experiences being hated. "Children seem able to deal with being hated," writes Winnicott, and "They can meet and make use of the ambivalence which mother feels and shows." What they cannot use is "mother's repressed unconscious hatred which they only meet in their living experiences in the form of reaction formation … At the moment the mother hates she shows special tenderness. There is no way a child can deal with this phenomenon" (quoted by Parker, 1997, p. 28).

There were times during the observation when this appeared to be what was happening, as Cathy's aggression was defended against by a manic excitement that mixed hatred and tenderness. At the end of May, when Wayne was eight months old, I made the following observation:

> Wayne is sitting on the floor, and pushes himself forward and gets down onto his belly, facing a toy car. He moves his arms, and his legs, but his belly is firmly fixed to the floor like a beached whale. He flaps his arms and his legs around, his head held up with a real look of effort on his face. He tries to move, but can't, and begins to get upset with frustration … Meanwhile Cathy is screaming at Gabriella to sit down or she'll wallop her. Andy looks up at me with a knowing smile, and laughs. From the hallway Martin starts crying, and Cathy comes in yanking Gabriella by the arm, saying "She's shut Martin's fucking arm in the door!" and starts to complain to Andy that the kids don't listen to anything she says while he just sits there doing nothing …
>
> Cathy picks up Wayne, pulls him close to her face, and smothers him in kisses, while Andy goes out to the hallway to sort out the other two. Cathy, meanwhile, starts playing with Wayne quite vigorously, turning him upside down, rolling him down her legs, jumping him up and down. He seems to be laughing, but when she stops he makes a complaining noise, which she takes as a sign to start again … [Eventually] he bumps his head and starts to cry.

How can Wayne deal with an environment such as this, one in which there is a loving, affectionate caregiver, but one who is struggling with massive feelings of hatred and aggression which are sometimes projected, sometimes sublimated, sometimes expressed directly or dealt with by a manic defence?

We have already seen some of the ways that Wayne responds to this environment, where his mother struggles with enormous feelings of anger and aggression, by becoming rather passive, or avoiding eye contact with his mother. Parens (1979) also speaks of infants who seem to displace their need for care (which is experienced as a dangerous demand on the mother) onto a need for food, which is a more acceptable one to the mother, although it then seems to confirm her sense of the infant as "greedy". This could be seen in Wayne's case, as he became an extremely fat baby. Cathy complained about how much Wayne ate while at the same time often responding to his demands on her, whatever they were about, by offering him his dummy or food—especially sweets. Yet her sense of him as overweight (as Cathy herself was) made him seem more helpless and dependent, further exacerbating her ambivalent feelings. At the beginning of March I made the following observation:

> Cathy sits Wayne on the sofa again, so that he can pick up a toy hammer by bending forward. When he does so she waits to see if he can sit himself up, but Wayne sits there, bent forward, unable to move. "He can't quite sit himself up, yet," says Cathy, helping him back into a sitting position … "He's too fat to sit up properly, aren't you fatty?" she says. Cathy picks up a toy gun lying near to Wayne, and puts it at Martin's head: "I'm going to blow your fucking brains out, punk!" she says, then turns the gun onto her own forehead and pulls the trigger four times—click, click, click, click. She hands Martin the gun, turning back to Wayne.

The sequence here seems crucial—first an awareness that Wayne is dependent on her (he can't sit up himself), then his greed (he is a "fatty"), which seems to arouse an aggressive fantasy, at first displaced onto Martin, and then turned back onto herself. Looking back at this observation, I was reminded of Winnicott's (1950) view that "[A] mother has to be able to tolerate hating her baby without doing anything about it … If, for fear of what she may do, she cannot hate appropriately when hurt by her child she must fall back on masochism, and I think it is this that gives rise to the false theory of a natural masochism in women."

As it came towards the end of the first year of Wayne's life, however, things were somewhat calmer, as if signs of Wayne's growing independence (he was crawling by nine months, standing at ten and walking soon after his first birthday) were something of a relief to Cathy. It was during the second year of the observation, however, that I could begin to see how the early experiences in Wayne's life were to be structured in his internal world and his own aggressive development, and it is to this that I now wish to turn.

The second year

In his essay on "Aggression in Relation to Emotional Development" (1950), Winnicott argues that from the beginning the infant is both aggressive and ruthless, although he believes that this does not necessarily imply a wish to damage the object. Given healthy development, however, this stage of "unconcern" or "ruthlessness" gives way by the second year of life to what Winnicott calls the "stage of concern". At this point the infant begins to be concerned as to the results of his instinctual experience and develops the capacity to feel guilty:

> A new feature thus arrives in the theory of object-relating. The subject says to the object: "I destroyed you" and the object is there to receive the communication. From now on the subject says: "Hullo object!", "I destroyed you!", "I love you", "You have value for me because of your survival of my destruction of you" (Winnicott, 1971c, p. 90).

But what if the object does not "survive" the infant's aggression, by which, Winnicott tells us, he means that the object retaliates? In "The Development of the Capacity for Concern", Winnicott (1963a) argues that "if there is no reliable mother-figure to receive the reparation-gesture, the guilt becomes intolerable, and concern cannot be felt". One consequence of this may be a form of splitting of the object into good and bad, which eases the guilt, but at a cost: the "love loses some of its valuable aggressive component, and the hate becomes the more destructive" (Winnicott, 1950).

At the start of Wayne's second year of life, his aggression was certainly more visible, whether it appeared as part of his exploratory activity and autonomous strivings (aspects of what Parens (1979) refers to as "non-destructive aggression"), or in a more explicitly hostile form. Cathy complained that Wayne tried to get everywhere now, climbing up onto the window ledge or playing with the stereo, and could not be stopped. She also told me about a visit from an uncle, who tried to frighten Wayne by giving him a fierce look, and how Wayne had responded the next day by scaring a young cousin of his who had come to visit, by pulling the same face and shouting at her loudly.

What also began to be apparent was a split in the way Wayne expressed his loving and aggressive feelings, the former often being directed towards Donna (mum's best friend), while the aggression or hostility was directed towards Cathy. At the beginning of January I arrived for a visit and found only Cathy at home. She told me that the children had all stayed the night at Donna's, and after a few minutes they arrived:

> Everything is fairly chaotic, the kids walking in and out of the living room, and Donna telling Cathy how well behaved they all were and that they ate well, slept properly etc. Cathy warns them that they'd better behave well with her today as well, and calls out "Wayne" to try and get him to come back in from the corridor … [After a little while] Wayne comes in, wandering over to his mum and taking a crisp that she offers him, putting the whole thing in his mouth (despite her telling him not to) and wandering out again. After coming in several times for a crisp, Wayne also goes over to Donna and puts his head in her lap a couple of times. The second time he does so I notice that Cathy holds out a crisp for him, as if to get his attention, then adds, when he comes and takes it: "You only come to me for food."

As an observer, this was a painful interaction to watch. Cathy's sense of having nothing "good" to offer her child was reflected in Wayne's split between Donna as a source of comfort and his mother as a source of food. The next time I visited this was taken one step further. On that day, Cathy came in with drinks for the children, but refused to give Wayne his until he sat on the sofa. She kept calling him a "bad boy", explaining to me that he is constantly pulling on the shelves, playing with the stereo, and breaking things, responding to her prohibitions with a cheeky smile:

> As she talks, Wayne continues to waltz around the room, being very charming and full of energy … Wayne goes over to his mum, and begins to slap her on the arm (smiling as he does so), and she tells him to stop. He climbs up onto her, and nuzzles his head in her chest. Then, it appears, Wayne starts to bite her, and she tells him to stop, calls him a bad boy again, and makes him get off her. He gets down, and goes back over to Donna, and nuzzles his head in her lap instead.

At this point Donna got up to go to the shop, and Wayne grabbed hold of her jacket, crying out for her not to leave. As he followed her out into the hallway Cathy called out, laughing: "She's leaving you, she's deserting you!" When Wayne came back in Cathy began to rough-play with him:

> The next fifteen minutes are a non-stop rough and tumble with first Wayne, then Martin, punctuated by Cathy's occasional insistence that they calm down, followed by her immediate re-starting of the rough play. She lifts Wayne up, turns him round, carries him by the legs, throws him through the air to give Martin kung-fu kicks, and rolls him up and down her legs. At one point Martin climbs on her back, and she throws him over her shoulder, pins him to the floor and puts her foot on his head so he can't move … Wayne, who is laughing and excited, runs out of the room, and Cathy runs out after him, shouting to him not to put his fingers in the electric points (20.1.98).

A vicious circle appears to have been established, where Cathy sees Wayne as a "bad boy" who will not behave, and he consequently enacts this, unable to internalize a "good" parental prohibition (he smiles when she says "no") or to integrate his aggressive feelings (biting) with his loving ones, which are split off and focused on Donna. It seemed as if Cathy's intense jealousy led her to tease Wayne with the loss of his loved object, perhaps reflecting her own sense of being "unloved". As Parker says of another mother in a similar situation: "She needed her child to provide proof both that she was able to love and that she was loved" (1997, p. 22). If such proof is not forthcoming, enormous feelings of hatred can be aroused.

Winnicott suggests that a mother must be able to tolerate these feelings of hatred, neither denying them nor retaliating. But on this occasion Cathy's manic activity, throwing the children about in an excited aggressive way, left Martin with a mild asthma attack and Wayne in a state of excitement which was hard to control. When Cathy refused to let Wayne have the asthma inhaler too, he provocatively went and sat on the window shelf. Cathy went over and smacked him, calling him a "bad boy" once again and left him to cry.

As spring approached Cathy's complaints about Wayne's bad behaviour increased, and with it her own sense of exasperation. When I arrived for the final observation before the Easter break I was told that Cathy was ill in bed, after spending a night in the emergency ward of the local hospital, having lost all feeling in one arm and developing terrible pains. For the remaining months of my observation Cathy's mystery illness continued, leaving her low on energy, sometimes dizzy, and with sustained headaches. During my visits she would give long accounts of her symptoms and the various tests that the hospital was doing (or failing to do) to try to understand the cause. In moments of vulnerability, Cathy spoke of her fear that "there was something" in her head, and that she might suddenly die and her kids would be left without a mother.

During this period Andy spent more time at home, Nan spent time looking after the kids and Donna continued to be a constant presence in the house. At one level Cathy's illness was a cry for help, a demand for the "supportive matrix" which Stern (1995) sees as a necessary part of the "motherhood constellation". Little was explained to the children, although it was made clear to them that they should not be too demanding of their mother, and their behaviour generally "improved", which meant silently sitting and watching videos. I found myself verbalizing for Cathy how frightening the illness was for her, and trying to help her think about how anxious her children must be about her state.

More than ever, perhaps, I wondered if Wayne's sense was of a mother who was not able to survive his "ruthlessness". In these months Wayne continued to be described as "wilful" and "spiteful" for the way he damaged things or refused to do what his mother told him. The dilemma Wayne was in seemed to be most poignantly summed up in an observation from the middle of May, when Wayne was one year and seven months old. Cathy had just left the room:

> Wayne gets up and looks like he might follow her out of the room, but Donna, who is sitting holding a cuddly toy, says to Wayne on his way past "Give teddy some love?", holding out the cuddly toy. Wayne pauses, looks at the toy, takes it and gives it a cuddle. Then he throws it on the ground. Donna says "Oh, poor teddy," and Wayne picks it up again and cuddles it, then throws it away again.

In this exchange, Wayne expresses both his loving and his aggressive feelings. But can these be brought together? Can the teddy (or the mother) to whom he "gives some love" be the same as the one whom he throws to the ground? And if they cannot be integrated, what effect will this have on Wayne's future emotional development?

Winnicott (1950) argues that when the loving and aggressive feelings are not integrated, "there cannot be a fusion except in a secondary way, through the 'erotization' of aggressive elements". On my final visit, when Wayne was twenty-two months old, this is precisely what seemed to be happening:

> After a while Wayne begins to play at climbing up the back of the sofa behind his mum's head. Cathy turns round and says "Stop that!", and Wayne giggles. "Get down!" she says, and when he giggles again she says sternly "Shall I slap you?" "Yeah," says Wayne, giggling, and she gives him a little slap on the hand. "Shall I slap you again?" she asks, and again he says "Yeah" and she does so. The third time this happens Wayne says "No", and Cathy grabs him by the shoulders and pulls him round from behind the sofa onto the floor. "Bad boooooy!" she says, as he laughs excitedly, and she starts to tickle his belly. She puts up her fists and says "Wanna fight?" He tries to punch her hands, giggling still, and Cathy pretends to box with him, giving him a push in the face.

Watching interactions such as this, which became increasingly common towards the end of Wayne's second year, what predictions might one make for his future development? Not only is the aggression becoming sexualized, but Wayne seems increasingly dependent on bodily excitement as a source of gratification. Yet as Winnicott points out, the "play of a child is not happy when complicated by body excitement with their physical climaxes ... any child with marked manic defence restlessness is unable to enjoy play because the body becomes physically involved. Physical climax is needed and every parent knows the moment when nothing brings an exciting game to an end except a smack which provides a false climax but a useful one" (quoted by Campbell, 1995, p. 218).

This description, which seems to describe so accurately a common pattern of interaction between Wayne and his mother, comes in a discussion of what Winnicott refers to as "pre-delinquent dependence upon bodily excitement", as a way of explaining how the "playful, provoking, self-willed attitude of a toddler" may be the forerunner of later antisocial behaviour (quoted by Campbell, 1995, p. 216). Is this a possible outcome of Wayne's aggression in relation to his emotional development?

Conclusion

Two months after finishing my observation, I returned to visit Wayne on his second birthday. Cathy opened the door of her council flat to me and led me into the living room where we always sat. She told me how she was still suffering from dizzy spells, piercing headaches, and occasional panic attacks. Wayne, she went on, is "trouble". He will never sit down and concentrate on anything—he is up every two minutes, pulling things down from the shelves, poking something into the stereo or climbing up somewhere he shouldn't be. Cathy says she can't leave him alone for a minute, and goes to sleep thinking "Wayne, Wayne, Wayne", then wakes up doing the same. Cathy also tells me that Wayne was taken to the health visitor for a regular check, and she was told that he is "hyperactive" and extremely destructive. There is mention of ADHD and perhaps seeing a child psychiatrist, if things don't settle down in a month or so. Cathy says it isn't as if he is one of those "neglected children", as he has been given lots of attention. Wayne's sister comes in and says that he is a "naughty boy", a phrase that Wayne himself uses when he comes in, giving me a big smile:

> He lies his head on Cathy's lap and rubs his nose with his finger, as he used to do when he was tired. But then he goes to the centre of the room and jumps about, then runs into Cathy's room and has to be fetched back from somewhere forbidden. When Cathy tells him off he slaps her on the leg and she slaps him back. At one point she shouts at him and he looks genuinely frightened, backing away saying "No", with a trembling lip.

The sexualized aggression that marks the interaction between Wayne and his mother seems to be a way in which both of them have come to deal with intolerably ambivalent feelings. As Winnicott reminds us, the development of a "healthy" tolerance of ambivalent feelings is not just a process that the infant goes through. It is essential for the mother too. Parker, developing Winnicott's ideas, describes different ways in which such ambivalent feelings can be dealt with by a mother:

> When manageable, the pain, conflict and confusion of the coexistence of love and hate actually motivate a mother to struggle to understand her own feelings and her child's behaviour. When unmanageable, the potential for ambivalence to foster thought and spark concern is overwhelmed by the anxiety generated when hate no longer feels safely "mitigated" by love (1997, p. 21).

As I came to the end of my observation, it seemed as if Cathy was finding such feelings "unmanageable", creating a situation in which she felt both attacked from within—the mystery illness—and was externalizing her aggression and finding it in her child. In turn, Wayne's loving feelings were becoming split-off from his aggression, which was increasingly dealt with by being sexualized.

Whether this solution would become permanent, I could not know. As an observer of this mother-infant relationship, I had to try to come to terms with my own ambivalent feelings too—feelings of anger and love, feelings of hope and real concern. There were times when I very much wanted to do something; others when my quiet attentiveness seemed to be the most important thing I could offer. In writing this paper too I struggled with how to make sense of what I had observed, and feelings of condemnation mixed with feelings of protectiveness and admiration. As Wayne and his mother had—and still have—to do, in writing this paper I hope to have made some of those ambivalent feelings a little more "manageable".

References

Campbell, D. (1995). From practice to psychodynamic theories of delinquency in adolescence. In: C. Cordess & M. Cox (Eds.), *Forensic Psychotherapy.* London: Jessica Kingsley.

Fonagy, P., Moran, G. & Target, M. (1993). Aggression and the sychological self. *International Journal of Psychoanalysis, 74*(3).

Freud, A. (1972). Comments on aggression. In: *The Writings of Anna Freud, Vol. VIII.* New York: International Universities Press.

Freud, S. (1905). *Three Essays on the Theory of Sexuality. S. E., 7.* London: Hogarth.

Freud, S. (1914). *On Narcissism. S. E., 14.* London: Hogarth.

Freud, S. (1920). *Beyond the Pleasure Principle. S. E., 18.* London: Hogarth.

Harris, A. (1998). Aggression: pleasures and dangers. *Psychoanalytic Inquiry, 18*(1).

Klein, M. (1957). *Envy and Gratitude.* London: Tavistock.

Mayes, L. & Cohen, D. (1993). The social matrix of aggression. *Psychoanalytic Study of the Child, 48.*

Mitchell, S. (1998). Aggression and the endangered self. *Psychoanalytic Inquiry, 18*(1).

Parens, H. (1979). *The Role of Aggression in Early Infancy.* New York: Jason Aronson.

Parker, R. (1997). The production and purposes of maternal ambivalence. In: W. Hollway & B. Featherstone (Eds.), *Mothering and Ambivalence.* London: Routledge.

Perelberg, R. (1995). Violence in children and young adults. *Bulletin of the Anna Freud Centre, 18.*

Phillips, A. (1988). *Winnicott.* London: Fontana.

Rayner, E. (1991). *The Independent Mind in British Psychoanalysis.* Northvale, NJ: Jason Aronson.

Stern, D. (1995). *The Motherhood Constellation.* London: Karnac.

Winnicott, D. W. (1939). Aggression. In: *The Child and the Outside World.* London: Tavistock, 1957.

Winnicott, D. W. (1947). Hate in the counter-transference. In: *Through Paediatrics to Psycho-Analysis.* London: Hogarth, 1982.

Winnicott, D. W. (1950). Aggression in relation to emotional development. In: *Through Paediatrics to Psycho-Analysis.* London: Hogarth, 1982.

Winnicott, D. W. (1960). Aggression, guilt and reparation. In: *Deprivation and Delinquency.* London: Routledge, 1990.

Winnicott, D. W. (1963a). The development of the capacity for concern. In: *The Maturational Process and the Facilitating Environment.* London: Karnac, 1965.

Winnicott, D. W. (1963b). Morals and education. In: *The Maturational Process and the Facilitating Environment.* London: Karnac, 1965.

Winnicott, D. W. (1964). Roots of aggression. In: *Deprivation and Delinquency.* London: Routledge, 1990.

Winnicott, D. W. (1971). The use of an object and relating through identifications. In: *Playing and Reality.* London: Routledge.

Intervention

CHAPTER TEN

Parent–infant psychotherapy: a new "real" relationship—"finding a way to be together"

Michela Biseo

In this chapter I will outline the work done in the Parent–infant Project of the Anna Freud Centre through the examples of weekly parent–infant psychotherapy of two mothers and their babies worked with over the course of the first year of life. These mothers, who came for treatment with their infant sons, can be seen to be located at the extreme opposite ends of the poles of relating, i.e., from withdrawn to intrusive. Either one of these extremes can be seen to be equally damaging to the developing infant's psyche and sense of "going-on being" (Winnicott, 1960b).

The technique and theoretical basis for the work practised in the Anna Freud Centre's Parent–infant Project has been extensively outlined (Baradon et al., 2005). Briefly, this approach to working with babies and their parents in the first year of life is based on a distillation of many theoretical strands: psychoanalytic theory, child psychotherapy, developmental psychology, attachment theory, and neuropsychology. Approximately half of the team members are, or have been, graduates of the Anna Freud Centre child psychotherapy training, and bring a clear emphasis on rigorous assessment and thought, pursuing the tradition of distinguishing pathology from normality and pinpointing areas of development that might be lagging behind. A tradition of valuing the developmental therapeutic aspects of psychotherapy is also intrinsic to the attitude and expectations of the therapists. Baradon and Joyce write that one of the aims of parent–infant psychotherapy would be: "The provision of new object experience to each of the participants in the treatment" (Baradon et al., 2005, p. 29).

Various theorists have attempted to pin down this extra-therapeutic aspect; whether termed the "real relationship" by classical Freudians (Greenson, 1968; Couch, 1999), or as a "something more" that is done above and beyond interpretation and the therapeutic stance (Lyons-Ruth, 1998; Morgan, 1998), or as child psychotherapists in the Anna Freudian tradition might have put it: the therapist as a "new developmental object". Hurry writes: "The interactions which take place within the therapeutic developmental relationship are essentially similar to those that ordinarily take place between the parents and the infant or child" (1998, p. 38).

In the therapies to be described, the role of the real relationship has also been an important and technically complex additional strand but it is intrinsic to the treatment of an infant-parent couple.

I will show that in the case of these two mothers, the need of the baby for an appropriate introduction of "triangular space" (Britton, 1989; Woodhead, 2004; Jones, 2006) aided and advanced by the therapy and "real relationship", resulted in the babies' and their parents' better capacities to mentalize and use reflective functioning (Fonagy, 2002). The goal then of the therapy was to help each pair begin to find the right distance between self and other, to enable parents to recognize their infant as a dependent person with a developing mind, and to maximize the potential for growth and the establishment of a "coherent" (Baradon et al., 2005, p. 26) or "true" sense of self (Winnicott, 1960b).

Variations to technique are highlighted in each of these case examples. In the first, by the use of an interpreter to make the work available to a non-English speaking patient, and in the second, by the incorporation of the use of video-filming in the therapy via a hand-held digital camera (used as outlined in Woodhead, 2006).

Parent–infant psychotherapy: a new "real" relationship?

> David arrives and is placed by mother on the floor of the therapy room. At a speedy crawl, he makes a beeline for the toys. However, rather than exploring them by looking or handling them with curiosity, he seems to bulldoze through and over them, not apparently aware of the collision of toys and his own crawling legs.
>
> I wonder if his aim is just to get away from his mother. I ask him, curious: "Where are you off to?" He glances up at me briefly, sits on his haunches, frowning a bit anxiously and bashes the stacking cups together. He then drops them, and crawls back to be closer to his mother.

Jeanine and David: a baby boy (four months) and his mother

The focus of the work with Jeanine and David was on their relationship; and one could say that the relationship was the patient (Baradon, 2002; Baradon et al., 2005). When Jeanine became pregnant her partner requested she terminate the pregnancy or he would abandon her. Jeanine refused as she was pleased to be pregnant, and had followed him to move to the UK from their country. Her community judged her as having brought shame on herself for being unmarried. She was left single, "cast-out" from her family and community, homeless, and pregnant. She did not speak a word of English.

A combination of devastating losses, her isolation, and vulnerability at being a first-time single parent seemed to hasten and magnify her fragile mental health into a state of almost psychotic breakdown.

In pregnancy Jeanine began to hallucinate and see and hear "ghosts"—she explained that they were "dead people" that appeared when she was awake and this worried her. After an initial month of weekly therapy, Jeanine allowed me to see how she was utterly gripped and imprisoned by paranoid ideas of harm and danger. Up till now Jeanine had had to use friends she had made through her network of native speakers from her home country to interpret for her. This made her reluctant to express her more primitive anxieties and states of mind, for shame that they too, might judge or abandon her.

Given the opportunity of a confidential space and, critically, the use of a specialist mental health interpreter, she began to disclose her really, at times rather florid disturbance, constant catastrophic rumination, and deeply depressed state. It is important to add that the interpreter was a man, of the same nationality as her. Jeanine remarked that she had previously found interpreters difficult but not this one; she had no objections to his gender. When I addressed the circumstances of our meetings, commenting on the lack of privacy with me as we needed the interpreter to understand one another, Jeanine said she did not mind this at all, rather she described herself to me: "… feeling as though I am in a cage. If I could find the door, then the words and feelings would come flooding out … and maybe they would never stop".

David was already nearly five months old, a fairly robust looking and solidly built boy. He was wary and would not approach me with his gaze until some time in the treatment. He had very big brown eyes that seemed often wide open with alarm, but he avoided making eye contact. I was aware of the need to regulate and soothe both of them, as well as a need to listen very carefully to what she told me in her words, but also in the way I saw her interact with her son. I was struck by Jeanine's capacity to derive a lot of comfort from her son, and at times my response to this was to wonder if he felt intruded upon. For example, she continuously and almost habitually caressed his head and hair.

She spoke of her wish to keep him safe and I commented that perhaps at times she believed he kept her safe (from the visions/ghosts) and she agreed. Gradually as her story unfolded, of rage and pain at being multiply rejected—by her family, community, and her ex-partner, it became clear that her feelings towards her son were also quite ambivalent. This was unconscious and conflictual, as she often stated how David was her reason for living. Indeed she gripped him tightly at these times and smothered him with kisses, whilst at other times she seemingly stared off into space and appeared to be unreachable. She would often focus on the "bad" world outside, potential dangers and accidents seen everywhere, and gradually I tried to link these "outside" fears to her internal bad thoughts and feelings.

Another important but almost unspoken contribution to the work was the mere presence of a third—the interpreter. Darling wrote that she approaches working therapeutically with parents, children, and interpreters as an encounter "which focuses on states of mind engendered in one (or both) workers, or on the relationship between them" (2004, p. 261).

Thus triadic reorganization with the (parental) couple in the room was happening throughout each session: the couple at times being therapist/interpreter, therapist/Jeanine, or at other times Jeanine/interpreter. It is my view that the bridging function of the interpreter enabled the triadic function to be very alive in the room particularly for David, as he saw in vivo a collaborative and fruitful intercourse whether in (two) language(s) or in play between the two couples that the adults made up. He also sometimes aligned himself with either the therapist or the interpreter in order to have a very different experience than the one he had at home with just his mother.

Woodhead (2004), writing about the role of the father in parent–infant psychotherapy, has stated that the paternal function (of the therapist) is to evolve "new relational opportunities … through triadic experiences conceptualized as dynamic trialectical processes" (p. 88).

It was clear that the genuine enjoyment that the interpreter could take in his playing with David was independently important to the use of the therapy by David, who experienced a benign, playful, and containing male presence weekly. I would speculate that the therapeutic couple made up of interpreter and therapist was experienced in the same way at times, as a parental couple.

One can assume that David was beginning to internalize this new experience. Indeed Britton (1989) writes of the extraordinary importance for the child in recognizing the link that joins the parents as a "limiting boundary for the internal world". He further states: "The capacity to envisage a benign parental relationship influences the development of a space outside the self capable of being observed and thought about, which provides the basis for a belief in a secure and stable world" (p. 87).

In a session from this time:

> David is placed inside mother's legs, seated together on the floor. Her arms are under his armpits holding him. He does not turn to her. She picks at David's body and clothing: pulling his sleeves up here, lifting his arm there, supporting him from falling to one side, then from falling forwards. She is gripping her hands around him like a corset. I have the impression of him as a floppy doll or puppet. Her attention to him is of the utmost alertness, and I feel an irritation rise in myself. David is trying to explore the bead and string rattle toy with extreme concentration and focus. Her picking gestures distract him, and interrupt his own spontaneity. He pulls the toy between both hands, hitting the floor with it—enjoying that bashing action and noise. He then starts shaking it, then mouthing the round end-beads and stringy parts between. As I watch her interruptions to his passionate explorations, I wonder aloud if she felt she had to hold him tight like that. She said if she did not he would surely hurt himself, either by falling and banging himself or by pushing the toy too far into his mouth and make himself sick or gag. She also complained that if only he would not put so many toys into his mouth "… so many germs".
>
> I ask Jeanine if here with me now, I can help her to let him go a bit. "Can you let your hands loose and we will make sure he is safe together?"
>
> She nervously agrees. She tells me that her friends all tell her she "panics too much". I support his body with my hands, talking to David: "We're going to let you come forward, down here, on your tummy." He successfully rolls onto his tummy with my hands to steady him. He holds the toy and mouths it. I move my face to make better eye contact and talk to him about being "down here on your tummy … it feels different here doesn't it?" I encourage mum to move her face so he can see her too. She asks me about his tummy, "Won't he get sore like that, or too tired?" She tells us she is not happy about the toy in his mouth "like that".
>
> I comment to David that "Mummy feels you are so far away!" She laughs nervously, and cannot control her need to scoop him back up now and does so, into a tight embrace—cheek-to-cheek. I say: "Even just that little distance felt like a huge empty desert between you." She nods.

> David did not resist his mother and was able now to sit supported by her body as before. He passed the toy he was still holding to the interpreter who passed it back each time with a smile and warm encouragement. David checked back with his mother, making eye contact, and played further to-and-fro games with the interpreter. I spoke to everyone about David's interest in the interpreter, but also told David directly: "I see how you check with mummy to see if this is allowed. Maybe you are asking Mummy: 'Is this game okay? Can I play with (interpreter)?'"

My attempt to use my countertransference ("irritation") to begin to understand how David might feel about the type of caregiving he was experiencing in that moment, prompted me to actively "scaffold" the baby's communications and age-appropriate developmental needs to mother. I suggested that they separate a little. I felt from this and further examples, that David had actively begun to turn away from Jeanine, and experienced her "picking" as intrusive and an attempt to deny their separateness. It seemed to interrupt his very "going-on-being" (Winnicott, 1960a).

It was also critical for me as David's psychotherapist to challenge Jeanine's belief that the world (here represented by the floor/toys/germs) is so harmful as to actively discourage her son's engagement with it. David's development was being observably restricted by the maternal psychopathology.

I verbalized to both of them the fear of being separate, and hoped to model that this can be achieved safely, without ending in catastrophic annihilation. David was thus allowed a brief new experience of feeling his body "alone" on the hard floor while mouthing pleasurably in the presence of we three adults. After this, in his return to mother's lap he seemed ready to use the other/the third as an object for a mutual game, while referencing mother for safety. This was also an example for David of the therapist (or the interpreter) being experienced as new developmental objects, offering a different way of being and playing.

At the same time this set up a moment of triadic functioning, in which the communication from his mother is that it is okay to play and enjoy the company of the other, and that mother approves and enjoys their pleasure too. Perhaps the paternal role of the therapist here is in accordance with Woodhead's (2004, p. 87) view and technique that: "… [my] introducing the Lacanian 'No' of the father … is to help them develop a more separated sense of self. My 'paternal function' is 'to woo the child and the mother away from too close a relation with each other' (Kramer & Prall, 1978), and to provide a shield from the mother's wish to keep her son in a state of symbiosis (Stoller, 1979)."

This might be confirmed also by the following very fleeting but affectively highly charged moment: after a holiday break, when collecting David and his mother from the waiting room, David greeted me with some warmth but greeted my translator colleague with a look and bodily gesture of openness and sheer joy. It seemed that David was expressing real love and enthusiasm at seeing this important man again.

The role of the interpreter/therapist as a "new developmental object" and with a "real relationship" to the baby seemed very alive at this time. Another technique commonly used in PIP of the therapist speaking directly to the baby (Baradon, 2005, pp. 58–59) is also illustrated by the above example. In this case, as everything I said had to be translated, it must have seemed to David that my words, suggestions, observations, and interpretations were coming to him (and to his mother) from the interpreter. I was aware of this, and made a point of maintaining eye contact with David when I spoke (or with Jeanine when speaking to her). The interpreter then translated and addressed my words, now in their native tongue, to the person (mother or baby, or both) as intended by me. I would suggest that this again strengthens the experience of the patient in the presence of the couple, who are relating and working together as a joined-up team.

Darling (2004) writes of the subtleties of such an interaction, how the psychotherapist is an interpreter of, at times, symbolic meaning into language, and this in turn is interpreted to the family in yet another "language" by the translator, in a collaborative working of two differently trained colleagues. In the case of working with a baby patient, the therapist's "interpretations" are not only psychoanalytic but additionally may for the first time represent to the baby and the parent the experience of the child as having a mind, and a mind that is separate from the parent's. Britton states the creation of this triadic space as being essential for the child as he then can assume a "third position … from which object relationships can be observed … for reflecting on ourselves whilst being ourselves" (1989, p. 87).

The difficulties of closeness and separateness that can be seen in the work outlined above are of course a combination of the physical and the psychic; for the baby needs the proximity of the maternal body for survival, but the availability of the maternal mind is vital for psychic survival and growth. In David's case, my hypothesis was that the maternal mind was experienced as intrusive. Through sensitive use of containing and regulating Jeanine's initially rather extreme states of mind, fears, and anxieties, my aim was to also regulate David's states. Through the encouragement of David's age-appropriate strivings for separation-individuation, my aim was also to allow this progressive pull to be met and matched by the mother's facilitation of her son's growing needs. Jeanine needed to be helped to lay some of her ghosts to rest through the unlocking of her "cage" as she so poetically said. In turn, this allowed her preoccupations to become less malevolent and with support to begin to develop some capacity to view her son as separate from herself. The additional aspect of the interpersonal relating that the four of us co-created contributed, in my opinion, an extra dimension to the burgeoning shapes and models of David's intra-psychic development. Thus the real relationships that David was co-constructing with each of us additionally aided his creation of a triadic space in his internal world. In the second example below, this space was co-created in a rather different way, as will be shown.

Tania and Dillon: the video as a third "eye"

> Tania and Dillon enter the consulting room. Dillon (three months) had been asleep in the pram on the way here but has woken now, though he is silent in mother's arms. We enter the room and sit. Tania tells me, rubbing her hand, that she has hurt it this morning: "It really is hurting." She places Dillon beside her, on a cushion on the floor, slightly propped up. His eyes are open and staring out at nothing in particular. His hands and arms are flung up in a startle-reflex position, but he is still. His legs are stiff. I greet him. He is motionless, frozen, and tense. He makes eye contact with me but I only sense his breathing increase, and his eyebrows raise even higher into a fearful expression and he looks away to the distance. He is completely still, silent and stiff as a board.

Tania, a young woman in her late teens, was referred to our service following her pregnancy from a rape. Dillon was already two months old when we finally met, having had several missed, cancelled, or rearranged appointments. For the first appointment, they arrived late and flustered. On collecting them from the waiting room, the pram looked dangerously laden with bags and instinctively, and precipitately, I peeled back a blanket as I could not see the baby beneath.

Dillon was lying on his back, wide awake, and seemed shocked. He was stiff, still, and frozen. I greeted them both. His big eyes were wide in fear. I felt that Tania too was tense and alert. I felt my role was to soothe them both, to contain their fears about coming here and perhaps having to tell a terrible story. In this first session Tania said to me that Dillon "cries and cries" if she is not holding him. The following session she attended alone, having left a "cranky" Dillon with her mother. We began to discuss this very recent traumatic event (the rape) as well as her letting me know of long-term sexual abuse in her childhood. In the telling, she was moved almost beyond tears, then silently sobbing and wretched. She agreed when I said I thought that she had needed to come alone to let me know about these terrible events and her terror that she could not be a good mother. I emphasized her courage, and also how she had thought of Dillon's needs and had wanted to protect him from knowing all this, and seeing her in this state. She spoke of how at home she feels numb mostly, and doesn't cry much. I held back from making links between her tears and Dillon's. She spoke of how she wished for Dillon to not be like her, for him to turn out different. She told me how here in the therapy, she wanted to look at how to be a mum, "*… but also how to be ME*".

I was concerned about how wary Dillon was with me in the following sessions. Tania would place him on the floor on the baby mat and he would hold his little body tightly tensed as he listened in silence to her speak. At the beginning of sessions he spent many minutes rigidly still, watching me or staring out. He was frozen and quiet, yet highly alert to noise, movements, or mother's mood changes. His alertness and tension highlighted his natural quizzical, rather sad/frightened expression. I felt I was seeing a baby with very precociously developing pathological defences, as those described by Fraiberg (1982). These withdrawal strategies are also known from research to be linked to insecure disorganized attachment patterns (Schore, 2010).

I attempted to help Dillon find a way-in to the talking by directly speaking with him. I spoke of his need for Mummy, for her to be close and help him take in the world around him. Tania spoke of how she would hand Dillon over to her own mother when he cried "too much" and we thought together about the meaning of this communication. I wondered to Dillon how it might feel: "Maybe you are too much for Mummy sometimes." She agreed. I wondered if at these times, Tania felt overwhelmed by his distress and all-consuming need for her, recalling her statement in the first session of him crying and crying to be held.

Tania reported her way of coping (which she also recognized as being historical with its roots in her childhood abuse) was to shut down, switch off, and walk away. I raised her awareness of Dillon's experience of her in this state. I spoke directly now to Dillon, asking if at those times he may feel frightened, like he seems here with me when he first arrives and has to sit so still and quiet. I wonder to Tania if Dillon may feel as she had done as a child in those awful moments of terror: lost and abandoned, frightened, and overwhelmed.

She was powerfully moved at the link between David's feeling unsupported by a grown-up carer and her own experience as a little girl. She spoke of her anger at her mother for not protecting her from abuse, and the need she had felt as a child to protect her younger siblings. Again she wept bitterly, remarking she never wept at home, it was "only here".

This type of intervention linking the affective experience which had defensively been split off in childhood from the memory of the trauma is as Fraiberg and colleagues (1975) describe in their classic technique of "hearing" the ghosts of the mother's tears as a baby so that the mother can begin then to hear her own baby's "here and now" cries.

About three months into treatment, I suggested that we use the video camera to help us reflect on Dillon's experience and give Tania a "third eye" (Woodhead, 2006). My hope was that she could become more aware and sensitively attuned (Zelenko, 2000; Jones, 2006) to the barely discernible ways in which Dillon was beginning to respond to or initiate contact with her.

They took to the camera with ease, and she loved to be filmed, showing a tender and lively playfulness for the camera that had heretofore been hidden. This alone proved beneficial to the pair, but I also used the film clips to view with her and Dillon in the subsequent sessions.

She was particularly delighted by a sequence I filmed of a nappy change:

> Dillon lay on the ground on a mat as Tania kneeled over him. Initially he turned his head to both sides: actively avoiding making any eye contact. She was silent, and I suggested that she talk to him about what she was doing. She did so easily now, lovingly. In a sing-song voice she called his name repeatedly in a stretched out musical way: "Di-llll-oooooon." Without her noticing, as she was busy wiping and cleaning, Dillon now was actively seeking out eye contact, trying to grab her eyes onto his. He waved his arms and legs as if to gain her attention, but he too (as she had been initially) was quiet.
>
> I draw her attention to it: "Look Tania, Dillon really wants to look into your eyes!" Tania looked. Dillon beamed, his eyes opening wider and smile spreading further, his whole body softening and seeming to open towards her. She responded with soft but lively tones, describing what she was doing and how he was now all nice and clean. I commented back to her as if from Dillon: "Oh Mummy, I love to look at you and have you so close!"

On viewing this clip together Tania was amazed, and very pleased at how active Dillon was in seeking out her eyes and a mutual looking/gazing. She said she would have "never seen that!". She seemed proud of her boy, and of herself. This example of the mother and infant being first in a mismatched state, then matching one another (mutual positive looking/smiling) is what Tronick (1989) named as "interactive repair". This cycle of disruption and repair is critical in developing a positive, secure attachment.

The "scaffolding" of the therapist's interjection (in which the therapist voiced the baby's positive attunement and heightened affective moment) attempted to aid the repair. Thus the therapist's intervention was within the realm of the mother-infant relationship, shoring up a fragile and newly hatching sense of shared pleasure; of positive accomplished mothering and of effective mutual engagement and synchrony. It highlighted Dillon's hunger and desire to see and be seen, to love her and be loved.

Discussion

As Anne Hurry (1998) has outlined, "Some classical analysts (Greenson, 1967) recognized the 'real' relationship to the patient rather than seeing it as an interference to the analyst's central role as a transference object." She highlights Anna Freud's own views on the need for the child analyst to be able to sort out the mixture and move carefully between the two roles of transference object and "new object".

Hurry's view of the developmental role is where therapists are at their most spontaneous: "… more evidently 'ourselves' than in our interpretive role". (1998, p. 53). Similar ideas emerged from the work of the Process of Change group in Boston (Lyons Ruth, 1998; Morgan, 1998). They highlight the "here and now" aspects of the real relationship. Morgan writes that the real relationship or "moment of meeting" which characterizes this is something that occurs "… often spontaneously, in some form of affective communication between therapist and patient … it is part of their mutual regulation so that the moment of meeting, with its "realness" for both therapist and patient creates a new dyadic state, a dyadic state of consciousness" (1998, p. 326).

In the first example, the spontaneity of my suggestion (informed by my countertransference) that David be allowed some freedom in his body and movement may have been experienced by David as a momentary freeing of some restriction which then allowed the to-and-fro game with the interpreter. He was permitted to be curious and relate to a third. David's experience of a mother who at times was lost to her anxious thoughts and fears, and at other times would cling to him like a life raft, is known to have detrimental effects. Beebe (2000) for example, has written about infant avoidance, where she argues that the infant co-constructs defensive strategies in the face of maternal intrusion or withdrawal. Beebe quotes a study in which at four months, the infants who would later be classified as insecurely attached (avoidant), look at the mother less.

This was more evident in my work and initial encounter with Dillon. In my peeling back the pram blanket to look for the hidden Dillon, there was a spontaneous enactment ("moment of meeting") which crystallized the theme of the work with this mother-infant pair: how to find the baby? Dillon had yet to find a place in his mother's mind. Perhaps his violent conception was partly the cause for the shame of wanting to keep him covered up and "out of sight", but of course there were older "ghosts" not least of which was Tania's childhood sexual abuse.

By filming the therapy sessions, Dillon's desire for Tania was visually captured/caught on film. This freeing of their mutual passion and love for each other was scaffolded by the presence of the therapist and the camera. They were thus open to new possibilities, to observe and view themselves from the position of the "third", and together with the capacity to make links and bring into consciousness some of the buried and dissociated affects Tania had been haunted by, their path was able to be diverted to a more normal one.

Schore (2010) has highlighted the impact on the developing infant's brain and thenceforth impact on intra- and inter-psychic relationships from maternal trauma and dissociative states. Both Jeanine's and Tania's capacities to begin to engage and regulate their babies' experience were extremely poor at referral and would have led no doubt to pathological outcomes for their babies. The interventions offered in PIP are an attempt to interrupt this and attempt to allow the mother-infant pair to see and get a taste of a more mutually satisfying way of relating in which negative and positive affects can be tolerated.

It is a unique time in family life and in a child's life to receive this type of therapy, and it is hoped that I have shown the profound influence it can have in raising the possibility for the infant, at least, of a different mode of relating and way of being.

References

Baradon, T. (2002). Psychotherapeutic work with parents and infants—psychoanalytic and attachment perspectives. *Attachment & Human Development*, *4*(1): 25–38.

Baradon, T. (Ed.) (2010). *Relational Trauma in Infancy: Psychoanalytic, Attachment and Neuropsychological Contributions to Parent–infant Psychotherapy*. Hove, UK: Routledge.

Baradon, T., Broughton, C., Gibbs, I., James, J., Joyce, A. & Woodhead, J. (Eds.) (2005). *The Practice of Psychoanalytic Parent–infant Psychotherapy: Claiming the Baby*. London: Routledge.

Beebe, B. (2000). Co-constructing mother-infant distress: the micro-synchrony of maternal impingement and infant avoidance in the face-to-face encounter. *Psychoanalytic Inquiry*, *20*: 421–440.

Britton, R. (1989). The missing link: parental sexuality in the Oedipus complex. In: R. Britton, M. Feldman & E. O'Shaughnessy (Eds.), *The Oedipus Complex Today: Clinical Implications* (pp. 83–101). London: Karnac.

Couch, A. (1999). Therapeutic functions of the real relationship in psychoanalysis. *Psychoanalytic Study of the Child*, *54*: 130–168.

Darling, L. (2004). Psychoanalytically informed work with interpreters. *Psychoanalytic Psychotherapy*, *18*(3): 255–267.

Fonagy, P., Gergely, G., Jurist, E. L. & Target, M. (2002). *Affect regulation, Mentalization, and the Development of the Self*. New York: Other Press.

Fraiberg, S. (1982). Pathological defences in infancy. *Psychoanalytic Quarterly*, 1(1): 612–635.

Fraiberg, S., Adelson, E. & Shapiro, V. (1975). Ghosts in the nursery: A psychoanalytic approach to the problem of impaired infant-mother relationships. *Journal of the American Academy of Child Psychiatry*, *14*: 387–421.

Freud, A. (1965). *Normality and Pathology*. London: Karnac.

Greenson, R. (1968). The real relationship between the patient and psychoanalyst. In: M. Kanzer (Ed.), *The Unconscious Today*. New York: International Universities Press.

Hurry, A. (Ed.) (1998). *Psychoanalysis and Developmental Therapy*. London: Karnac.

Jones, A. (2006). How video can bring to view pathological defensive processes and facilitate the creation of triangular space in perinatal parent–infant psychotherapy. *Infant Observation*, *9*(2): 109–123.

Lieberman, A., Padron, E., Van Horn, P. & Harris, W. (2005). Angels in the nursery: the intergenerational transmission of benevolent parental influences. *Infant Mental Health Journal*, *26*(6): 504–520.

Lyons-Ruth, K. (1998). Implicit relational knowing: its role in development and psychoanalytic treatment. *Infant Mental Health Journal*, *19*(3): 282–289.

Mahler, M. S., Pine, F. & Bergman, A. (1975). *The Psychological Birth of the Human Infant: Symbiosis and Individuation*. New York: Basic Books.

Morgan, A. (1998). Moving along to things left undone. *Infant Mental Health Journal*, *19*: 324–333.

Schore, A. (2010). Relational trauma and the developing right brain: the neurobiology of broken attachment bonds. In: T. Baradon (Ed.), *Relational Trauma in Infancy: Psychoanalytic, Attachment and Neuropsychological Contributions to Parent–infant Psychotherapy*. Hove, UK: Routledge.

Tronick, E. (1989). Emotions and emotional communication in infants. *American Psychologist*, *44*: 112–119.

Winnicott, D. W. (1960a). The theory of the parent–infant relationship. *International Journal of Psychoanalysis*, *41*: 585–595.

Winnicott, D. W. (1960b). Ego distortions in terms of true and false self. In: *The Maturational Processes and the Facilitating Environment* (pp. 140–152). New York: International Universities Press, 1965.

Woodhead, J. (2004). Shifting triangles: images of father in sequences from parent–infant psychotherapy. *Infant Observation*, *7*(2): 76–90.

Woodhead, J., Bland, K. & Baradon, T. (2006). Focusing the lens: the use of digital video in the practice and evaluation of parent–infant psychotherapy. *Infant Observation*, *9*(2): 139–150.

Zelenko, M. & Benham, A. (2000). Videotaping as a therapeutic tool in psychodynamic infant-parent therapy. *Infant Mental Health Journal*, *21*(3): 192–203.

Applications

CHAPTER ELEVEN

"Silent scream"—work with a traumatized immigrant mother and her infant with a severe neurological disorder

Sheila Levi

Introduction

The title "Silent scream" depicts the experience of a mother-infant dyad, deprived of their most useful tool of communication—crying. A crying baby depends on having a sensitive listener (Music, 2011). So, what happens when a baby is physically so damaged that he cannot cry, or even make a sound or move, and is cared for by a mother with a traumatic history filled with her own screams and cries with no one to hear them?

Furthermore, it is through successive phases of separation-individuation that the child forms self- and object-representations from the images of his own and his mother's satisfying bodies (Sandler & Rosenblatt, 1962; Jacobson, 1964; A. Freud, 1965, 1967; Joffe & Sandler, 1965). But these satisfactions depend on the intactness of sources of pleasure, of the pleasure-giving organ and of the need-satisfying object (Kestenberg, 1971a, b). As Anna Freud observed: "Any single defect in the individual's inborn equipment suffices to throw the entire developmental course into disarray, far beyond the sphere where the damage itself is located" (1981, p. 92).

In this chapter, I will explore the impact of a major defect, an absence of "organ pleasure" in the context of Sami, a neurologically disabled infant who will never be able to walk or talk—and his traumatized, culturally dislocated mother, Mrs M. Even though Sami is biologically two-and-a-half-years-old, I refer to him as an infant as it best describes him. For his mother, separation appeared to be intolerable and often experienced as a "catastrophic threat" (Mahler & Furer, 1963). While normally by his age the achievement of upright locomotion initiates a period of elation during which the toddler joyfully explores the world around him (Mahler et al., 1975), this was not applicable for this little boy. I will attempt to demonstrate the mother's desperate need to keep her baby as an extension of herself not only in response to her own painful feelings but also due to his significant physical impairment which kept him arrested in passive levels of infantile development. I hope to show how I was able to modify my expectations and technique to suit the needs of this particular mother-infant dyad, and to establish a psychoanalytically informed mother-infant psychotherapy in which meaningful change and growth could take place.

This was outreach work from an NHS setting and I was expected to engage this "hard to reach" mother, Mrs M, who was struggling with social isolation, mental health problems, housing loss, and deprivation and multiple cumulative traumas, while parenting her two young children, one with special needs. She had little sense of belonging to a community, and due to fear, language, and cultural deficits could not engage with the available services. As she failed to attend her son's medical appointments, social services were already involved in accompanying her to all hospital sessions. Mrs M did not accept any of my colleagues' offers of psychological support-group sessions for parents of children with special needs.

It is possible that Mrs M was struggling to come to terms with her predicament, and might have been worried that her precarious defences would make her feel vulnerable in a group setting, particularly when that group was about emotional functioning rather than anything concrete like physiotherapy. Considering all these factors, I decided to make a home visit which Mrs M accepted. During that visit it became clear that she was preoccupied with urgent practical matters to do with her family's day-to-day survival in circumstances of little autonomy and agency. It was not that she denied needing help in thinking about herself and her children's emotional well-being, but that she needed this help to come to her in a concrete way. Thus I offered her mother-infant psychotherapy in their home setting.

I believed that my reliable, non-intrusive, and attentive stance while seeing this infant and mother together in their home setting would contain the latter's anxieties. Furthermore, verbalizing and clarifying the mother's experiences in relation to her baby would help her to feel more in control (Katan, 1961), and enable her to be able to think about her baby as a whole person, beyond his debilitating special needs. In other words, it was my impression that within the therapeutic developmental relationship Mrs M could be empowered to cope better with her situation.

The basic principle of mother-infant observation as described by Rustin (2002) seemed applicable—remaining receptive and calm in the presence of the baby and mother, so as to be able to take in their different states of mind as well as the feelings they evoke in the countertransference, a key element of this work. Perhaps due to a lack of provision of such support in her own early life and/or because of the current adverse circumstances, Mrs M seemed to experience difficulties in her "auxiliary ego function" (i.e., providing the necessary scaffolding, reflective function, and mentalization), which meant that her resources were focused on physical survival rather than psychic development (Fonagy & Target, 1997; Target & Allison, 2011). I was inspired by Baradon and Joyce's (2005) application of the contemporary model of mentalization in parent–infant psychotherapy, defining the aims of such therapy as enhancing parental functioning and promoting the infant's developmental moves. Thus I understood my role in terms of "mentalizing the unmentalizable" in the context of Mrs M's predominant mistrust of all authority figures, possibly due to her history of multiple, chronic trauma. This type of "developmental psychotherapy" has been achieved at the Anna Freud Centre for many years (Hurry, 1998).

The ongoing question present from the beginning of the work was: "Who needs to soothe and who needs soothing?" In the coming pages, I will attempt to describe the hurdles encountered in the separation-individuation process when so much had gone wrong from the very beginning for this traumatized mother-infant dyad. I will explore the role of home visits as an alternative way of working with such vulnerable cases, and using a multidisciplinary team in the creation of the "third". After presenting the background, I describe our work, transference and countertransference issues, the child's needs and their impact on the mother, and finally the mother's own mental health needs and their impact on her mothering.

Referral and work process

When Sami was two years old his mother was referred for psychological support in parenting due to prolonged and significant difficulties in establishing a working alliance with the multidisciplinary team of mental health workers and other professionals who had offered support. Burdened by her son's disability, Mrs M was refusing to cooperate.

Sami was diagnosed with septo-optic dysplasia when he was eight months old. As a result of this congenital malformation syndrome his brain had formed differently, particularly in the midline. The bridge between the hemispheres and the nerves between the back of his eyes and brain were underdeveloped. The cause of the condition was unknown, presumably genetic. From Sami's MRI scans, doctors predicted severe problems with learning and future development.

His first two years of life were spent in and out of hospital with breathing difficulties related to his epilepsy and lung infections, and because he needed to be fed artificially. Sami's body movement was severely restricted. He could move only his eyes, and his feet from the ankles; and, though he could open and close his mouth, he did not utter a sound. His sight was partially impaired.

I visited the family weekly at their home during the initial six months. As treatment progressed, I continued my visits fortnightly for three months, and monthly for the last three months.

Sami's mother had emigrated from the Middle East to the UK several years ago and did not speak much English. As I speak her native language the multidisciplinary team hoped that I could engage her more effectively regarding baby care issues. At the time I was primarily concerned with her relationship with her baby. Later on, I became aware that her difficulties in adapting to the host country were reflected in her difficulties in collaborating with the team.

The aim of my involvement in the early phase of our work was to act as an auxiliary ego to the mother, helping her to articulate her view of her circumstances, without undermining her parental position and authority. At times, she was gently challenged and encouraged to develop ego skills and competencies. I invited her into an attitude of curiosity about the child, and about her maternal role, which in turn strengthened her reflective function. This emerging capacity allowed her to develop a therapeutic alliance with me. It was vital for me to be part ofa network of professional colleagues.

Family background

Sami lived with his mother and eight-year-old brother Yusuf in a two bedroom, second floor council flat with steep stairs and no elevator. The family depended on income support. Sami's father was not involved in our work, as he had a job in a different city in the UK and offered no support. Both parents were born and raised in the same province of a Middle Eastern country. During their high school years they fell in love and married soon after, aged eighteen and nineteen respectively. As the eldest child in her own family, from a very early age Mrs M was allocated the task of looking after her bedridden mother, which she resented deeply. She recalled with shame how she chose to neglect and ridicule her mother during that time.

Mr and Mrs M immigrated to the UK in 1996. Their first son Yusuf was born in their home country, and Sami was born in the UK. According to her initial report, her husband deserted the family because of Sami's handicap and related medical needs. However, further explorations indicated that there were marital difficulties even before Sami's birth. Mrs M emphasized the damaging effect of the father's repeated failures in various business projects which had resulted in the family's frequent moves. Sami's birth and his severe handicap strained the relationship to breaking point.

Mrs M firmly believed that the emotional and financial stress she experienced during the pregnancy had damaged her baby. According to her account, her husband had run an entertainment parlour in their home country. He was accused of letting members of a terrorist group use the facilities, then was arrested and tortured for four days. During that period, the mother reported that she was sexually assaulted by two police officers, while two others guarded the door. The couple did not talk to each other about his torture or her experience. Possibly Mrs M was ashamed of the sexual nature of the assault and frightened of being blamed for it. These traumatic events led to their decision to migrate to the UK. They perceived migration as a necessary step to remain alive, even though it resulted in the death of all positive feelings towards each other. Instability, insecurity, and numerous relocations ruled their family life. Mrs M became depressed with suicidal ideation, and even after eight years in the UK, she had to depend on antidepressants during her pregnancy with Sami.

Beginning our work

First home visit

I found Mrs M, a tired-looking lady with pretty features in her thirties, alone in their small and simply furnished council flat, located in a remote and poor area of London. The flat was clean and tidy with enlarged framed family photos on the walls. She seemed puzzled to find out that I speak her mother tongue fluently even though my name and surname sound Western. Mrs M informed me that Sami was in hospital undergoing yet another operation to change his naso-gastric feeding (through his nose) to a tube to feed him directly to his stomach. Also, to stop his reflux, the surgeon was going to bind his stomach with a "metal string". When I wondered aloud how Sami might be feeling in hospital, mother told me that he was actually "happier there", as there were so many things wrong in his body. In a way, she felt that he belonged in hospital rather than home. I was unclear about her reasons for not being with him during the operation, and wondered to myself whether she also believed that the medical team were better able to take care of his needs than her. Possibly as the mother of a severely impaired son she had more intensely ambivalent feelings about her boy. Perhaps she needed a break from her daily contact with her impaired child when the medical team took over his care during his hospitalization, and to use the session with me to deal with her trauma of coming to terms with the diagnosis and having to mourn the loss of a "perfect" baby.

Mrs M told me that over the last two weeks Sami had visited the hospital eight times, and five weeks ago, had needed to go to the emergency clinic due to inability to breathe. She communicated her anger towards the medical team freely, saying: "Once you become dependent on them they start giving appointments without [providing] understanding. Therefore I do not believe in them. At first doctors told me that there was no cure for him. So why do they treat him now?" The pain and frustration of living with her son's life-threatening chronic illness and constant intrusive medical interventions seemed too hard for her to come to terms with. Perhaps my home visit also frightened her, feeling that I too would become another intrusive, critical professional. She often projected her feelings of hopelessness and uselessness onto the multidisciplinary team. It is understandable that before this mother could grieve her losses, she would need help in coming to terms with her rage and disappointment.

The second visit

> When I rang the bell there was no answer for a minute or two. Soon after I rang it the second time, I heard footsteps down the stairs to answer the door. It was the mother looking a bit surprised when she saw me. She told me she'd forgotten all about our meeting even though it was on her mind the day before. She invited me in and informed me that she was in the middle of changing Sami. I asked her to continue with what she was doing, and said that I would be joining her after taking off my shoes as it was the custom in this house. I watched her go up a narrow and steep staircase leading to their living room. There were two bedrooms on either side of this area. I found Sami in his mother's bedroom where a double bed was placed in the middle of the room and a crib was pushed against the wall next to her bed, presumably as a safety measure as one of its side barriers was missing. Mother excused herself for the mess in the house even though the room and the living room looked tidy. Sami was lying on the bed wearing only his nappy while his long, lifeless legs were dangling over the side of the bed, looking unfocused towards the ceiling, with a smile on his face. Mother was telling Sami what a "cheeky pet" he was and how he wanted to play but only Mummy could understand that. She tickled him and his smile became more prominent but his eyes remained unfocused. Sami's seemingly normal-looking body and his handsome features belied his severe immobility. Mother dressed him in comfortable clothes and carried him to his special chair in the living room. She sat in her usual armchair next to him, and I sat diagonally across from them on the sofa. Mother began telling me of the developments in her life since our last session. …

Early work

During the initial stages of our work together, Mrs M was furious that she had been abandoned by her husband, and seemed to lack family support, even from her home country. She described the first five years of her marriage as calm and happy. But then they moved to London, and the last five years of their relationship were filled with her husband's business failures, arguments between the couple, and then Sami's birth followed by medical complications. She told me that when her husband had been around, she could not concentrate on her children as he was very demanding of all her attention. She described him as irresponsible for choosing a new life for himself, and firmly believed that he had left them due to her intense involvement with the baby, which left no space for him. She complained about the unfairness of her predicament and the constant pressure from the medical profession to bring Sami to so many check-ups and intrusive physical interventions with no "'cure"; instead, a constant battle to avoid further damage now and in the future. She often felt unsupported and criticized. I encouraged her to acknowledge the tremendous losses and dislocations both she and her husband had experienced, saying that she was the stronger parent to remain with the responsibility of taking care of her damaged son. Gradually she began to replace her anger with more awareness of their respective mental states.

In the course of our work, she became more aware of her mood changes due to depression around that time, and reflected on how they might have contributed to pushing her husband away. She started taking into account the impact of losing their home country and work opportunities, and of experiencing the loss of their anticipated "healthy" infant, as well as their different styles of dealing with trauma. Consequently, she decided to accept Sami's father's sporadic visits, which she had banned in anger before our work had commenced. Visits to their home enabled Mr M to see both his sons. Mrs M began communicating to me a longing that her husband would get "bored" with his lifestyle in the end, and come back home.

Mrs M's experience with her eldest son seemed positive, and Yusuf had made a good adjustment in general. He was able to verbalize his need for his mother's attention even though Mrs M felt she was having difficulties in satisfying it. She often chose to send Yusuf out with the social worker when she came, never using this support to spend time with Yusuf while his brother was cared for. As our work progressed, Mrs M began telling me about Yusuf's ongoing sleep difficulties since birth, refusing to sleep in his own room and sharing her bed. As a result, she was feeling more and more "suffocated" by her two sons with no breathing space for herself. She then went on to tell me that she felt upset to hear from Yusuf that he preferred to be with his father: "Yusuf sees only 30% of his dad's life but he idealizes everything about his dad. But he does not take Yusuf as much as he wants; always has excuses for him."

Traumatized and displaced migrant

When I met Mrs M she spoke hardly any English and only had friends from her motherland. She expressed strong identification with a damaged person. In a way, she had felt abandoned even before she left her home country—both by her mother, and then by her society. She mentioned having a sister in London but their relationship seemed to be an ambivalent one. When I arrived, she always sent away any visiting friends and family, but kept her sons. We were of a similar age. Even though we originated from the same country, she came from a rural background and I from an urban one. I think that my being a different sort of a migrant from the same generation at times created competitive transference feelings in Mrs M. She often communicated her fear of being treated by professionals as a person no one really listened to, and as a result of them supporting each other, she was the one blamed and left out.

Not knowing the British culture and way of life, she felt very paranoid. She often mentioned suspicious thoughts regarding the intentions of social workers, nurses, and doctors whom she saw as authority figures critical of her mothering and intending to remove her sons from her care. It is hard to say how much of this was due to her cultural marginality, to actual behaviour by professionals at times of conflict, and/or her poor command of English. Mrs M was also offended by her mother-in-law who suggested handing over Sami to social services and limiting her contact with him to once a week or even once a month as it seemed impossible to cope with his care. She also claimed that doctors in a prominent hospital in London had offered to terminate his life during one of his hospitalizations. It is unlikely but not impossible that the team may have felt relieved if the child were to die given that the family refused to cooperate in his treatment. But these claims could also be projections of her own unconscious wishes onto others, indicating her great difficulty in coming to terms with mothering a child with such severe handicaps, and, at times, perhaps understandably, finding such short cuts appealing as a way out of her misery.

Disability in babies and young children evokes powerful and disturbing feelings in everyone. Professionals were accusing Mrs M of failing to use the support she was offered to look after Sami. Faced with the helplessness of Sami's condition, it seemed as if adults were reminded of their own frailty and mortality (Stoker, 2011). I believe, consequently, not only his mother but also most of the professionals in the team at times found anger an easier emotion to cope with than the extreme helplessness and sadness they were all experiencing in response to Sami's severe handicap. A closer look indicated that those professionals who had concrete tasks at hand built a better relationship with her, whereas others with no clear tasks had serious problems in relating to Mrs M.

It is also likely that Mrs M felt overwhelmingly responsible for Sami's impairment. A few times, she voiced thoughts related to her use of antidepressants during pregnancy as a possible cause of the damage in Sami. At the same time she denied the difficulties she was going through as the mother of a son with severe disabilities. As she did not know what to expect from Sami's future, she was battling with herself to avoid thinking about it but also at times appeared to be frightened of her own exaggerated expectations. For instance, she once told me that she was expecting Sami to grow up and be constantly attached to all sorts of machines in his room in order to survive. By contrast, at times I heard her saying that Sami was not as disabled as the doctors believed, and he would walk when he was six or seven years old, and have girlfriends when he grew up. Initially, her denial was so strong that she even refused to receive the disability allowance in spite of the family's great financial strains. It is understandable that she was feeling tremendously anxious about what the future held, and struggled with a sense of isolation with the problem.

As Sami was unable to speak, his mother naturally relied a great deal on his non-verbal communication. She often told me that she could understand Sami by just looking into his eyes. My observations indicated that she kept Sami in a contented state mainly by satisfying his bodily needs, stimulating him physically, and talking to him in a loving way with good eye contact. It is known that the impact of severe, accumulated trauma causes difficulty in distinguishing between the external world and the internal world of fantasy. This is an inevitable risk in such a situation for any mother, but perhaps more so for this mother due to her own traumatic experiences. Thus she was prone to see in Sami's eyes not his state of mind but her own projected feelings. According to *Burlingham* (1972, 1979) in babies who are born blind, attachment to the object world is delayed; once formed, it remains longer on primitive levels; motility matures later than normal and remains restricted, and prolonged dependence interferes with the unfolding of aggression. Verbalization suffers from a gap between words and their meaning; superego formation bears the mark of the initial differences in object relationship. In short, Sami's severe disability alongside mother's mental health issues might have complicated further an already difficult process.

Once I tried to link his mother's anxiety with Sami's repetitive action of opening and closing his mouth as if he were screaming with no sound. I believe Mrs M took it literally, as a confirmation of her fears. She chose to say that Sami was tired, and took him to his bed to sleep rather than engaging with me in thinking about his "silent screams" and her own fears. After that incidence she kept Sami in his bed during my visits, claiming that he was tired. I still do not know what this idea of a "silent scream" represented for the mother; whether she unconsciously perceived such a scream as a retaliation—by her mother's "ghost" in the form of Sami's disability, or the toll of her own depression on her damaged creation: "Look what you have done to me. You gave birth to a monster." Despite her best intentions, at an unconscious level, perhaps Sami represented a threat to her feminine creativity, and she could not engage with explorative thinking. It was obvious that this "silent scream" was a very frightening experience for Mrs M as it evoked her own "silent screams" of the past and those now, in the present. At that point in time she dealt with it by shutting it out rather than hearing.

Development of our work: learning to register and express emotions

With time, the magnitude of Sami's developmental delay became more obvious and his mother's depression seemed to be increasing. She appeared frightened of her own and Sami's anger without being consciously aware of it. She talked about being scared of dropping Sami down the stairs at a time of panic, and of Sami's biting his arm. Mrs M often mentioned her anxiety that one night Sami would scream and frighten Yusuf in his sleep. She also admitted that once Sami's doctors had told her to expect to find him dead in his sleep one morning, and she did not want Yusuf to find him. For that reason Mrs M kept Sami's crib in her room instead of letting the boys share a room. Mrs M's state of mind reminded me of Baradon and Joyce's idea of "fear of mutual damage" when a parent carries (conscious or unconscious) powerful destructive feelings towards the baby and experiences him as potentially harmful, associated with attachment difficulties. "Parents in this referral category find the boundaries between thought and action frighteningly fragile, and therefore need to constantly monitor the well-being of their baby … These parents are in a state of vigilant hyperarousal much of the time" (2005, pp. 37–38). Niedecken (2003) writes about the unconscious grandiosity in carers who try to protect the damaged and disabled infant from society's death wishes. Even an utterly committed carer's omnipotence is tested at some points, which then lead to overwhelming feelings of helplessness and anxiety. I believe Mrs M was also feeling overwhelmed and at risk of splitting, mistrust, and wishes of abandonment that might undermine her provision of care for Sami.

Mrs M complained about her practical problems relating to housing not having been responded to. Her situation increased her sense of isolation and feeling trapped at home.

She told me in a panic that her key worker had "caught" her having left Sami alone at home. Social services were alerted. We tried to understand and go over the incident together. Apparently, that morning Mrs M had overslept because she did not hear the alarm clock, and as it was so late had decided to leave Sami behind, in order to get Yusuf to school on time. She was aware that the worker was coming to collect Sami for his hospital appointment that morning, i.e., she expected a professional's visit. It became clear that she was actually seeking punishment by setting up the conditions for her negligence to be found out. Might she also be unconsciously hoping for them to take him into care? Perhaps Mrs M was particularly disappointed about the significant developmental delay in Sami, who showed no sign of separation anxiety and settled easily with strangers. Her fear of his lifelong dependency possibly contributed to her acting out by abandoning him. I also linked this to her possible disappointment in me, for having to end our previous session abruptly because of her visitor without confirming our next appointment, until she called my secretary in a panic right after this incident. This interpretation helped her to express her anger towards me more openly, and we were able to make links between her intense feelings and her acting out. Mrs M told me that I was the only support she had, and she felt anxious when I had not called her to make an appointment. She acknowledged her difficult life and her wish to ease her relations with others, and said she found talking with me helpful. In other words, feeling neglected by me, she was communicating her sense of being dropped by me, and dropping her needy son from her mind that morning. This mother had already told me previously how she was scared that as a result of her neediness and stressfulness she might lose others' interest in her. On this occasion we were able to focus on her need to keep my own interest alive by raising my concern regarding her parenting ability at times of stress.

In one of my visits, Sami was ill and sleeping in his crib. Mrs M greeted me with tears in her eyes. She communicated her state of mind and impossible position with a moving metaphor: "I feel like I am in a restaurant's kitchen to prepare food for six families. But I am only given three or four potatoes and the owner of the restaurant comes in and scolds me." Perhaps at that point it was difficult for her to perceive even my own visit as something supportive, rather than critical. Soon she added that there are people more needy than herself, and even at the most difficult times she did not ask for help. "If I ask for help, they will have evidence that I am not a good mother. But at the same time I feel in a big chaos and frightened to lose my ability to cope. I need some concrete work around my needs."

The next session the same themes, deprivation, and harsh treatment from the workers whose support she depends upon, came in the form of a different metaphor: "… as if I am naked and expecting from the services a thin jacket to cover myself and not getting even that. I am so frightened to die from cold."

My process notes from our eighteenth session show that at those times, Mrs M really could not believe that social and medical services were trying to help her. Furthermore, due to her difficulties in English she often avoided communicating her immediate needs to the agencies involved.

> Mother opened the door with tears in her eyes. She told me that she found Sami's blanket edges being gnawed. She was convinced that there was a rat in the house and it had tried to climb up to Sami's crib last night. She cried, telling me that Sami would not be able to

> protect himself if it entered into his bed. She urged me to help her concretely as she was beside herself. I wondered whether she had reported the incident to her key worker or to the landlord. She decided to call the landlord and tried to explain what she thought had happened. I realized her limited ability to express herself in English. This seemed to make her even more nervous and she kept laughing. I doubted that her landlord managed to understand the urgency of the situation.

She ended up having depressed periods where she lost all her hope and trust in support around her and became suspicious of the professionals instead of realizing her part in it. Such a comment from me immediately brought up an intense anger towards her key worker, Ms S. I responded to her with a metaphor of my own to express my understanding: "It sounds like you are trying to tell me that you and Ms S are supposed to carry a heavy burden together. The task is so difficult that you find yourselves arguing instead of cooperating. Perhaps that is more tolerable than doing the day to day carrying."

I believe that in these states of mind Mrs M experienced all her objects leaving her, or not satisfying her, and felt there was no one there for her. Her murderous wishes were very close to the surface and it was clear that she could not be pleased by the professionals until they were pleased with her. She only cooperated when she was taught to do specific tasks, and needed a clear definition of these and of realistic plans in order to function to help Sami. Mrs M as well as the professionals used the same mechanisms of projection and blame; both sides were not happy with each other. In this state of mind I believe for Mrs M guilt feelings were not the main issue as she was externalizing with limited ego strength. She required a realistic, concrete programme, agreed upon and supported by all involved. Consequently I suggested a family support meeting between Mrs M and all the professionals dealing with her case. She hesitated at first and communicated her fear of not coming across as having "clear thoughts" in such meetings. But she worked on it and managed to organize the issues in her mind that she wanted to address. After the meeting, she told me that she was able to use my presence as a reassurance in managing her anger during the meeting. Her housing needs, Sami's medical and educational needs, respite services, and management of her debt to the gas company were all discussed and for each item an action plan was agreed to support this mother.

The child's needs and their impact on his development and interaction with his mother

According to Anna Freud, "The separation-individuation phase of the second year of life is negotiated successfully only in cases where there is perfect synchronization between three factors: motor development which provides the means for the infant's physical departure from the mother and for his rejoining her; the ego's awakening wish for exploration and adventure; the mother's readiness to grant the child a measure of independence. If any of these influences comes in too early, or lags behind the others, development is interfered with and the infant, instead of advancing, misses out on an important step" (1981, p. 116).

In her writings about "The role of bodily illness", Anna Freud (1952) stressed how hospitalization separates the child from the rightful owner of his body at the very moment when his body is threatened by dangers from inside as well as from the environment. On the other hand she also emphasized the importance of the gradual mastering of various bodily functions such as independent eating, independent bladder control, bowel evacuation, etc., marking for the child highly significant stages in ego development, as well as advances in detaching his own body from that of the mother and possessing it at least in part. Loss of (or inability to develop) these abilities means an equivalent loss in ego control, i.e., a pull back towards the earlier and more passive levels of infantile development. This case demonstrates the many challenges encountered when ordinary development is jeopardized by severe neuro-developmental abnormality, and their impact on the mother's and the child's way of being and relating, especially when the requirements of the phase of separation-individuation can not be met.

Mrs M once gave an account of a very desperate situation she found herself in with Sami when the use of cortisone caused diarrhoea in him and he actually made a sound at 2 a.m. When mother came to check him she saw his face becoming purple and she began trembling uncontrollably while Sami became restless in her arms. She said that she began praying to God that this would not be an epileptic fit as her main fear was of frequent epileptic fits requiring daily hospital visits. In her state of heightened anxiety mother felt so stressed by the needs of her extremely damaged baby that she could not resist intervening physically, and injected him with cortisone. Possibly at that moment, burdened by guilt about past damage as well as the anticipated guilt for present damage, in her reparative attempt to become the rightful "owner" of her son she acted out as a superhuman.

Transference and countertransference

I found Sami an attractive-looking boy and on one hand empathized with Mrs M's need to preserve him. On the other hand, the extent of his disability created a strong sense of sadness in me due to his bleak future. I found that my observations focused more on the mother than the child, as sometimes this was probably too painful for me. Somehow Sami's survival made me feel sorry both for him and for his mother. Exposed to chronic unpredictability with such a severely impaired son, Mrs M's unconscious desires were easily evoked. What was most difficult to bear for her, as well as for me, was not only the intensity of the internal conflict that his severe impairment triggered in her, but the fear that it would continue into the future. As Stoker notes: "Unconscious and unacceptable wishes risk eruption and it is this that upsets our equilibrium, pushing us into defensive positions of omnipotent reparation or feelings of failure and helplessness" (2011, p. 101). My therapeutic engagement with her supported her in becoming aware of these feelings and managing them. I also found ending my visits difficult, especially as during the last minutes Mrs M began talking about important issues. An example from my process notes of our eleventh session:

> After I informed her that we had reached the end of our time and got up to leave, Mrs M began telling me that she likes massaging Sami's body in order to help his blood circulation. She soon began talking about her worries regarding her own health and anxiety about being unable to take care of Sami if she lost her own health. This theme was quickly followed by

> Yusuf's resentment of Sami's getting more love and care from their mother. Anxiously, Mrs M continued talking about not wanting to be dependent on the medical team and instead trying hard to sort out Sami's medical difficulties herself by palliative measures.

Seemingly my leaving at the end of the sessions reverberated with her sense of abandonment by her mother and her husband, alongside reactivated dependency needs. She often managed to end the sessions with a remark regarding the "uselessness" of professionals, thus casting me out. Reflecting disappointment of her own hopes for her baby, perhaps she was communicating her strong feelings through projective identification, by making me feel as frustrated and useless as she felt regarding Sami. Similarly, maybe in response to feeling deprived of normal expectable patterns of interaction with her child, Mrs M was testing me to see how much I cared about her, and how much I could take. I felt that my ability to maintain interest in our work was fundamental in keeping hope alive for the woman, who may have been depressed all her life (Alvarez, 1999).

Mother's mental health needs and its impact on her mothering

Mrs M's account of her own bedridden mother's dependency on her children made me think both of the vulnerable adult in the hands of children, and the absence of a capable, responsible adult in the background. As a child, being denied her own dependency needs, and with her need for guidance, Mrs M understandably could not tolerate her mother's dependency. Although she could not communicate this to me, when her mother died, she most probably felt that her own internal, and at times even external, attacks (through mockery) were responsible for the death. Her mother's depression became part of herself, with no expectation of being alleviated. Mrs M's mental state, rape, and actual experiences of exile, and loss of motherland and mother tongue, complicated her ability to come to terms with the further significant trauma in her life, i.e., the loss of her imagined healthy baby son, and the need to care for a damaged one:

> After I rang the bell twice, Mrs M opened the door, excusing herself for having fallen asleep. It was almost midday. I found Sami sitting in his special chair attached to his feeding tube, and the TV channel of their home country on. Mother began wiping the top of the table saying that for the last few days she always wanted to sleep even if she did not need to, and neglected the housework (3rd visit).

In the child's file I had seen a psychiatric report from the mother's previous GP, and found out about her suicidal ideation and depression during her pregnancy with Sami, before she knew about his disability. I understood how traumatized she was, with her multiple traumas like an overhanging black cloud. This area, which we never discussed in our work, at times made me feel uncomfortable; but also, being aware of her past history made me listen to her with real concern.

Mrs M needed help in integrating her internal object relations before focusing on the impact of her losses. For instance, she initially agreed when I suggested getting a psychiatric assessment as her depression had become more prominent. Possibly at that moment she perceived me as someone with good intentions. But in the following session, she angrily rejected the idea, saying that she was "not crazy". I think that during my absence I became a "bad" person, perhaps for abandoning her in her needy state. Thus in her mind anything I suggested became "bad". Simultaneously, most probably her experience of herself also fluctuated between "good" and "bad". Instead of perceiving herself in need of support, in her intense anger and sadness, she considered herself as "crazy".

Mrs M's defensive manoeuvres functioned either to deny the existence of her mental states or to project them onto others in an attempt to get rid of them. As these defences inhibited three-dimensional creative reflection there was always a risk of concreteness in her thinking. For example, when Sami was having an epileptic attack she immediately thought of him as a dying child, and felt frightened that she might kill them both by throwing herself and him down the stairs. One way of denying the painful reality of Sami's condition is by remaining in a merged state with him, i.e., seeing him not as a separate being but as an extension of herself.

However, there were advances. Late in our work, during the review meeting:

> Mrs M reported that she had ups and downs—at times she felt very depressed and cried a lot, but said these times did not last long any more and she was able to pull herself together pretty quickly. She told me that now she was able to spend "fun time" with Yusuf which both fully enjoyed. For instance, last weekend Yusuf and mother went to the cinema to see a Spider-man movie—having popcorn and Coke, laughing and enjoying their time together. She also registered herself for gym classes, in addition to attending an English school the following academic term, in her free time when Sami would be at his nursery school.

Evaluation of our work

Mrs M was sceptical of authority figures. Being sexually assaulted by the police whose job is actually to protect the citizens had been doubly horrific, and confusing. Nonetheless, she resolved to do it differently, and instead of identifying with the aggressor was able to show compassion. Similarly, she alleged that the older generation would have her abandon her much-damaged baby but she chose to keep him. Perhaps her growing ability to cooperate with the multidisciplinary team was another indication of her capacity to repair the damage done to her.

I believe that talking with me helped Mrs M to normalize her reaction to her difficult predicament. Gradually, she became more able to accept her anxieties about losing control and being unable to take care of her children during such states. Focusing on the near future and immediate plans around Sami helped Mrs M to feel more tolerant and capable as a mother. She discovered and accessed the available special educational services for Sami, and felt more supported in caring for his needs. She began to use respite services provided for Sami in order to have fun with Yusuf, and even to visit her home country after many years. I think our work also helped her to feel less traumatized and more at home in the UK. She started voicing her need to strengthen her ties with the host country by learning English and acquiring a driving licence. Also, after a long wait, she was informed about the social services' decision to provide the family with more appropriate accommodation. As the agencies involved responded in a supportive manner, Mrs M became increasingly interested and motivated to reach out, to ask for help, and make use of what was on offer. To impress me further, during one of our last sessions, she spoke for the first time about the multidisciplinary team as her "big family" whom she found supportive in Sami's care. She said she considered herself lucky in having such support to facilitate her ability to mother Sami and Yusuf as a lone parent in a foreign country. As Mrs M moved from a paranoid stance to a more trusting one, the state became a caring parent instead of an intrusive one. Our work had helped her to change her persecuted identity from victim in an alien country to a person who felt supported and able to open up while starting to feel at home.

According to Selma Fraiberg and her colleagues (1975), a mother cannot hear her baby's cries unless somebody hears her own cries. In this case, Mrs M could not let herself acknowledge her son's traumatized state until she felt that the traumatized child inside her was recognized. By speaking in her mother tongue the silence surrounding this family's experience—perhaps the silent scream—slowly became articulated. It could even find expression in English as the language of her new country, which now began to feel motherly to her. I believe that, perhaps for the first time, she felt heard and understood without fear of being judged or persecuted. My speaking her language and being well informed of the social and political undercurrents of her homeland as well as those of her host country encouraged her towards more open communication and trust in me. Finally, as an immigrant myself, I felt privileged to put to use my psychotherapeutic experience and skills, in my mother tongue, for the benefit of a less fortunate migrant.

Follow-up

In Mrs M, unresolved trauma and loss contributed to the overwhelming impact of her son's disability, alongside the re-evocation of insecure attachment experiences from her past. Anna Freud's (1965) notion of "developmental help", fostering a new and different emotional experience informed my understanding. In our work together I applied techniques such as those suggested by Baradon and Joyce (2005), aimed at clarification and extending the patient's sense of efficacy in communication. Similarly, although this was not psychotherapy per se, I was inspired by Alvarez's (1999) suggestion of a psychotherapeutic technique which is flexible and active, highly attuned to the moment, and takes into account all possible aspects of the relationship, not only during its dynamic moments but also in terms of the results of this relationship on the patient's individuality.

Soon after my visits came to an end, Sami, aged three and a half, began attending a special school. Both children now receive respite services after school, which have enabled their mother to attend English classes. In addition to getting her UK driving licence she bought a car. Social services have provided the family with more spacious and functional accommodation, tailored to meet Sami's daily needs. After my home visits came to an end, Mrs M also participated for six months in a psychotherapeutic group that I ran for migrant mothers of similar background with disabled children. Since then there has been no further contact with the family, which I believe is an indication of their better adjustment and not needing to be referred for further psychological input.

References

Alvarez, A. (1999). *Live Company: Psychoanalytic Psychotherapy with Autistic, Borderline, Deprived and Abused Children*. London: Routledge.

Baradon, T., Broughton, C., Gibbs, I., James J., Joyce A. & Woodhead, J. (2005). *Practice of Psychoanalytic Parent Infant Psychotherapy: Claiming the Baby*. London: Routledge.

Burlingham, D. (1972). *Psychoanalytic Studies of the Sighted and the Blind*. New York: International Universities Press.

Burlingham, D. (1979). To be blind in a sighted world. *Psychoanalytic Study of the Child, 34*: 5–30.

Fonagy, P. & Target, M. (1997). Attachment and reflective function: their role in self-organization. *Development and Psychopathology, 9*: 679–700.

Fraiberg, S., Adelson, E. & Shapiro, V. (1975). Ghosts in the nursery: A psychoanalytic approach to the problem of impaired infant-mother relationships. *Journal of the American Academy of Child Psychiatry, 14*: 387–422.

Freud, A. (1936). *The Ego and the Mechanisms of Defence*. London: Hogarth.

Freud, A. (1952). The role of bodily illness in the mental life of children. *Psychoanalytic Study of the Child, 7*: 69–81.

Freud, A. (1965). *Normality and Pathology in Childhood: Assessments of Development*. Madison, CT: International Universities Press.

Freud, A. (1967). About losing and being lost. *Psychoanalytic Study of the Child, 22*: 9–19. Freud, A. (1981). *Psychoanalytic Psychology of Normal Development*. London: Hogarth.

Hartmann, H. (1939). *Ego Psychology and the Problem of Adaptation*. New York: International Universities Press, 1958.

Hurry, A. (1998). *Psychoanalytic Monograph No. 3, Psychoanalysis and Developmental Therapy*. London: Karnac.

Jacobson, E. (1964). *The Self and the Object World*. New York: International Universities Press.

Joffe, W. G. & Sandler, J. (1965). Notes on pain, depression and individuation. *Psychoanalytic Study of the Child, 20*: 394–424.

Kestenberg, J. S. (1971a). Development of the young child as expressed through bodily movement. *Journal of the American Psychoanalytic Association, 19*(4): 746–764.

Kestenberg, J. S. (1971b). From organ-object imagery to self and object representations. In: J. B. Mc Devitt & C. F. Settlage (Eds.), *Separation-Individuation: Essays in Honour of Margaret S. Mahler*. New York: International Universities Press.

Music, G. (2011). *Nurturing Natures*. New York: Psychology Press.

Niedecken, D. (2003). *Nameless: Understanding Learning Disability*. Hove, UK: Brunner Routledge.

Rustin, M. (2002). Observing infants: reflections on methods. In: L. Miller, (Ed.), *Closely Observed Infants*. London: Duckworth.

Sandler, J. & Rosenblatt, B. (1962). The concept of representational world. *Psychoanalytic Study of the Child, 17*: 128–145.

Stoker, J. (2011). Difference and disability. In: M. Z. Woods & I. Pretorius (Eds.), *Parents and Toddlers in Groups*. London: Routledge.

Target, M. & Allison, E. (2011). Conclusion. In: M. Z. Woods & I. Pretorius (Eds.), *Parents and Toddlers in Groups*. London: Routledge.

B. UNDER FIVES

Clinical work and applications

Overview

CHAPTER TWELVE

Overview of theoretical and clinical applications, and current developments

Angela Joyce

Child psychoanalysis at the Anna Freud Centre has been at the cutting edge of developments in the theory and technique of clinical practice over many decades, and psychoanalytic work with children under school age has a long and impressive history there. The papers in this part reflect both the continuity and the changes that have taken place, whether for young children in the toddler group setting, or individual clinical work—either at the Centre itself or in the National Health Service setting of child and adolescent mental health clinics. The quality of the work described in these accounts is indicative of this impressive tradition.

The children described here reflect changes in referral patterns for treatment, which has gradually encompassed those whose early lives had been marked by experiences of what might now be called "relational trauma" (Baradon (ed.), 2009). These experiences, in which the quality of the earliest relationship does not meet the relational needs of the young child (Cramer & Brazelton, 1991), are now recognized to affect the trajectory of ordinary development in ways that challenge the efficacy of classical psychoanalytic techniques. Nonetheless, it is notable that the range of references cited in the following chapters includes authors from the 1960s and 1970s such as Margaret Mahler and Erna Furman, as well as Anna Freud, in addition to recent work, especially on the developmental aspects of the clinical process such as *Anne Hurry's* seminal book *Psychoanalysis and Developmental Therapy* (1998).

Contemporary psychoanalysis at the Anna Freud Centre, as evidenced by these papers, builds on the foundations of classical authors who had recognized the variety of problems prompting parents and others involved in the care of children to bring them for treatment. This variety was delineated in Anna Freud's framework for diagnosis in her Provisional Diagnostic Profile (in *Normality and Pathology in Childhood*, 1966c), where she enumerated six levels of functioning. These ranged from (1) basically healthy development through (2) a transitory phase of disturbance, (3) a neurosis or character disorder, (4) atypical development (including borderline, delinquent, and psychotic children), to (5) an underlying "primary deficiency of an organic nature or early deprivation" distorting development. Her last category enigmatically referred to "destructive processes at work which have effected or are on the point of effecting a disruption of mental growth" (p. 147).

This framework indicates how Anna Freud revolutionized the traditional way of understanding psychopathology. She maintained that disturbance was to be understood from the standpoint of normality: if the trajectory of normal development could be mapped then its deviations or pathologies could be better understood and treated. This also reflects her view of the aims of a psychoanalytic intervention for a child: to restore the pathway of normal development. Although this risks a normative straightjacket on the notion of development, it seems to be a more creative way of understanding when and why things go wrong that manifest themselves in the variety of symptoms presenting for treatment and then to see how to work with them, by having a yardstick of the range of ordinary familiar development.

Alongside her Diagnostic Profile, Anna Freud (1966c) famously elaborated a variety of Developmental Lines along which such normality could be tracked. These then could indicate relative harmony in the well-developing child or disharmony across a range of indices in a more troubled child.

A major contribution to the techniques of psychoanalysis has developed out of this differentiation of levels of disturbance in children. Classically, psychoanalysis had privileged the interpretation of internalized conflict that the child suffered, made evident through neurotic symptoms such as phobias. These children were assumed to have had good enough early development, founded upon satisfactory early relationships, where sound mental structure had been established, allowing for these conflicts to emerge via a structured ego and emerging superego. This way of understanding children's development was shared by Donald Winnicott (1977) who, like Anna Freud, was alert to the ways in which the parental and family environment of the child had a profound impact upon its emotional development.

Children who had not been so privileged began to present for treatment with "the step from private practice to the opening of consultation centres and clinics for children, where a whole mass of unsorted case material arrived and claimed the analyst's attention" (A. Freud, 1966c, p. 151). Steven Ablon, an American analyst and long-time friend of the Anna Freud Centre, wrote in 2001 of the changes that followed the publication of Anna Freud's *Normality and Pathology in Childhood*:

> In addition to treating children with largely neurotic difficulties, child analysts explored ways of treating children with more severe developmental problems. They responded to what children in analysis seemed to indicate was helpful technically and what characterized therapeutic action in child analysis ... These features include greater awareness of object relations, identifications, introjects, and relational and interpersonal factors. In addition, technical considerations involving enactment and action, pre-Oedipal foci, affect, uses of the countertransference, and the therapeutic action of play have become important considerations first in child analysis and subsequently also in adult analytic technique. Many of these developments are present in the work of Anna Freud and were subsequently extended and elaborated (2001, p. 27).

One of Anna Freud's closest colleagues from the original War Nurseries, *Hansi Kennedy*, was also one of the first trainees in child psychoanalysis at the Hampstead Clinic. She was interested in understanding developmental disturbances based on compromised initial construction of the personality. Following Anna Freud's concepts of the Developmental Lines, Kennedy and her colleagues created a form of analytic treatment for impaired development termed "developmental help" or "developmental therapy" (see Miller & Neely, 2008). The work Kennedy began in her studies of children suffering from developmental disharmonies continued at AFC after her retirement in 1993. Anne Hurry, her colleague and long-term staff member, described "developmental therapy" in her 1998 book as "an opportunity for change through a relationship fine-tuned to the patient's developmental needs" (p. 34).

In a review of some of Anna Freud's remembered comments from seminars and meetings published after her death in 1983, she is quoted as saying on the subject of ego defects evident in children with uneven psychic development:

> It is terribly important in discussing differences between defect and conflict that we hold no brief for either. We do not share the view of people who think that everything should be one thing or the other; we merely make the attempt to sort the matter out objectively. The main point [...] was to create a difference in our own minds between the original building up of the personality and the later involvement in neurotic conflicts. [...] how can the first part, the building up of the personality, be modified? Of course we would like to think that the ego defects can be undone. However, I am pretty convinced that they *cannot*. When we analyse a person, the whole process is really aimed at that person's ego, at widening the scope of the ego's influence, at helping that person deal with the internal conflicts and what is left over from the earliest experiences. Can we apply that formula to the building up of the very structure which we expect later on to perform the task? We can probably apply it to certain ego defects and not to others, and it would be for us, in practice, to find out where this can be done and where it cannot. As you know, this runs counter to the analytic theory which says that if only you can revive the early experiences in the transference, you can then, in the very revival, modify the consequences. I don't believe that, not for the earliest ones, not for the basic ones. But this is, of course, an open question (1983, p. 125, emphasis added).

She was more optimistic about the efficacy of such aims for treatment in younger, pre-latency children than for older children, believing that the limitations wrought by the realities of the passage of time in the developmental process have to be recognized. This was in line with the classical view that the Oedipal situation (aged between three and five years) organized experience so that the consequences of earlier development were no longer so susceptible to modification and change. "You can't have an eight year old and rectify what has happened at the age of two. But you can often get a three year old or a four year old and rectify what happened at the age of one or two" (A. Freud, 1983, p. 126).

Retrospective research, carried out by Mary Target on the records of analytic treatment at the Centre up to the early Nineties, certainly could be said to support this contention as the most successful outcomes for analysis were for younger pre-school children (Fonagy & Target, 1994).

Anna Freud was alert to the complexities and challenges of treating children with developmental disturbances, regarding the technique and setting needed for work, i.e., helping a child's ego to make certain distinctions, or to acquire capacities, such as keeping the image of the absent person in his mind, or distinguishing between what happens in his mind and in his body, as "not a once weekly technique. If anything it has to be more intensive than child analysis: certainly not less intensive" (A. Freud, 1983, p. 126).

For a long time the Hampstead Clinic had held a view privileging intensive treatment with frequent sessions. In 1991 Hansi Kennedy (Target & Kennedy, 1991) described it thus:

> We consider that daily contact with the child is desirable to gather the maximum amount of material and maintain the interpretative work, to keep the analytic material within the bounds of the consulting room, to deal with the anxieties mobilized and not to place too great a burden on the child's environment. We believe that daily treatment enhances the efficiency of the therapeutic work and this is especially true of the treatment of under-fives (p. 25).

The two clinical papers in this part describe work in the AFC tradition of analyses conducted intensively (four times weekly), taking account of the developmental difficulties evident in these children. All three children described could be said to be disturbed or at risk of disturbance at the third or fourth level of Anna Freud's framework. They reflect disturbances in ego development, object relations, and superego formation. The issues described include impulsivity, poor affect regulation, and a profound level of mistrust of those caring for them. Both Ray and Ella were referred because of uncontrollable aggression: Ray, aged four, because his violent behaviour had led to his expulsion from nursery school; Ella bit children, ran around with things in her mouth, had no sense of danger, pushed others out of her way, had difficulties concentrating, and was unaffected by punishment or praise. Both these children as well as Ari in the toddler group setting had suffered early losses through the exigencies of modern life: maternal return to work, migration, sudden weaning. The significance of these events as real losses experienced by young children is often underestimated; it is usually only in these kinds of clinical accounts that the child's predicament in suffering their consequences is closely examined. Such papers afford us the opportunity to recognize the emotional costs, and the kinds of interventions that can make such a considerable difference to the lives of these children and their parents.

Such clinical work demonstrates the innovative application of classical psychoanalytic technique together with the adaptations that emerged out of applications to work with children with developmental disturbances. As Hedde Evers puts it, her young patient "needed a combination of interpretative and developmental techniques that are now recognized as characteristic of the Anna Freudian approach to child analytic work" so that she was "able to revisit and work through developmental areas that had remained unresolved and consequently distorted and obstructed her ongoing development".

This connects with another concept of critical importance in this expansion of analytic treatment: that of the significance of the analyst as a new developmental object for the patient. Evers reminds us of Anna Freud's (1966) view that "Children have a hunger for *new* experience, which is as strong as the urge to repeat." Anna Freud believed that the therapist functions as a new object to the child, and is only used as a transference object to repeat disturbed areas of development. She observed that "In child analysis the interpreting object is also a new and developmental object, and that distinguishing and carefully moving between the two roles are essential elements of child analytic technique."

Specifically developmental techniques were aimed at promoting ego development that was out of sync with other aspects of the child's functioning. Evers mentions the naming and verbalizing of affective states, the clarification of cause and effect, and for this child, support in toilet training. She says that many times in the work Ella required "developmental holding and relating"—the provision of a setting that had hitherto been unavailable to her. Ray's treatment also utilized these kinds of interventions. Both authors show how the analyst's capacity to play and to promote playing in their young patients is central to their emerging coherence and developing sense of self. Both emphasize that at crucial times in these children's treatments, words, and particularly interpretations were not a panacea. Rather akin to Winnicott's notion of holding (1960e), a predominantly non-verbal "being with" rather than "doing to" is provided in this aspect of the work. Both papers demonstrate the "primordial panic" that these children were prone to in the absence of a sufficiently reliable internalized good object. Both Ray and Ella were subject to acute narcissistic rage as their identifications with badness superseded the possibility of anything more benign. Both analysts had to bear the brunt of this in their affective responses. As Anna Freud said, "Most children put a strain on the analytic model. Deprived children more than others" (A. Freud, 1983, p. 126). They also put a strain on the analyst treating them.

A sine qua non of work with children is applied analytic work with their parents. Although only passing reference is made in the two clinical papers, nevertheless the importance of this work in parallel with the analytic treatment of young children has long been recognized, reflecting the complexity of factors seen to contribute to the children's difficulties. Federica Melandri's treatment of Ray took place at the Anna Freud Centre where the tradition of the therapist of a young child also seeing his parents was maintained. She comments that this work was "essential in helping mother acquire some understanding of her child's normal needs". Seeing Ray's mother weekly she was able to observe that her organized defences against painful affects were impeding her capacity to respond empathically to Ray's distress. Parent work enables both the ordinary needs of a child plus his disturbances to be better understood by the parent.

In the NHS setting where Hedde Evers treated Ella, another child psychotherapist saw Ella's mother. The father found it difficult to attend regularly although he did make it for the termly review and school meetings. Pressure on resources meant that the weekly meetings could not be sustained and the reduction to fortnightly was felt in the child's treatment. These are major issues for the provision of services for children in the public sector as the complexity of factors that create the child's difficulties invariably includes the relationship with the parents.

The chapter by Justine Kalas Reeves is set in the AFC toddler group service, a feature of the Centre since the early days of the Hampstead Clinic. In that setting the building blocks of parent-child relationships are the focus, affording an opportunity for early preventive work when "sub-clinical" disturbances emerge. The little boy who is the subject of this paper was already in some considerable trouble when he began to attend, with his mother, aged fourteen months, presenting with an autistic-like repertoire of defences and withdrawal. Like the children in the two clinical papers, Ari had also suffered a major loss in his first year of life: his mother had returned to work four days a week when he was nine months old and a nanny had taken his place. This presents dilemmas which are very common these days, put succinctly by Ari's mother to the toddler leader: "As a working mother I sometimes find it difficult to juggle my work and a healthy relationship with him [Ari]." Justine uses the considerable experience of Erna Furman to illuminate the consequences for the child whose mother leaves him (by going back to work early in the toddler period or before) rather than being there in order to be left: "When mother is not there, the harbour is gone and venturing out feels less safe and less fun." As well as being deeply personal issues for families, political issues, including the duration of maternity leave, are raised by these observations. The contemporary challenge to parents, whose investment in their children risks being curtailed by the exigencies of modern living such as the demands of the workplace and their own professional fulfilment etc., is deeply conflictual. It is hard not to be seen to be against women's freedom to work when the arguments are put from the point of view of the child. What these papers show us is that whatever the political arguments, children experience and feel the consequences of such decisions and are marked by them.

In the toddler group setting similar processes can be observed as were noted in the individual work with Ray and Ella: the provision of new object experience for Ari where the toddler group staff are interested in his inner reality, and for his mother, able over time to imbibe their example, as they modelled ways of relating to the young children. Again, play and its manifold benefits so often affords the locus for the developmental process to be apparent. The toddler group setting facilitates playing between adults and children, between the children and even between the adults, and this toddler and his mother are certainly shown to have benefited from their attendance over the two years.

Finally, in their chapter, Hillary and Tony Hamburger movingly describe the culturally sensitive application of psychoanalytic concepts to Ububele Umdlezane Parent Infant Project and other facilities in a mental health centre catering to a deprived and under-resourced South African township. Their various interventions offer a "thinking space" for pre-school children and staff—a minute resource in the face of considerable need. However, as they convey, a little goes a long way to reap almost unimaginable results in interventions with young children, reclaiming them from the abyss of abandonment that they feel threatened by.

From these closely observed psychoanalytic interventions, it is possible to understand what lies behind the presenting symptoms of violence and impulsivity, withdrawal and lack of pleasure in these children. The nature and degree of anxiety that they experienced, in the absence of adults able to attend adequately to their emotional needs in ways that could be sufficiently supportive of their development, is apparent. The inner worlds of these children are woefully deficient in expectations of others as helpful objects enabling them to have a healthy narcissistic investment in themselves. Instead, problems of poor self-esteem and a fragile capacity to manage powerful feelings hold sway. All these children were at severe risk of not just distorted and disturbed development, but also of living lives that would be impoverished of real satisfaction and pleasure, in reaching a measure of their potential, and of having relationships which would be substantial and satisfying.

As the result of these kinds of psychoanalytic treatment, in the tradition begun by Anna Freud and developed by those who worked closely with her and others that have followed on, these young people have considerably more chance of living their lives with satisfaction.

References

Ablon, S. L. (2001). The work of transformation: changes in technique since Anna Freud's normality and pathology in childhood. *Psychoanalytic Study of the Child, 56*: 27–38.

Baradon, T. (Ed.) (2010). *Relational Trauma in Infancy: Psychoanalytic, Attachment and Neuropsychological Contributions to Parent–Infant Psychotherapy.* Hove, UK: Routledge.

Brazelton, T. B. & Cramer, B. (1991). *The Earliest Relationship.* London: Karnac.

Fonagy, P. & Target, M. (1994). Who is helped by child psychoanalysis? A sample study of disruptive children from the Anna Freud Centre. A retrospective investigation. *Bulletin of the Anna Freud Centre, 17*: 291–315.

Freud, A. (1966). *Normality and Pathology in Childhood.* London: Hogarth.

Freud, A. (1983). Excerpts from seminars and meetings. *Bulletin of the Anna Freud Centre, 6*: 115–128.

Hurry, A. (1998). *Psychoanalysis and Developmental Therapy.* London: Karnac.

Miller, J. M. & Neely, C. (Eds.) (2008). *The Psychoanalytic Work of Hansi Kennedy: From the War Nurseries to the Anna Freud Centre (1940–1993).* London: Karnac.

Target, M. & Kennedy, H. (1991). Psychoanalytic work with the under-fives: forty years' experience. *Bulletin of the Anna Freud Centre, 14.*

Winnicott, D. W. (1960). The theory of the parent–infant relationship. In: *The Maturational Processes and the Facilitating Environment.* London: Hogarth and the Institute of Psychoanalysis, 1965.

Winnicott, D. W. (1977). *The Piggle.* London: Hogarth.

Clinical

CHAPTER THIRTEEN

"Learning to love"—a story about a young girl's analysis

Hedde Maartje Evers

Introduction

Describing the emotional experience of two year olds parting from their mothers, Anna Freud and *Dorothy Burlingham* noted that when separated from her "the child suddenly feels deserted by all the known persons in his life to whom he has learned to attach importance ... His longing for his mother becomes intolerable and throws him into states of despair ... Observers seldom appreciate the depth and seriousness of this grief of a small child" (A. Freud & *Burlingham*, 1974, pp. 182–183). This understanding had developed from their observations of young children in the Hampstead War Nurseries, later to become the Anna Freud Centre.

Ella was a little older, four years old, when she first came for treatment—a year of once a week psychotherapy, followed by two years of four times weekly child analysis, then one final year of twice weekly treatment. The focus of this chapter will be on the two years of intensive analytic work when Ella was aged between five and seven years old.

Early days

On referral Ella was a petrified, defiant, provocative, and out-of-control little girl who had been expelled from two nurseries for biting other children. This symptom began when she was only nine months old, apparently in response to the separation from her mother on going to a crèche. By the age of four Ella had become an outsider, was feared and avoided by other children, and defied adults to the point of despair. Ella feared closeness, despised vulnerability and need, and turned to hatred to defend herself against loving feelings, sadness, and helplessness (Isaacs, 1934; Fairbairn, 1942). She longed deeply for her mother yet was overcome with angry resentment and deep uncertainty about her own lovability. Separations had remained intolerably painful. Her case presented a puzzle—what was it in her early years that had created her terrible dilemma?

On meeting Ella for the first time, she impressed me as a muscular child who avoided eye contact. With her still toddler-like build and puffy pink ski coat she bore some resemblance to a tiny tank. Her complexion was light brown and the many strong features in her small face made it look a little crowded. She had large brown eyes, lavish lashes, and curly dark hair in two pigtails. She shared her impression that the colour of her skin was somehow related to the wild and angry feelings that left her feeling so bad and unlovable and made her want to "get rid" of herself. She also showed an acute awareness of differing shades of skin tone in her family, telling me that she and Daddy had brown skin, and Mummy and her sister Mae, yellow. She added that I, Hedde, had yellow skin too. Ella went on to demonstrate the strength of her impulses or drives and the way she felt taken over by them. From her belly button she attempted to extract a wild and overwhelming blood-curdling entity which she called "The Weird" and who she passionately tried to chase out of the room. In her assessment sessions, Ella also communicated intense feelings of uncertainty and dread of not being loved and held onto well enough, and of being lost. She had set the scene: these themes would continue to play a very central role in the four years of work that were to follow.

Background information

Ella came from an intact family. Both parents were of mixed Afro-Caribbean and white ethnicity. Ella was the first child for her mother and the third for her father, who sired two children in his young adulthood. In the father's personal life and family line, there was a history of risk-taking behaviour and difficulties with authority. Ella had a younger sister Mae, who was three years her junior. At the time of referral, Mae was almost continuously taunted and hurt by Ella, who would wake her from her sleep with a loud shout, pinch her, or push her over. The parental relationship seemed under strain, with Ella's mother feeling unsupported by her husband and overwhelmed with the care for the children, and challenging Ella in particular. Ella was born full term with an emergency Caesarean as she did not descend. Little is known about her mother's experience of becoming a mother and of Ella's early days. Mrs X remembered her daughter as a beautiful, clever, and well-loved baby who breastfed satisfactorily and weaned herself at six months. Ella was nine months old when she started day care and her mother returned to work. Mrs X remembered that "Ella didn't cry at this point but bit other children instead." But on reunion she was clingy and at bedtime cried desperately, sometimes until she became sick. Ella's biting, which had apparently started in response to separation from her mother, led to a first referral to a local child and family centre when she was fourteen months old. There were no additional developmental concerns.

When almost four, Ella was referred again. Her parents now described her as "spiteful, extremely defiant, disobedient, and hard work". A particularly worrying symptom was that Ella would run away, often towards a dangerous road. At her new nursery Ella had continued to bite objects and children. She had no sense of danger and seemed unaffected by punishment or praise. Ella required continuous one-to-one support to keep herself and the other children safe.

Techniques

This account of Ella's treatment will show her difficulties in allowing herself to be vulnerable enough to feel dependent, and to hazard the true relatedness and love that she so craved. These were gradually explored and understood as she worked through central developmental conflicts that had been left unresolved. Her four-year-long psychoanalytic treatment was characterized by a combination of traditional psychoanalytic technique (using interpretation of transference and resistance to address areas of conflict) and developmental techniques, aimed at treating areas of delay and deficit (Edgcumbe, 2000). There were times and areas in Ella's treatment that specifically required developmental holding and relating. This included the use of techniques such as verbalization of feelings, clarification of cause and effect (Hurry, 1998), and importantly, supporting her toilet training. Held by this combination of interpretative and developmental techniques, now recognized as characteristic of the Anna Freudian approach to child analytic work, Ella was able to revisit and work through developmental areas that had remained unresolved and consequently distorted and obstructed her ongoing development.

Once weekly therapy

Initially Ella had started non-intensive, once-weekly therapy. Soon she was also given a diagnosis of attention deficit hyperactivity disorder and a provision of twenty hours of individual support at nursery. During those ten months of therapy she showed the depth of her passionate and desperate longing for a maternal object who would be able to take her on and survive her intense hunger and need—a longing that filled her with shame and humiliation.

As the first summer holiday break approached, Ella felt increasingly unwanted and unloved. She ran wild with fear and anger, did all she could to prove that no one could contain her, and began to soil, apparently to discharge feelings of rage and disappointment with her maternal love objects (Anna Freud, 1966d) and to punish them. With this new symptom, Ella had moved to the next developmental expression of aggression: the soiling of the anal phase. Her parents were shocked and it was in this context that they welcomed the start of four times weekly analysis from the next academic year.

Intensive work

In her first analytic session in September, Ella, now five, made a brew of tissues, glue, and water coloured green with ink. She called it "the Land of Doom" and spoke about wild beasts that would come and kill us, and about how my heart would be filled with "doom". It would be like monsters, all monsters in my heart. She brought a bit of green tissue to her mouth and gave me one to hold in my hand. I spoke about how maybe we could slowly start to talk to these monsters a little, maybe if we held them well, they wouldn't need to go so wild. She reclaimed the snippet and looked at it carefully. Then she said that it was no longer the Land of Doom, but the "Land of Bravery and Courage and Fear". Ella was very frightened of the part of her that felt like wild beasts and monsters and its perceived potential to kill all loving feelings. In this first analytic session she showed her worries about the destructive impact of her aggressive impulses and, then, having felt held and understood, was able to share a sense of hope about our joint venture.

The first year of analysis: feeling small and horrible

Ella's first year of analysis might be described as an intense reliving and re-enactment of pre-Oedipal conflicts, at the painful heart of which lay Ella's fundamental uncertainty as to whether she was wanted and desired by her mother, and, in the transference, by me. I felt very protective and accepting of her as a much younger child, possibly sensing that despite her large and loud efforts at defiance, and in line with her ongoing primitive omnipotent defences, Ella could not yet bear to feel too separate as this made her feel very unheld and, literally, run wild with fear (Symington, 1985). A large amount of oral and anal stage material was poured out in this first year, yet Ella was also very controlling and often prevented me from speaking. Hence, it might take many sessions for an important interpretation to be delivered in full.

One of Ella's most dangerous symptoms at this time was a passionate state of panicky running away from her mother, often towards a busy road. Enacting in the transference how very bad and unheld she felt, she did what she had always done and ran. Actually keeping her with me, physically safe and unharmed, was an all encompassing task. Her running out reminded me of a young toddler darting away from the mother in the "practising" phase of the separation-individuation process (Mahler, 1972a, 1972b), both in "turning passive into active" the "losing and re-finding the love object" and in confirming that she still is and wishes to be connected to mother, hopeful that mother on her part still wants to catch her and gather her up in her arms (Mahler, 1972b). Ella's running did however seem to communicate a sharp question of physical and emotional survival: did her mother love her enough to make sure to scoop her up or would she allow Ella to "get rid" of herself and be killed?

Wild and dangerous running about and acting out characterized the end of many sessions and would continue to do so for a good while longer, especially around breaks. At such times Ella seemed to experience that her existence would end unless she could feel connected to and loved by her mother, and me as a maternal object in the transference. Overcome by fears of annihilation typical of earliest babyhood, fear of object loss and loss of the object's love, she was plunged into states of utter helplessness and panic noted by Yorke and colleagues (1989). Separations also infuriated her and seemed to unravel any tentative fusion of libidinal and aggressive impulses that might have occurred during the session. At such times Ella defied and rejected her objects and could find solace with no one. In endangering herself, she seemed to swing between suicide and murder, her aggression alternately directed towards herself and towards her object, as noted by Anna Freud (1972b). In the transference I was the mother who could not take care of her.

During this period, Ella often played the mother and designated me as the little girl. As the mother, she was full of disdain, reluctantly providing care while deeply resenting her child. She told me I was a dependent little girl: "Horrible poo poo horrible." She sent me, the little girl, away. She said she hadn't liked me when I had been in her belly. She said I was dependent and when I wondered what that meant she said "small and horrible". I spoke to my little girl feelings and she said she knew, because when she had been little ... She quickly stopped herself and told me about when she had me instead and how she hadn't liked me "dependent and horrible". I was sent away to sit on the other side of the room and Ella commanded me about stating that she was "your royal highness" and "your majesty".

I spoke about my sad feelings and about how very worried I was that my mummy didn't want me enough. Ella was ruthless in her condemnation of her own feelings of dependency and loss, and when sensing them, would usually resort to primitive omnipotent defences. Symington (1985) noted that fear of dependency reflects an underlying and early primitive fear of unintegration. Infantile feelings of helplessness are so unbearable for some children because they echo early experiences of feeling unheld, prompting the child to find a "second skin" to hold herself together, as in babyhood, to prevent an experience of falling to pieces (Bick, 1968; Winnicott, 1965). For Ella a quick turn from feeling small, needy, and unwanted to imperious majesty, was one way of trying to re-find her omnipotent armour.

She commented on a "mucky mushy" feeling in her tummy to describe the experience of her libidinal longings, nevertheless beginning to be drawn into the transference, adding that it was as if mummy was "teaching" her to be a baby again. She tried to keep her longings at bay by keeping me at a distance as she shut me up, hit out, and ran away, yet showed her oral hunger for a bountiful maternal object by always getting more water and trying to fill herself up with stolen sugar and biscuits, all to no avail.

Toilet training revisited

In correspondence with the typical dual libidinal and aggressive cathexis of bodily products in the anal phase, Ella's entire attitude towards the object world was characterized by ambivalence, the simultaneous existence of strong feelings of love and hatred towards the same object. Without toilet training having been emotionally mastered, libido and aggression had remained un-fused. As a consequence she was left prone to violent mood swings between love and hatred and unable to control aggression within her object relationships. She showed the typical anal phase tendencies towards hostility, domination, and provocation of her love objects (A. Freud, 1966d). Ever since before the first summer holiday separation, she had continued on occasions to use excrement as a weapon to express rage and disappointment within the object relationship, as described by Anna Freud. Ella's soiling and later, exhibiting her excrement, further appeared to imply urgent questions of love and hatred: would she be able to provoke her objects to agree with her self- impressions as a disgusting "poo girl", so dangerous that she needed to be kept out and flushed away, or could they survive her attacks (Winnicott, 1968) and take her on in a new relationship between little girl and a mothering object? (Green, 1998).

In an apparent effort to re-work what had been physiologically approached but not emotionally mastered and consolidated, Ella revisited her toilet training, now in the Clinic with me as both a new developmental object and a maternal object in the transference. Months followed in which developmental help aimed at supporting Ella to master toilet training formed the centre of our work. Every session there were times of us urgently needing to run to the toilet and on a few occasions Ella decided to wee or poo in the room, usually close to the end of a session, when the approaching separation caused her to feel suddenly deserted and angry, illustrating Anna Freud's (1966d) observation that toilet training remains vulnerable to reversal in times of disappointment in the object until it finally becomes an autonomous ego and superego concern. Interpretations were rare in this realm in which developmental help prevailed, aiming to support Ella in actually mastering her toilet training.

Ella was spiteful and relentless about smelly and messy bums, she screamed and swore profusely whilst on the toilet. Her struggle with her excrement was acutely painful as she felt it to be the very proof of her badness and horribleness. In this first term of work she saved her poos for her sessions. Over time, she began to act more calmly and as her poos and wees were more reliably done in the toilet, she also began to create some order in her toys: crayons in one cup, felt pens in another.

Softer feelings

Alongside and supported by her emotionally mastering toilet training and the accompanying binding of aggression with libido, the end of sessions were no longer felt to be as disastrous as before. Now that Ella was better able to experience feelings of love and concern for her objects and no longer only overcome with hatred and the accompanying panic around object loss and retribution, she could approach the rhythm of the separation and reunion. She shouted at the top of the voice "Hee!" to which I would reply with a firm "Wow!" and Ella would shout "Dee!" (pronouncing the phonetic syllables of my name), after which I would say: "Ella is calling me." So we continued until Ella added "Always come and go," and allowed me to speak about how difficult it was for her to go and believe that she would come back to see me again. After this session, she had suddenly appeared behind the receptionist, saying "I have lost Hedde, can you help me find her?", thus indicating a growing sense that I *could* be found again. It appeared that here, Ella began to experience me as an object that had survived both her oral hunger and her anal phase attacks and hostility, and had neither gotten rid of her as a "disgusting little poo girl", nor changed in quality or attitude nor retaliated. The destruction she feared had not happened and I could now be used in reality (Winnicott, 1969; Posner et al., 2001).

We were a few months into the first year of work and the initial storms began to abate. Softer feelings and gentler experiences appeared slowly and hesitantly. Ella began drawing love hearts, which was to become a dominant activity in the months to follow. Love hearts appeared for Mummy and Daddy, linked with lines, although sometimes a heart looked as if cut. When the Christmas holiday, the first break since Ella had started analysis approached, Ella wished to take away my breasts with her to keep during our separation. When not allowed inside my blouse, she said she wanted to run away and allowed me to speak about how she runs away when she is frightened that she will be left alone. And that now with the holiday, she was thinking of going first, before I could. I went on to speak about how much she felt she needed my "boobies" for comfort now, with the holiday, when she felt small and lonely. She went on to fabricate a pair of paper scissors, adding "for when things get out of hand".

Here Ella showed both the intensity of her desire to take away enough nourishment from me in the transference as the maternal object to appease her hunger over the holiday, coupled with her concern about harming me with her hungry bites and wish to protect me by making paper scissors that could not do damage, should her aggressive impulses get the better of her.

The spring term

The return after Christmas was complicated by Ella missing sessions due to an overseas family visit as well as a new rule I set specifying that the session would end if she tried to run around the building. The Clinic's tolerance around Ella's behaviour had plummeted. *Prior to scheduled interruptions and holidays, interpretations of her anxiety often failed to contain her.* With Ella's running having been experienced and understood in the first term of work, it did moreover also seem technically appropriate to now try and put some boundaries around it. The aim was to help Ella stop her panicked defensive manoeuvre by giving her a chance to experience adult containment, especially at these times that she felt all alone, utterly defiant, and without any sense of inner containment whatsoever. Both the interruptions to her treatment and the new rule were experienced by Ella as confirmations of her being bad and unlovable. Although she now reliably used the toilet, her conviction that poo was proof of inner badness gained intensity in this context. In her material, more indications gradually appeared of Ella perceiving her skin colour in a similar way.

Two months into spring term Ella's parents decided to start her on Ritalin (methylphenidate) which reportedly produced significant positive changes at school and at home. However, in her analytic sessions, no such clear change in Ella's behaviour was witnessed. Over the next months of Ella's analysis the poignant theme continued around how wanted she was or was not, whether she could "be" in my heart, whether there was any chance of this, given the competition around, and increasingly, whether I could love a brown baby and girl. She drew many much embellished little blonde girls in lovely dresses and would aggressively shout over me when I tried to address her disbelief that I could like a brown little girl. She made many cards—offerings, especially to her mother which would invariably say: "I love Mummy—love Ella", to which I commented: "To Mummy I love you and please Mummy love Ella too". Ella persisted in telling her family members how much she loved them and in her sessions produced endless cards to the same effect. The meanings of this were manifold: I understood Ella's declarations of love as courageous first experimentations around daring to offer her love and braving having her offerings out in the open, to be received, left dangling or rejected. Yet Ella was also able to be remarkably cruel verbally and in particularly cutting tones. The intensity of her aggressive impulses, her magical omnipotent beliefs about their killing power, the angry responses she managed to provoke in her objects, as well as her struggle to overcome her aggression in the service of love and belonging, contributed importantly to the endless nature of Ella's declarations of love for her family over this period.

Just prior to her sixth birthday, she worked hard on another card for Mummy, telling me that Mummy had asked her for one before everything would "come Ella's way" on her upcoming birthday. I commented on the effort she was putting into it and if only Mummy could see all that. I added that sometimes Ella may feel she needed so very much to tell Mummy that she loved her and to do things for Mummy because she was so scared that sometimes she was "too much" for Mummy. She nodded and continued her diligent work. On her actual birthday she was subdued, tried to be a good girl, could not enjoy the special birthday attentions coming her way, and felt compelled to share everything with her parents and Mae. She made many sad offerings to me from one of her birthday gifts—a girly sticker book. For the first (and only) time, she went outside the room "to pass wind", which Daddy had said was the polite way. Once she was back inside, I spoke about her wish to make Mummy, Daddy, Mae, and me very happy with her by sharing, and doing what she thought we'd like, so that we would all be pleased with her on her birthday. She passed a little wind and studied my face, then she went outside again, but asked to be allowed to open the blind on the door so that she could see me. She stood there outside the door for a little while, then said that I now needed to come as she needed the toilet. From inside there she asked in a very small voice "Hedde, are you going away?"—a complete turnaround of her earlier defensive imperative commands for me to go away and revealing the underlying anxiety. It appeared that her birthday was a day of uncertainty about how welcome she was and had been, and whether she was worth loving and keeping. In my countertransference, I felt full of sadness.

Separations and reunions and the question of the possibility of an ongoing and loving connection had continued to be primary areas of work in the first year of analysis. By the end of this year, Ella was increasingly able to experience feelings of sadness and loss, and less driven to act them out. However, endings, especially prior to and after holidays, remained unbearable at times, and Ella acted out feeling unloved and thrown out of my heart by trying to endanger herself on the staircase, attempting to defy my intention and efforts to keep her safe. Before the summer holiday, she screamed out how much she hated me, that she never wanted to see me again, and would never make a card for me. In her last session prior to the break she did, however, arrive looking beautiful and feminine with a flowery dress and prettily done hair. I felt moved at her having dared to take the risk to make herself beautiful for me, and with this, to convey both her desire for my loving feelings and maybe also the beginnings of a feeling that she could be a lovely and lovable girl. In this session Ella screamed a bit, felt a little sick, complained about the table "pricking" her tummy. I empathized with her pain, the hurt feelings about us not seeing each other for some time. She had brought in her own soft toy dog to hold onto, and made a card for me that said "To Hedde, thank you for being nice to me". She mumbled "nice, even in the beginning" seemingly referring to stormy earlier times when she had felt herself such a horrible girl. She went on to bump her head while hiding under a table and was able to tell me I had hurt her feelings. I said I knew I had, by going away. She added "Hedde, I don't like you." I was impressed with her ability to stay with me and not run wild, amid feelings so intense that they could be seen chasing over her face like storm clouds. On saying goodbye in the waiting room, Ella wrapped her arms around my body. Her mother told her kindly that after the holiday everything would go back to normal.

The second year of analysis

On her return, Ella brought different concerns, indicating developmental advances. It appeared that the gradual developing of a safe and reliable way of relating, and her mastery of toilet training in this context, had helped her develop a larger degree of structuralization. In this new year the emphasis of our work would be on Oedipal themes, femininity, and family. With this, Ella's thoughts and feelings about the colour of her skin and being lovable and loved were gathered in and worked through on a deeper level. Although her mother was Ella's main Oedipal rival, she was now also able to face her feelings of jealousy towards her sister a little.

Ruby and Daisy

Ella left drawing behind and now often played with soft toys. At the beginning of the autumn term, she told me to get the toys out, adding sharply "Not the brown doll!" As I took up her worry about my having spent my holiday with a "light" baby, and her uncertainty about whether I was happy enough to be back with her, my brown girl, she was infuriated and told me that she was "mixed race" and not brown. She was more enraged when I said that she seemed to feel that there was something bad about brown but that I didn't think that. Ella shouted: "If I see a brown person I will hit him!" and told me "I will hit you!" It has been noted that "Racial difference is probably as powerful a trigger and container for the projection of unacceptable impulses as we have in our culture" (Holmes, 1992, p. 2). Ella, feeling herself to be the bad dark girl in her family, tried desperately to disown all that felt unacceptable to her, especially her aggressive feelings, by finding others, darker or different, that she could project into.

Alongside her increasing Oedipal preoccupations, pre-Oedipal pain continued, and influenced Ella's Oedipal experience, most notably in relation to her mother's role. This situation of different developmental levels (pre-Oedipal and Oedipal) overlapping, illustrates Anna Freud's understanding that progress can vary, with a child advancing more on some developmental lines while struggling to do so on others (A. Freud, 1966d). In this second year of analysis rivalry with her sister Mae over her mother's love could be addressed more directly, with Ella feeling that Mae was more loved as the mother's lighter child. Both themes—rivalry and colour—entered her play, which featured endless competitions between two baby dolls, one brown, which Ella named Ruby and one white that she called Daisy. For months Ruby and Daisy with their competing families and teams were at the centre of Ella's play. She was wrapped up in her family constellation, which included a multitude of Oedipal rivals: her lighter mother, her father's adolescent daughters, and their respective mothers. Although somewhat fazed, Ella was set on becoming "the one" for her daddy.

To win her father and become his favourite, and in an attempt to be mother's better loved light child, Ella continued to forcefully disown the dark part of her mixed ethnicity, which she used as a depository for all she felt undesirable and bad. I spent many weeks in identification with this experience in my role as Ruby as the poor, unattractive, bossy, greedy, and envious girl, whose hopes for better times were sometimes tantalizingly raised, only to be crushed. Experiencing Ruby's unfair treatment, the way she would always lose in races, blunder at every modelling contest, never get any of Daisy's pile of sparkly shiny trinkets, nor the favourite room, or the preferred daddy bear for a father, there were moments in which I, in the countertransference, just felt like giving up. Meanwhile, Ella continued to try to identify with her "white" side which she apparently associated with prettiness, goodness, and lovability. She always played the part of Daisy who, apart from being popular, rich, and pretty, was also terribly nice. Ella ate white chocolate and revealed a fantasy that her skin underneath the surface was white. She thought about Michael Jackson's change of colour and sometimes scratched her own skin to make white marks or to obtain pink skin coloured plasters.

However, by the middle of the autumn term, Ella began to mix up the dolls' names, apparently indicating some change in her ruthlessly clear division between the two dolls' fates and colours. Consciously she now divided her difficulties between the dolls as she explained: "Ruby has a condition: she wants what other children have. Daisy has a condition too: she cannot sit still on the carpet."

Themes of rivalry around a maternal object, doubts about her availability and capacity to love two children at once, issues of darker and lighter children, and specifically Ella and her sister Mae, were now increasingly brought into the transference. Ella briefly changed Daisy's name to Hanna (the name of another, white patient I saw on a three times weekly basis), whom she had seen in the waiting room. As Ella pondered once more about the division of rooms in the doll's house, I spoke about her wondering whether there would be enough room in my heart to really like and love more than one child. A few weeks later, Hanna featured again and this time I talked about Ella's fantasy that Hanna came here too and got more and the better aspects of me. I added that I thought Ella had really started to take so many toys from the waiting room to make sure that Hanna wouldn't get any, nor be the best. Ella told me to shut up and to never speak about it again. To my relief, after weeks of having experienced Ruby's ordeal, Ella now suggested a tying up game later in the same session in which the light dolls and soft toys were passionately tied up and taken to "the place of embarrassment". I spoke about her need for all other and especially lighter children to disappear so that she could feel the best and needn't worry about competition. I also commented on Ruby wanting the light girls to feel how she had felt for so long: embarrassed, sad, and unhappy. When it was time to end, Ella cuddled Ruby, bringing her to her face, then caringly put her into Daisy-Hanna's favourite dolls' bed. Looking back at me, she said, "I bet she had fun today!" I said it had been Ruby's day of revenge. Ella nodded.

In a review meeting that same month, her parents reported that Ella was now feeling better about herself and her mother. She also got on better with Mae, whom she had marvelling at her appearance, indicating developmental advances towards the phallic Oedipal realm.

Femininity and the colours of Oedipus

Ella's impressions about the colour of her skin, which had been such a central depository for pre-Oedipal pain and doubts around her mother's desire and love, also impacted on her Oedipal aspirations. Apart from needing to come to terms with the parental relationship, and her mother's mature female body for which she would have to wait until puberty, Ella needed to find a way to integrate her feelings about her skin tone into all this. Given the fraught insecure pre-Oedipal relationship between Ella and her mother, and their current relationship only just beginning to improve, becoming her mother's Oedipal rival was a daring pursuit to take on.

In her analysis, in an effort to get away from her humiliated feelings about being a child, Ella had Ruby and Daisy be teenagers. She also seemed to hope for revelations about the mature female body and relations between men and women, through my input into Ruby's role. Anything belonging to small children was jeered at and for a while there was a lot of girlfriend–boyfriend material with dancing, undressing, and kissing in corners, which sometimes got Ella rather excited. She continued to work on themes around the colour of her skin, deciding it was "golden". She told me she had many colours inside her, adding "also black!", at which she shot me a sharp glance. Some weeks later she exclaimed in despair: "Hedde, even *you* are light!" In a rush she added that both Mummy and I were "light", and "against" her. She came up and pressed me angrily and insistently: "Do you like mixed race skin? Is there anyone with mixed race skin that you don't like?" I said that I couldn't think of anyone right now but that what she really wanted to know is whether I really liked her, with her mixed race skin. She pressed on, demanding "Which side are you on?" I said that I was on her side, but that she wasn't feeling so sure of it.

Following this exchange about skin colours, love, and loyalty, Ella was freed up to be openly more curious about female bodies and began bringing her own Barbie dolls, as well as a cousin's action heroes. Ruby and Daisy proved very curious girls and peeked as Barbie had a bath. By the end of the spring term, Ella, now seven, had light and dark dolls peek under each other skirts, and when I commented on her curiosity about grown women's bodies and whether they were the same with different colours, Ella rebuffed me saying that she knew everything she needed to know as she had seen Mummy in the bath yesterday. I asked her whether she'd had a good peek and she said "Of course, Hedde." She repeated that she knew all she needed to know as she had seen Daddy naked too and his willy. She said she had seen Mummy getting dressed, and then quickly moved to the back of the dolls' house where she had previously discovered an opening that was otherwise hidden from view. She took a piece of dolls' house furniture and moved it in and out of the opening a few times, before quickly moving back to decorating the dolls' house.

Ella also increasingly brought her Oedipal rivalry, part of her current relationship with her mother, into the transference, as she sang, first quite gently: "Listen to me and not to Hedde pee!" She looked at me and grinned. Then she made her lines for me a little worse and assured me that she didn't mean it and liked me really. She urged me to continue my drawing and sang its praise: "Like you, like a flower, like a rose." I commented that she had gotten a little worried about whether things were still good between her and me, and now wanted to say nice things, having become worried about having told me "too many nasty" things. In response she continued: "Ella is like a flower, like a rose; Hedde is like a rat, stinks of poo, has boobs like rat bags."

A period followed in which she often could be very jeering and denigrating, and the transference turned negative. It is telling that with me having been so identified with Ella's feelings about her disowned and repudiated aspects, which she had linked to darker skin, it took me a while to reach full realization of the role of my actual white skin colour as an object of tension, hatred, envy, and hurt. In the transference, I, with my white skin, seemed to have become like the enviable white Barbie doll and lighter mummy, an idealized, never achieved object (Holmes, 1992) by which Ella felt painfully excluded. It was now possible to take up Ella's hatred for me as big, white, and in charge, especially at the end of sessions when she felt like a "thrown away" little dark girl, thus allowing the analysis, that had come to feel rather stuck, to move on.

In the course of the spring term, I added, at Ella's request, a light and a dark Barbie doll to her toys: the light one after persistent pleas and the dark one with her tentative agreement.

The brown Barbie, whose part I played, initially befell largely the same fate as Ruby. Ella spent weeks dividing favourite items in order of gradations in skin tone, with the palest of dolls getting the best of all. Yet two months later, she named "my" brown doll Emily, her own middle name. Gradually life looked up for Emily; she got a prince, though initially still only with white Barbie in the bin. Yet one day at the start of the summer term, Ella asked me at the beginning of a session whether Emily wanted to be the pretty girl today. Then, when Ella had things suddenly turn difficult again for Emily in her play, I had Emily be sad and concerned, wondering whether this had happened because of her colour. Ella told me that Emily now liked her colour. I answered yes, but it was strange: at times when Emily felt good, she liked her colour but when she felt thrown out and left alone, she didn't. And at those times, she thought that if only she could have a light skin, all her troubles would be gone. I said that they wouldn't, it would be just the same. Ella came to sit very close so that our bodies touched. She allowed me to continue about how people looked different from the outside, the colour of hair, skin, and eyes, but that on the inside all people looked the same and could feel the same things. Ella sat listening quietly and said tentatively "All people have feelings." I said "Yes, people of all colours have the same feelings: happy, excited, sad, angry, and big feelings."

A few weeks later, Ella took Emily from my hand and had her excel in gymnastics. Overcome with happiness, she exclaimed: "See! All that jealousy and it wasn't even necessary! She is just as good!" By claiming "Emily" for herself, Ella seemed to show that she had overcome her persistent good-bad, love-hatred, light-dark cleave. For Ella, with the ability to have mixed feelings, came the possibility to feel loved and loving and at ease with the colour of her skin.

It was agreed that Ella was now ready to reduce her sessions and become more embedded in education and school life, the area where the emphasis of her latency development should be. After the summer she settled well in twice weekly treatment as well as in primary school.

Conclusion

Ella's big problem when she started treatment was her fear of loving relationships in case she should find no one to love her and receive her love, and feel alone and hated. She defended against her fear of desertion and loss by running away and being spiteful, hateful, and aggressive, thus inviting hatred and rejection. In wondering what aspects may have contributed to Ella's painful dilemma, Burlingham's (1967) observations about the young child's profound perceptiveness of his mother's "surface as well as her depth" (p. 774) seem particularly instructive. Burlingham describes how direct observation of his mother's affects towards him allow the child knowledge of what happens in the mother's consciousness, whereas perceptiveness of attempts to deny emotion, defences, and inhibitions, especially indications of repressed impulses on which the mother's character is based, lead the child to conclusions about her unconscious functioning. Drawing conclusions from what he has observed about his mother's feelings towards him, the child bases his actions on this understanding and follows where she leads him, responding to her seduction and seducing her in turn. It may very well be that Ella did understand aspects of her mother's more complicated and mixed feelings towards her, and experienced them very deeply. As frustration increased, she may have responded to possible masochistic elements in the mother by hurting and humiliating her. Ella did have a well developed capacity of knowing exactly what would hurt someone most deeply. In the case of her mother, one important aspect seemed connected with exposing her mother and spoiling an ideal external presentation, thus also drawing attention to what was not good and painful underneath. Ella's struggle appeared so very centred on her relationship with her mother that, interestingly, the birth and existence of her younger sister did not seem to have a major part in the development of her difficulties.

Finally, I would also like to mention Anna Freud's (1966d) understanding that if a child's relationships have, in reality or imagination, not managed to result in a balance in which love can control hatred, aggression becomes destructive (Edgcumbe, 2000). Despair and fury at not being able to feel secure in her mother's love may have contributed to an impaired amalgamation of libido and aggression in Ella (Mahler, 1972b). In order to try to protect the loved mother from her growing destructive omnipotent rage, Ella seems to have split the object world into good and bad, taking the bad all upon her darker self to protect her lighter mother (Fairbairn, 1943). It is important also to note that Ella seemed to have a constitutional vulnerability from her father's side, in whose family ADHD-like symptoms were common. A propensity to an excess of aggressive impulses may have contributed to the problem by frightening and intimidating Ella's mother, causing loving impulses to be easily outbalanced. Anna Freud (1949a) felt that for overly aggressive children the appropriate therapy should be directed at the "defective" side, that is the emotional libidinal. Where there is severe early deprivation in object relationships, the close, intimate relationship with the therapist, and the libidinal attachment that comes with this, may help the child move to higher and more appropriate levels of libidinal object relationships within the setting of child analysis. This movement could be followed in the work with Ella as she worked through aspects of complex object relational experiences of the oral, anal, and Oedipal stage before arriving at the latency level. What also could be observed in Ella's analysis was Anna Freud's (1965) notion that children have a hunger for *new* experience, which is as strong as the urge to repeat. She believed that the therapist is only used as a transference object to repeat disturbed areas of development and otherwise functions as a new object to the child. Anna Freud dedicated a lot of thinking to the use of transference in child analysis. Contrary to what is sometimes understood, she believed that there usually *is* significant transference involvement in child analysis (1965, 1980) and noted that children, like adults, repeat through regression, and enact around the analyst their object relations from all levels of development. Distinguishing between the concepts of "transference involvement" and "transference neurosis" (1980), she doubted the possibility of a full transference neurosis in child analysis as the objects are present day objects (even in matters of the child's past) and not the past or fantasy objects of the adult transference neurosis. She noted that in child analysis the "interpreting object" is also a new and developmental object, and that distinguishing and carefully moving between the two roles are essential elements of child analytic technique. In the work with Ella, I negotiated these two roles and the correspondingly different types of interventions.

In ending, a last aspect that I would like to mention is the way play was used in Ella's analysis. There were times in which Ella's play was, in the original classical way, used as an opportunity for interpretation of unconscious conflict. In the Anna Freudian tradition, a child's play has increasingly been understood as intrinsic to her growth, as her own way of discovery; a metaphor expressing realization of the potential within herself and her relationships to others and hence more meaningful to her than the adult metaphor of interpretation (Hurry, 1998).

In my work with Ella, it was important for me to know when to just *be* with her as she worked on self discovery and attempted mastery of her impulses in the service of onward development. Sometimes she was so scared that my words would make her frighteningly lose control that I needed to be quiet for extended periods of time. Very often it was only after a good period of playing or drawing together, that Ella could bear to hear and make use of interpretation, which then would often provide relief, helping Ella to move on. This is in line with Anne Hurry's understanding that "effective interpretation often begins by offering hope in the context of the developmental relationship between patient and analyst" (1998, p. 73), and demonstrates the interwoven nature of interpretative and developmental work in the child analytic process.

References

Bick, E. (1968). The experience of skin in early object relationships. *International Journal of Psychoanalysis, 49*: 484–486.

Burlingham, D. (1967). Empathy between infant and mother. *Journal of the American Psychoanalytic Association, 15*: 764–780.

Edgcumbe, R. (2000). *Anna Freud: a view of development, disturbance and therapeutic technique*. London: Routledge.

Fairbairn, W. R. D. (1943). The repression and the return of bad objects (with special reference to the "war neuroses"). In: W. R. D. Fairbairn, *Psychoanalytic Studies of the Personality* (pp. 59–81). London: Tavistock, 1952.

Freud, A. (1949). Aggression in relation to emotional development: normal and pathological. *Psychoanalytic Study of the Child, 3*(4): 37–42.

Freud, A. (1965). *Normality and Pathology in Childhood. Assessments of development*. London: Karnac.

Freud, A. (1972). Comments on aggression. *International Journal of Psychoanalysis, 53*: 163–171.

Freud, A. & Burlingham, D. (1944). "Reports on the Hampstead Nurseries". In: *Infants without Families and Reports on the Hampstead Nurseries 1939–1945*. London: Hogarth, 1974.

Green, V. (1998). "Donald": the treatment of a 5-year-old boy with experience of early loss. In: A. Hurry (Ed.), *Psychoanalysis and Developmental Therapy*. London: The Anna Freud Centre & the Psychoanalytic Unit at University College London.

Holmes, D. E. (1992). Race and transference in psychoanalysis and psychotherapy. *International Journal of Psychoanalysis, 73*: 1–11.

Hurry, A. (1998). *Psychoanalysis and Developmental Therapy*. London: The Anna Freud Centre & the Psychoanalytic Unit at University College London. Isaacs, S. (1934). Rebellious and defiant children. In: *Childhood and After* (pp. 25–35). London: Routledge & Kegan Paul.

Mahler, M. S. (1972a). On the first three subphases of the separation-individuation process. *International Journal of Psychoanalysis, 53*: 333–338.

Mahler. M. S. (1972b). Rapprochement subphase of the separation-individuation process. *Psychoanaytic Quarterly, 41*: 487–506.

Posner, B. M., Glickman, R. W., Taylor, E. C., Canfield, J. & Cyr, F. (2001). In search of Winnicott's aggression. *Psychoanalytic Study of the Child, 56*: 171–190.

Sandler, J., Kennedy, H. & Tyson, R. L. (1980). *The Technique of Child Psychoanalysis, Discussions with Anna Freud*. Cambridge, MA: Harvard University Press.

Symington, J. (1985). The survival function of primitive omnipotence. *International Journal of Psychoanalysis*, *66*: 481–487.

Winnicott, D. W. (1965). The maturational process and the facilitating environment: studies in the theory of emotional development. *The International Psychoanalytic Library*, *64*: 1–276. London: Hogarth & the Institute of Psychoanalysis.

Winnicott, D. W. (1968). The use of an object and relating through identifications. In: C. Winnicott, R. Shepherd & M. Davis (Eds.), *Psychoanalytic Explorations*. Cambridge, MA: Harvard University Press, 1989.

Winnicott, D. W. (1969). The use of an object. *International Journal of Psychoanalysis*, *50*: 711–716.

Yorke, C., Wiseberg, S. & Freeman, T. (1989). *Development and Psychopathology: Studies in Psychoanalytic Psychiatry*. New Haven, CT: Yale University Press.

CHAPTER FOURTEEN

"A long journey from catastrophe to safety"—the analysis of a violent boy

Federica Melandri

Introduction

This paper is an account of my therapeutic relationship with Ray, a young boy who used violence to communicate and to relate to others. It traces Ray's struggle to establish trust and begin to internalize "benevolent enough" objects, strengthen his ego, and develop a capacity to symbolize.

Referral

Ray was four and a half when his mother, Ms K, referred him to the Anna Freud Centre on the recommendation of his nursery school, who were so concerned about Ray's behaviour they asked his mother to remove him from the nursery until she had come to see us. However, this arrangement soon broke down and Ray was permanently expelled from nursery, as his disruptive behaviour and violence towards children and staff had escalated. The staff felt unable to handle him as he lashed out, pushing, scratching, kicking, and biting children and teachers alike. Often his attacks seemed unprovoked and inexplicable.

In the nursery Ray would also become very frustrated and aggressive when attention was given to another child, sometimes asking to be cuddled and hugged by the teacher. During the same period he was thrown out from a Saturday morning drama class for kicking a teacher and his mother was told not to bring him back.

Ms K was also concerned that at home he became disruptive if a visitor came and would not let them speak. Outings with him were very difficult too. On one occasion Ray threw a ruler with force across a shop when mother was talking to a male shop assistant. On another occasion, when visiting a market and his mother tried to persuade him to buy something he did not like, he threw things from the stalls to the ground and then ran away brushing objects from their shelves as he ran.

Ms K described Ray as a precociously bright little boy, who until then had not been in any trouble but had only been loving and affectionate. She claimed that he had friends and was immensely popular at nursery. At home, as long as nobody else was there, he would amuse himself with digital clocks and calculators. She was puzzled about this sudden change which, in her opinion, coincided with several changes of teachers and their move to a new home.

Only later in the treatment did we hear of Ray's occasional soiling and regular bed-wetting.

Background information

Ms K has several siblings, all of whom live in London although originally from a foreign country. Her relationship with her older sister has always been difficult as, according to Ms K, her sister is "narcissistic" and prey to violent anger. Ms K's own mother is also described as having similar characteristics and contact between them is now rare. Ms K works from home, running her own business.

Little is known about the father's history and background. Ms K reported that they met and became friends at university. They went out together a few times, until he went to the US for further study and work experience. He returned about ten years later, proposing that they had a more serious relationship, and soon after Ms K became pregnant with Ray. As soon as he heard of the pregnancy he broke off the relationship and for a while there was no further contact between them. Nevertheless, Ms K reported that the pregnancy was enjoyable and the birth easy and unproblematic. Ray was breastfed for a few months and everything seemed fine. Only later in the treatment did we hear from her about Ray's violent rocking and head-banging as an infant and of her own social isolation, lack of family support, and possible unrecognized depression.

When Ray was born Ms K was persuaded by a family member to make contact with the father's family, as Ray had the special status of being the first-born son of the first-born son. The paternal grandparents in turn persuaded the father to become more involved and he re-established contact. Ray and mother spent some time with him in the US and he would visit them in London occasionally. He stopped paying maintenance when Ray was three years old and mother took him to court. Court proceedings continued throughout the years of Ray's analysis. The last time Ray saw his father was a few months into his treatment, when he came to London for a short and very disappointing visit. Some contact was maintained with the paternal grandparents who came occasionally for short, unplanned, and unsatisfactory visits from their country of origin, which left both Ray and his mother angry and confused.

The first year

Starting analysis

Ray started his four times a week analytic treatment on his fifth birthday. He was a big boy with a charming and contagious smile, who immediately involved me in his lively imaginative play, containing many of the themes that, as the treatment unfolded, I came to understand to be at the core of his difficulties.

The conflictual mother-child relationship, and her inability to respond to his affective experience in a sensitive way were played out in a scene where Oscar (a soft toy seal) got pushed away and shouted at when asking to play. Yells to "cheer up" were thrown at him after being threatened with "I'll smack you!" I was to observe mother's incongruous affective response to Ray's feelings many times throughout his treatment.

The sense of this mother and child's enmeshment, and their need for a third to come and rescue them was also played out in the very first session. After several scenes in which mother and child were stuck under a cushion and nobody could help free them, Ray noticed and got excited by three cushion strings spread on the couch that looked to him like the number three. Only then were the mother and child couple freed in the play. Indeed, the arrangement of seeing mother once weekly alongside Ray's intensive treatment somehow put me in the role of third for Ray and his mother.

In the first weeks of his analysis, together with his playful, engaging, and imaginative play I was struck by the compulsive quality of his pedantically counting the steps to and from the treatment room, and by the defensive quality of some of his games.

Ray's capacity to engage with his object was, I felt, permanently threatened by an inability to modulate his loving and hating impulses, and to regulate his affects. His maladaptive attempts to control them by means of rigid defensive manoeuvres was translated in the therapy into repetitive and controlling play. When these defences failed he would resort to violence.

Although I did not experience the powerfulness of his full-blown aggression until the weeks preceding our first Christmas break, I had a taste of it in our fourth session when Ray began to find it difficult to leave the room at the end of the session. His disappointment, rage, and anxiety about ending turned quickly into manic, excited shouting and clowning, and when his attempts to seduce me did not lead to the hoped- for extra time, he quickly turned to retaliatory attacks.

His very low self-esteem and lack of object constancy made it extremely difficult for him to hold on to the belief that we could survive separation and be reunited the following day. At the end of each session he would regularly scream: "Help, help! I'm falling" while holding precariously and dangerously to the banister on the stairs.

Occasionally he would add that he was falling down the toilet, conveying his fears of being left because of his poor value. Ray presented as an anal child at the mercy of his inability to control his body and his impulses, especially at times of heightened anxiety. He was constipated and on laxatives for a long period of time.

Omnipotence and helplessness

Ray would adopt an omnipotent stance and order me around, trying to ward off his feelings of being out-of-control and helpless. I noted:

> Following a session in which he soiled himself and wanted me to clean him up, he brought Action Man to his session, and declared that it never got hurt. He threw it around and then

decided to wash the floor of the room because "Action Man was sitting on the dirt". In the same session I informed him that we were going to have a break at Christmas. He did not seem to respond to this information until the following day when his anger exploded. When I did not comply with one of his wishes he unexpectedly and violently shouted at me: "Go away stinky girl/boy." He looked transformed, shouting wildly at me from the top of the stairs: "Go away, I hate you!".

I was shocked and shaken by the power of his rage but managed to remind him that we should not get hurt. However, as a punishment, he violently pushed me into "a cage with the tiger" and tried to bite my hand. He then just licked it and pretended to eat it declaring that it was good. Feeling his terror, I playfully enacted a panic scene in which, now that I did not have my hand, I did not know how to fix the book that he had previously broken, and that we were in the process of repairing just prior to his anger exploding. I told him that I needed his help to do so and Ray accepted this. While going back up to the therapy room he switched off all the lights and cried with deeply felt sadness that he was "blind and lived in the dark" and could not see any more. I spoke of the anger that blinded him and his fear that his rage and aggression would drive all of his friends away including me. In recognition he hugged me at the end of the session, and repeated this scene several times in the following week. Games of hide and seek followed as well as attempts to control my comings and goings by elaborate games, which we referred to as "controlling machines". Ray used different baby toys which he found in the waiting room. These had big buttons to press and he would use them while going up the stairs to our therapy room on the top floor. As he pressed the buttons he would shout "Stop!" or "Go!" to me. Usually it would take a long while to reach the room.

In the last session before our first Christmas break I found Ray sitting on the stairs playing with a calculator. Pretending that it was a digital clock he was pressing the numbers 4.05, 4.06 … (the starting time of our session) desperately trying to be in control of our time together before we parted. He mentioned Daddy while pretending to make phone calls in a disorganized sort of way and then "collapsed" on the floor. I took up in the transference his feelings of sadness for the imminent break and his fear that I, like his daddy, would not return.

The wish for the father

In the weeks preceding our first Christmas break Ms K told Ray that his father would come and visit during the holidays. In the treatment we spent several sessions waiting for the electrician (which at times Ray would call the magician) to come and fix the light in our room. His wish for a powerful paternal figure, who would come and fix things, was so vivid and blurred with reality that at the end of the sessions Ray would look sad and disappointed about the electrician not having shown up, and I could verbalize for him how hard it was to be waiting for someone so special and not knowing whether and when he would arrive.

As noted, the father's visit was short and very disappointing, taking place soon after the Christmas break. Ray had great expectations and planned to try hard and control his temper, telling his mother that they should not get upset with Daddy. However, the father stayed only half a day and then fell asleep when Ray wanted to play toy trains with him. Ray went into a rage, hit him, and threw the trains at him. Later in the day while accompanying him to the airport Ray would not talk to his father and refused to kiss him goodbye.

In the therapy sessions that followed there was no direct mention of the father's visit, only a maladaptive attempt to control events through repetitive playing with trains, naming and counting them. This was followed by all sorts of catastrophic events, which left us feeling helpless. Again Ray made use of his magical thinking to get us out of trouble and made a phone call to the magician who was asked to come and fix things while Oscar (his soft toy seal) was cast in the role of the naughty boy with whom Ray refused to play. By the end of the week he told me he felt terrible but when I tried to link his feelings with the father's last visit he lashed out and hit me.

> The following week when Ray spoke of the animals waiting and waiting I could link this with his long wait for Daddy. He shouted that he did not have a Daddy, he "only had a Mummy", but later, he told me a bit more about his Daddy who went away travelling. Only in displacement could I address his feelings of hurt and abandonment and provide some containment for them. He let me take care of his soft animals "all hurt and bleeding" and put sellotape bandages around their hurting paws. We took them to the doctor who spoke warmly of their need for care and love and looking after. Ray asked me to repeat the doctor scene again and again—"What did the doctor say?"—as if he could not really take in my words.

Any direct link to, or interpretation of the reality of his loss were felt by him as an attack to which he would respond with aggression. I had to choose my words and what to address very carefully. He often experienced interpretations as an assault on his fragile sense of self and he would defend against them with all his might.

Phallic moves

Ray was a regular bed wetter. Often in his first months of analysis he wanted to play night scenes in which he would go to bed, be scared, and come to my bed, curling into my lap, enjoying the intimacy of the contact. He would refer to floods, bad dreams of sharks that would eat him up, especially following incidents in which he had been aggressive towards me. He would also often play by the sink and make a mess on the floor. Alternatively we could spend entire sessions on endless journeys on trains. Ray would make train noises, and open the door at regular intervals to announce which underground station we had reached and which line we could change to. His knowledge of the London Underground system was remarkable. He could either be a very effective and knowledgeable train controller or a messy, violent, and out of control baby.

> Five months into his analysis we were playing a night scene. Ray had wet the bed and put the bed sheets (the bedspread which covered the couch in our room) in the washing machine and we were waiting for them to be washed and dried. He said that the drier would take twenty minutes and he counted the minutes by pressing the phone buttons twenty times. He then threw the phone away in anger declaring that it was broken. He pushed away all my attempts to attach meaning to this communication, and left the room, running into another child patient

> who was all wrapped up in an identical bedspread. After his initial puzzlement he returned to the room where he wanted to do the same. He wrapped himself in the bedspread and began to jump on the couch, waving his arms about and becoming very excited at the prospect that he could fly. With his eyes shining with delight he jumped and jumped shouting "I can fly!" He wanted to go around the clinic to be admired by everyone but contented himself with his mother's admiration, mine, and that of his soft toy animals. Indeed, we spent a few sessions admiring Ray's beautiful wings and newly acquired ability to fly high. His sense of pride, pleasure, and joy in this simple game was quite astonishing and made me wonder about the profound lack of normal parental pleasure Ray may have experienced from his primary carer.
>
> The emotional unavailability of his mother was immediately played out when, tired of jumping, he wanted to rest: he became the Mummy, while I was cast in the role of the little boy. I had to ask Mummy to play with me, and Ray, now pretending to be the Mummy typing on the computer, would say no, she had to work. She (he) threatened to put me outside the house as I protested that it was no fun to be playing alone. Then at bedtime a fire came and made a mess of the room and of Ray's beautiful wings. Catastrophic events such as bombs and earthquakes followed, from which we had to flee.

Ray missed the following week for his mother was ill and could not bring him to his sessions. When he returned he was enraged that my magic wand had not "magicked" him back, and after repeating the flying game, made a mess of the room, throwing furniture in a pile and becoming violently excited and out of control. The week was marked by wild behaviour, and my efforts to contain him intensified his terror that I, like his father, would abandon him, or, like his mother, I would stop caring for him. I felt terror and despair.

The monster and the boy

On the last session of this stormy week Ray was for the first time able to represent in play the predicament he was trapped in:

> He came upstairs for his session and started playing by the sink. The water was coming and a man could not get out as his foot was stuck. The story became mixed up with another convoluted one and I could hear Ray whisper to himself: "I will be good today, not like yesterday." He then picked up the nailbrush and the towel holder and made a show for me. The show lasted the whole session. Ray was engrossed and kept my interest alive by maintaining eye contact throughout his narration.

The nailbrush became a little boy and the towel holder a monster. The monster was trying to get the boy and eat him up. There were big chases and fights all over the room. The boy would try to call the police but would get stuck in the wire. The boy would get inside the cupboard and the monster stuck in the door. The monster would chase and the boy would run. At one point the monster changed his mind, he became good and the boy became naughty. He changed his mind again and the monster turned very mean and the boy was good. The story became more and more dramatic with loud terrified screams from the boy, which now on top of the cabinet was fighting the monster and everybody could hear his screams "all over England, all over London, and all over New York!" The story ended in the sink where both monster and boy died, and this was the end of the show.

Although Ray was beginning to be able to symbolize the terrifying shifts in his sense of identity as a "monster/boy" he was still unable to control himself. As the second break approached at Easter his aggression and out-of-control behaviour escalated. Among violent attacks on me, Ray would repeat the monster and the boy show again and again with loud metallic bangs from the monstrous towel holder and loud terrified screams from the nailbrush boy.

On our penultimate session before the break and at the height of his anxiety Ray soiled himself and quickly turned into a train, which would keep me waiting on the platform for long stretches of time.

> One day, soon after the Easter break, Ray arrived twenty minutes late for his session and was enraged. He shouted: "Go away!" as I approached him in the waiting room. When I wondered about the reason for his anger he shouted that he came from New York and continued "Go away, go to Camden!" (the borough he lived in). As I puzzled over his need to push me away after such a long journey from New York, Ray stopped to ponder over this but then became contemptuous and aggressive pushing me away again. From the top of the stairs he declared defiantly that he was on the plane where I could never catch him. "Go away, go to Camden!" He spat down on me, laughing manically as I verbalized my confusion and disappointment. He ran to the therapy room and barricaded himself in by putting all the furniture against the door. As I forced my way in, I playfully expressed my surprise at finding a stranger in my room. He told me that he was stealing, but then, a bit scared of my pretend anger he said: "I am Ray don't you see? This is my face, my tummy and my sticker."
>
> Having regained some sense of reality he accepted my link to his father's past visit and his disappointment and sense of rejection. He showed me a map he was carrying to which he now wanted to add my house. He told me that Dad didn't know where they lived as he had travelled away and that they had to find a new daddy. Before ending the session he wanted me to keep a tiny piece of paper on which he drew the map of his house and accepted my interpretation of his wish that unlike his daddy I would know where Ray was. I was struck on this occasion by Ray's identification with his abandoning father and his projection of the painful feelings of rejection onto me.

Ray's third break in therapy was approaching soon, as he and mother were going abroad. In the last two sessions before the break Ray cried inconsolably, expressing for the first time his overwhelming sadness at the prospect of parting from me. Moving from uncontained anxiety to tears, it seemed that Ray was beginning to learn to say goodbye.

On this occasion it was striking to notice how difficult his mother found it to acknowledge and accept Ray's expression of feelings. "What's in your eyes? Stop being silly …" she kept on saying about his tears. It was noticeable in my weekly meetings with Ms K how her strongly organized defences against painful affects were impeding her capacity to recognize and respond empathically to Ray's feelings of distress.

When Ray returned from the holiday he had been in treatment for eight months and appeared more contained and more able to communicate his conflicts and his affects through displacement or symbolization. He made up a story of a broken cuckoo that needed fixing. But like Ray, it felt damaged beyond reparation and could not be mended. "Nothing in this world could fix it," he announced in despair. But later in the session when an ant appeared, Ray reassured me that it was not a red "bitey" one but a black friendly one. We would have moments of togetherness in which we would do the alphabet, as Ray began to bring some of his schoolwork to the sessions, having started attending primary school. There were still stormy times but the intensity seemed to have lessened and Ray began to behave more like a little boy than a monster.

The second year

Catastrophic events and the return of the monster: "Did I kill my father?"

Ms K and Ray returned from their summer holiday in New York on September 10, 2001. There had been no conscious attempt to make contact with the father who lived there, but one could speculate that mother's choice of location was driven by a powerful unconscious wish to find him or be found by him. Characteristically, she did not make the link for herself or Ray.

Ray returned to the clinic smiling broadly and proudly showed me his new T-shirt with the New York skyline printed on it. He also had a present for me, a New York baseball cap, which he wanted me to wear. The following day New York was attacked. Mother was so shocked and shaken that she could not leave the house nor bring Ray to his sessions for three days, leaving me feeling quite worried for them.

Following this event and also prompted by a change of teacher at primary school, Ray's behaviour in school, at home, and in the therapy deteriorated dramatically. He trashed his classroom, the head teacher's office, his bedroom, and the therapy room. He attacked the teachers, mother, and me. His anxiety and aggression were uncontainable and the school felt at a loss about how to understand and help this child. I had to network closely with the school to provide them with some understanding and containment and they welcomed this.

Ray's preoccupation with the Twin Towers tragedy was evident in the sessions with me where his attempts to represent the disaster in play seemed just to escalate his anxiety and aggression. Alternatively he would resort to the mindless train game where he could bounce on the couch for the length of the session making train sounds that would send him and me into a trance-like state—I had to hold on tightly to my mind to retain my capacity to think.

This went on for nearly two months. A very dramatic session with mother and child seemed to provide a turning point. In this session Ray became enraged with me for not allowing him to play a game which I thought was dangerous. After attacking me, he ran down to the waiting room where he attacked his mother, who reacted first with indifference and then with fury. I could witness their sado-masochistic exchange and feel the extent of Ray's despair. He looked like a wild animal trying to escape from life-threatening danger but having no safe place to run to. His sobbing was difficult to bear. Mother could not provide any form of containment for his primordial panic. As he attacked her she did not attempt to stop him but would look at him with contempt and scornfully ask me, "Do you think he is normal?" I felt I had to be quite firm to stop this and address their mutual feelings of despair and anger. They left the clinic calmly at the end of the session holding hands.

The following day Ray came to the room eagerly wanting to repair a picture he had broken. He then organized a dinner party. He set the table most creatively and prepared delicious dishes. He then went down to the waiting room and invited his mother to join us. He was very much in touch with his wish to make reparation and show his gratitude for the good therapy food. He had also a touch of humour when he said: "Mind the pepper because it's hot," and pretended to accidentally drop too much in my plate.

> A few weeks later I arrived late for one of his sessions. The receptionist told Ray that I was stuck in traffic, and when I arrived I found him in the waiting room playing calmly with a toy dashboard pretending to drive. He looked calm but I could feel his anxiety about my being late once we reached the treatment room. He was at a loss as to what to play with. After a while he asked me if he could "make" New York. He lay a blue towel on the floor as "the ocean" and put some pieces of train track next to it. He looked at me with uncertainty. "Let's pretend that these are the World Trade Center," he said, putting down two wooden blocks. We needed trains and cars to make the traffic. I said that very terrible things had happened in New York, as he began to move the trains, leaving the cars to me. He switched the light off and the room went dark. It happened to be November the 5th, Guy Fawkes Night, and there were loud bangs from fireworks outside the building. In addition, the continuous obsessive bleeping of the toy dashboard contributed quite a dramatic atmosphere. We heard the sound of a plane flying over. Ray asked me somewhat anxiously if it was going to crash.
>
> He took the cushions that had some long strings dangling down and shook them, declaring that it was raining in New York. He shook them more forcefully over me and I said that it was a storm and felt very scary. Several times he held up a yellow plate, "the sun" and a blue plate, "the moon". This alternated with big clouds and storms passing over New York. Suddenly, he took a toy plane and crashed it over New York and then he threw all the chairs and tables over it. We stood in the semi-darkness looking silently at New York in ruins before us. I said words about the sadness of it all, adding that, although I could not do anything to save New York, I wanted to help Ray feel better. Ray volunteered to help me tidy up the room and then we walked downstairs in the darkness together, as he switched all the lights off.

The New York event provided a context to represent Ray's catastrophic anxieties and fear of annihilation, echoing his terror that his omnipotent anger would bring destruction beyond reparation. His panic that his anger had killed his father in the most violent way intensified before holiday breaks, when there would be some reference to New York.

A new narrative

Having been able to represent this catastrophic scenario safely seemed to free Ray from some of his panic, allowing him to relate to me in a very different way and express some of his worries. My weekly notes at this time read:

> This has been an important and productive week in Ray's therapy. I feel that Ray is actively engaged in the therapeutic process and that the quality of his relating to me has shifted

> dramatically. We have been engaged in meaningful dialogues most of the time and Ray has produced little stories accompanied by colourful drawings that vividly illustrate some of his conflicts and fears. He has also been able to listen to some of the stories I produced to illustrate my understanding of his difficulties and provide some solution to his conflicts. Ray's progress had been confirmed in a network meeting held in his school. The teacher outlined an improvement in Ray's behaviour and an increasing ability to tolerate frustration and delay gratification. The school had been alerted to Ray's psychological difficulties and great anxiety. They implemented a series of rewarding strategies by which Ray obtains a sticker whenever he is able to comply with the school requests (sitting still, listening without disturbing, etc.). He has joined a little group of children that receive individual attention and has responded positively to it. He has not displayed any of his aggressive outbursts in the past few weeks and his behaviour has generally improved. Some concerns remain: he is sometimes overwhelmed with joy and excitement when rewarded and has a tendency to go and hug other children. Being large for his age he has involuntarily hurt them. However, on one occasion he showed some concern by bringing the child to the teacher and explaining that it was an accident. This seems to confirm that Ray is also gaining some understanding of social situations. His academic abilities are still under average.

During this period Ray introduced me to the Mr Men characters which provided a route to talk about different feelings, conflicts, and difficulties. Mr Grumpy and Little Miss Helpful were our main characters. The stories Ray told were strikingly lacking the presence of a benign and concerned object, which could provide if not resolution, at least some relief. His stories always had dramatic and terrifying endings.

Although at this stage in his therapy he was starting to relate to me as a "new developmental object" (Hurry, 1998), his fantasies were still coloured by powerful and archaic anxieties. However, as the second Christmas break approached, Ray drew a shop with all sorts of goods in it and aisles "for people not to get lost".

The following year and a half of analysis was a roller coaster. Progress was fragile and often short-lived. Holding on to the good therapist in his mind proved difficult for Ray. Whenever something threatened his omnipotence I could suddenly turn into a bad object, which he would attack mercilessly, having lost sight of any good bits of me. Painful affects felt especially catastrophic and annihilating and had to be defended against with all means. He would shout "You are saying sad things again!", or "You are making me mad!", before attacking me, if I dared make an interpretation at the wrong time. His magical thinking was deeply rooted in mother's mystical vision of the world, proving a powerful obstacle to my attempts to help him move to a more realistic sense of himself and others. He experienced a mistake in his work as a narcissistic blow and would fall apart in front of my very eyes. The speed of his regression was such that I felt that I was working with a borderline child and that part of my work was to help him build up more adaptive defences and support his ego to help him achieve a more grounded sense of reality and of himself (see Alvarez, 1992).

Alternatively, we could get stuck in obsessional activities, which would keep us mindless and safe. Ray's interest in the Underground system transformed from pretending to be a train or a train controller into drawing the Underground map. He (and I) drew maps of the London tube system endlessly. Locating the stops and knowing where the "meeting points" were was immensely important to Ray. Indeed, at times it felt that it was the only way to provide him with some sense of safety and control. Slowly, I was able to help Ray move, for instance from reproducing the tube map rigidly in every painstaking detail, to being able to draw fantasy maps where we could make up fanciful names of imaginary lines and stations.

Thus firmly held in his analysis, Ray made steady progress in school and began making friends. Parent work proved essential in helping his mother acquire some understanding of a child's normal needs. As a single mother who worked from home, she herself had a restricted social life, and struggled to provide her son with a normal range of appropriate social experiences. They would often spend weekends and holidays alone, sometimes at home in total isolation for days. Ray watched TV or played his repetitive games while his mother worked on her computer. Several times Ray expressed the belief that the Anna Freud Centre was a place where children came to play when they did not have anyone else to play with.

Ray's hunger for emotional nourishment was clearly expressed in the sessions where oral themes dominated. We often had feasts and banquets, dinner parties with all sort of goodies—a different food for every day of the week. He would start each analytic session devouring the biscuits and gulping down the drink provided by the receptionist in the waiting room. Overcloseness and enmeshment in this mother and child couple seemed to cover up and compensate for their emotional deprivation and social isolation.

Two and a half years into her weekly work with me mother had an important dream. She had just told me about spending the weekend at home because she had to work, and how Ray played by himself making a city and watching television. She thanked him for being so understanding. As I talked about how difficult it was for Ray, and how badly he tried to convince himself that he liked playing alone, she recalled a dream in which she is looking at a woman who is in a room with bars. She can see Ray in an adjacent room lying on a bed. He tells her: "I am alright, Mum," but she feels strongly that it is *not* all right. "He doesn't know, he cannot know! But she [the woman] has to know and do something about it. She is his mother." She woke up feeling very sad.

> The same day I felt deeply disturbed by Ray's state of mind in his session. He made us write identical lists of letters and then we paused. After a while I asked what the game was about. He laughed in a way that chilled me, "Nothing, it's a game of nothing, it's called nothing," he said. I wondered out loud what we were not playing when we were playing nothing. Ray violently shouted at me: "Fussy!". Feeling that he was falling apart I felt his terror. It followed a game of hang-man where his first word was "United States". Later he drew a picture with three characters, which he called funny, dumb, and angry. I introduced sad, which he immediately equated with: "Mad, crying baby wha wha," scribbling tears excitedly all over the page and the table before throwing it away, exclaiming with anger and contempt "Stupid!".

In the absence of an object that could help him make sense and "digest" his internal experience and provide what Bion (1967) called "alpha function", Ray's internal experience seemed to turn persecuting and maddening, and he needed to push his terror violently into others. The only way to feel safe seemed to be to turn numb, and empty the mind of all contempt and desire. This appeared to be the function of the "nothing game".

Ending analysis

Ray's analysis ended prematurely due to my becoming pregnant and later taking maternity leave for about a year. He reacted with disbelief at the news first: "Is this April's fool?", and then with anxiety. Instructing me on how to get to Harrods to get a nice toy for the baby he began to quiz me compulsively about train interchanges. His preoccupation with my baby (which toys and food to buy) and his resorting to the old "train game" seemed to serve the purpose of containing both his anxiety and his aggression towards the baby and me. However, Ray was also able to express some of his feelings playfully and appropriately when he pretended that we were going to the funeral of Oscar's (his soft toy seal) granddad. After a long train journey we arrived at the grave where Ray gave a long and articulated mournful speech thanking the granddad for the help he received and expressing his grief for the loss. With deep-felt sadness we then proceeded to the burial and while doing that I reminded Ray that we could always remember the time together and keep it in our hearts.

Coming back: Ray today

Ray is now a big boy who has just turned ten. I have been seeing him in once weekly psychotherapy for about a year, after a long break in his therapy. Ray is settled in school and is now in year five. He is popular, plays sports, and has been taken off the "watch list" for children in trouble. Some concern remains, as he seems sometimes to be lost in his own world and is easily distracted. Ray comes willingly to his sessions and on several occasions has asked whether he can carry on coming until he is fifteen or eighteen, somehow sensing that adolescence may be a difficult time for him. He has never been violent again but he clearly remembers that he had been, and has been able to talk about those times with some humour and appropriate distance. He has also expressed some concern about losing control, but he can now be articulate, using words instead of actions. One of his favourite topics and games is "transport for London". He knows now that he uses this game defensively and recently said "Let's play something trainy, brainy, and un-painy."

Ray is often preoccupied with catastrophic events, earthquakes, tsunami, wars, and the like. In his accounts, real events mix with fantasy in the construction of the most terrifying scenarios. He identifies with his mother's mystical and fatalistic view of the universe, although at times he seems to think of it as "a bit mad".

On the eve of his tenth birthday he asked me how long he had been coming to therapy. When he worked out that he was five when he first came, he remembered that he was very angry then. He told me that he had two reasons. The first one was that his father left him, didn't care or love him and the second one he will never tell. It has to do with God and still makes him cry at night.

Conclusion

I have always been struck by Ms K's account of Ray as a little boy. When his mother was working he would entertain himself by matching the time on the clock with his blocks and could do this for hours, or he would look down from the window to the nearby station for the trains passing by. This vignette seemed to graphically capture his mother's emotional absence and Ray's attempts to regulate his emotional states by tuning in to the only moving objects around him, such as the ticking clock and the passing trains.

This image corresponds to Schore's description of a relational growth-inhibiting early environment by contrast to a growth-facilitating scenario.

> This caregiver is inaccessible and reacts to the infant's expression of emotions and stress inappropriately and/or rejectingly and therefore shows minimal or unpredictable participation in the various types of arousal regulating processes. Instead of modulating she induces extreme levels of stimulation and arousal, very high in abuse and very low in neglect. And because she provides no interactive repair the infant's intense negative states last for long periods of time (2001, p. 205).

Ray's play and preoccupation with clocks and trains stemmed from an attempt to regulate his intense feelings of anxiety. It was striking to observe how quickly he was able to shift to his regulating "device" when his sense of self felt threatened. When he was not able to do so, he seemed to lose his grip on reality, as anxiety escalated to the point that only left attack as an option.

Working with violent patients has been described as walking on a "tightrope" where fear, danger, and safety are central issues, for both patient and therapist. As psychoanalysts Parsons and Dermen suggest, "The violent child desperately attempts and fails to find some sense of safety and stability. Being unable to process and contain his anxieties, he cannot think, only act" (1999, p. 337). The therapist has to continue to think and to process what is happening in the room in a way the child cannot. By addressing "his bodily enactments as concrete expression of his emotional states, the therapist can provide one of the functions of the protective shield" (Parsons & Dermen, 1999, p. 337). This helps the child begin to process his internal experience.

In this analysis I had to learn to respect Ray's need to use his magical devices to provide himself with the sense of safety that my interpretations could not always offer. On the contrary, interpretations often seemed to expose the vulnerability that he so desperately tried to defend himself from experiencing.

It has been a long journey together but Ray now trusts me and, more importantly, he trusts himself. Recently, with pride he told me how he managed to cross "a big busy road" on his own. This I heard as a metaphor of his newly acquired ability to feel safe and in control both internally and externally.

References

Alvarez, A. (1992). *Life Company: Psychoanalytic Psychotherapy with Autistic, Borderline, Deprived and Abused children*. London: Routledge.

Bion, W. R. (1967). *Second Thoughts*. London: Heinemann.

Hurry, A. (1998). *Psychoanalysis and Developmental Therapy*. London: Karnac.

Parsons, M. & Dermen, S. (1999). The violent child and adolescent. In: M. Lanyado & A. Horne (Eds.), *The Handbook of Child and Adolescent Psychotherapy: Psychoanalytic Approaches* (pp. 329–345). London: Routledge.

Schore, A. N. (2001). The effects of early relational trauma on right brain development, affect regulation and infant mental health. *Infant Mental Health Journal, 22*(1–2): 201–269.

Applications

CHAPTER FIFTEEN

A depressed toddler and his mother reunite in the toddler group

Justine Kalas Reeves

Introduction

Below I shall describe how a depressed toddler and his mother grew to interact more pleasurably during their two-year membership of an Anna Freud Centre toddler group. While in many group settings there may only be resources to intervene when children are causing distress to the group through screaming, hurting, or taking toys, in our small setting we are able to intervene in cases such as the one of this sad little boy, prized by the other mothers for his ability to sit alone with picture books or to play with Duplo figures for long periods. Through our psychoanalytic frame of reference in both observing and thinking about this mother-toddler dyad, we were able to help them prevent further distance in their relationship—a process I shall describe below.

When this little boy came to our group at fourteen months, he frequently was observed sucking his hair while rubbing his ear to soothe himself. Ari overate in an automatic way, handfuls of raisins making it to his mouth without measure. He avoided his mother as well as other adults and children. His mother told us that Ari slept upwards of fifteen hours per day. We were curious to understand his solitary activities and avoidance of people. Though we felt very concerned when our attention went to him, we were just as likely to overlook him due to his quiet, studious nature in a group full of other robust, energetic, and sharing-averse toddlers. His mother was a young, pretty, and fashionable professional woman who appeared well put together—an appearance that helped hide her long-standing feeling of not being amply looked after and cared about. Fortunately, we were able to help them acknowledge how painful the emptiness between them felt, and to encourage their reunion.

Premature and superficial separation

Ms B stayed home with her son for his first ten months, at which point she returned to full-time work in patent law. She rhapsodized about Ari's first year, though her lack of detail did convey that there were difficulties she found hard to articulate. Ari's mother described her return to work as something she needed for herself, but was tormented by her mix of relief, sadness, and guilt, and called home often to check in with the nanny. It seemed that this mother was neither ready to leave her infant son nor able to be apart from her consuming work. Unable to articulate these mixed feelings, she left Ari before the toddler phase would impel him to leave his mother through the normal "excursions and returns" (Winnicott, 1966) of toddlerhood. Then, alarmed by her son's withdrawal and self-soothing symptoms, Ms B took the advice of her general practitioner and came to the AFC toddler group. On her intake form, mother wrote "As a working mother, I sometimes find it difficult to juggle my work and a healthy relationship with my son."

"Special time" at the toddler group

Ms B saw the toddler group as their "special time together" in the week. Both mother and child suffered from the lack of a co-constructed mental link to one another during the long days that mum left the house before Ari awoke. We speculated how difficult creating such mental links must have been for mother, whose own mother, an important politician in her city of origin, had also hired a nanny to raise Ms B and her two siblings. On the one hand, mother resisted the "ghosts" of her past by staying home with her son for ten months, yet was unconsciously led by them in minimizing both her significance to Ari as well as his to her at the time she returned to work (Fraiberg et al., 1975). Both were in a state of unacknowledged, undigested mourning at the start of their participation in the toddler group. According to Ms B, instead of helping to bring mother alive to the child during her absence, Ari's nanny took over the mothering role (see Furman, 1989), echoing what had happened to Ms B herself in her infancy. To compensate, Ms B put enormous pressure on herself and on Ari to make the toddler group a perfect experience.

Early days in the toddler group

Ari was fourteen months when he first arrived in the toddler group, one week after having taken his first steps. He was observed thus:

> [Ari] looked scared and lost. He sucked his hair and thumbed his ear for a long time and gave me a desolate feeling. He looked withdrawn. There is a strong contrast between Ms B, so lively and talkative, and Ari, who came across as very floppy, less held together than Sally (the sibling of another toddler) who is only seven months old.

Ari was an adorable, fair-haired toddler, with stunning but hidden pale grey eyes, more comfortable exploring a toy than people's faces. His withdrawn state indicated his real grief over the loss of his mother at a time when he needed his mother to "be there in order to be left"

(Furman, 1982). Mahler and her colleagues (1975) noted that if the mother is absent, even for a short period of time, the young toddler tends to become sober, "low-keyed", turned inwards, perhaps trying to evoke an internal image of his mother to feel safe (cited in Zaphiriou Woods & Pretorius, 2010, p. 22). On their second visit, Ari clearly remembered the group, smiling and vocalizing more than on the first visit, but still appearing passive. It was observed: "Ari does not walk confidently and he seems easily discouraged; he would rather crawl. He seems very slow in his responses and lacking in initiative."

Despite being in the "practising phase" (Mahler, 1975) when typically a toddler feels "the world is his oyster" (Greenacre, 1957), Ari kept his eyes down, did not persist in his new physical skills, and looked blank when a child took one of his toys. Though his mother stayed with him throughout the morning's toddler group, we speculated that Ari had become depressed after she returned to work and that this dampened his drive to explore. As Furman has written: "When mother is not there, the harbor is gone and venturing out feels less safe and less fun" (Furman, 1989, p. 63). We imagined that without his mother to admire all his new skills, he, too, could not experience the wondrous highs of toddlerhood. On their fourth visit, when Ari was sixteen months old, we observed:

> Mother carried Ari to the swings and pushed him gently. Ari sat passively in the swing, eyes at times half closed. Mother spoke excitedly about the sun and how nice it was to be outside but Ari responded little save for an occasional smile. Mother then put Ari on the slide, moving him up and down it several times. Ari seemed like a lump. Later that same day, mother told the leader that her husband worked long hours. She said at times this was a burden, as she felt it her sole responsibility to ensure that Ari gets "the best". She [said] that when father is home, Ari ignores mother, sighing "Daddy is for fun."

Mother's concern that she alone was responsible for giving Ari the "very best" hinted at her abiding sense of inadequacy and guilt, not to mention unconscious anger at Ari for having profound needs that competed and conflicted with her own. Despite efforts to draw her into playing with Ari, Ms B often stood back, observing Ari's play with the assistant, as on this day when Ari was seventeen months:

> The assistant handed Ari two balls; he took one in each hand. As she handed him a third, Ari put one down the toy chimney in order to take this third ball, and said "Ball". Mother watched with a big smile then pulled Ari to her and said, "Sorry, but I just have not had enough time with Ari yet. I just love being with him. I am mad about my son." The assistant commented on their precious time together at the toddler group, and mother said that they had had to rush from errands that day so there had not been any "cuddle time" for the two of them.

We began to notice how hard it was for mum and Ari to play together, and wondered how it felt for Ms B to watch him play with the assistant. We also wondered how it felt for Ari to miss his mum so much while she was at work, and then be enveloped by her with declarations of love when together, with no thread between the two experiences. We began to notice that her hugging would occur in moments when she appeared to feel at a loss herself, not sure how to interact with her son, or when she felt competitive with one of the leaders. We also observed in ourselves how eager we were to provide Ari with a playmate, manically plugging the lonely feeling that existed both between them and in each one of them.

Ms B became attached to the leader with whom she spoke with urgency each week about her frustrations in managing motherhood, work, and running the household. Trying to help keep the link between Ms B and Ari alive during the long days apart, the leader wondered if mother could visit or speak with Ari during the work day, and also suggested showing Ari her place of work. A couple of weeks later, Ali's visit to Ms B's workplace was described thus:

> Ari started shouting and playing with pleasure, and mother felt uncomfortable that his noise level might be disturbing her colleagues who might question her commitment to work. Finally, she became so anxious she decided to leave. Ari became very upset by this and screamed louder. In the lift were two senior colleagues and mother imagined they were thinking, "Come on girl, can't you separate from your son?"

Mother projected onto her colleagues her denigrated view of mothers with their toddlers as noisy, interfering with real adult work, but then felt persecuted. Having taken the suggestion of the leader to try to see Ari before departing for work, mother reported feeling more fluidity between her two roles when she had more time with her son each day. The following week, Ari, now nineteen months, sucked on his hair and rubbed his ear nearly the whole toddler group. He went over the bump between the two rooms in the toy car repeatedly, while Ms B told the leader that she had a panic attack earlier in the week, not sleeping or eating in anticipation of a presentation at work. She had told Ari, "Mummy is ill," and gave no further explanation for being unavailable. For Ari, having special times with mummy alongside feeling dropped left him confused and empty, and we linked his self-soothing symptoms to these very disparate experiences.

In the autumn, we observed that mother was more attuned having spent a month together in the country over the summer break. Ari's language was coming along, and he now loved to jump vigorously on the trampoline, something unimaginable in their first term in the group. Then, in October, mother casually reported she was working longer hours as she filled in for a colleague. She reported "loving" her increased responsibilities at work, and reasoned that Ari did not need her as much now. When we linked his recent higher mood to the summer, reminding Ms B how much he was affected by her comings and goings, she felt guilty, then sad, as if it felt impossible to love her son and her work at the same time.

Ari's hide-and-seek play now increased, and his play with the little bus, the mode of transportation mum used to get to work, revealed that he was thinking about the vehicle that took his mother away and delivered her back:

> The assistant and Ari each took a bus for a ride until reaching the Duplo house. The assistant showed him how to open and close a drawer. Ari spent a long time opening a drawer to put a little red car in, then took the car out, placed it in another drawer, closed it again and repeated this many more times. He was focused but withdrawn and seemed sad. Mother was anxious and left him for long periods playing alone with the leader or the assistant, during which time Ari fell several times, resulting in crying and being picked up by mother.

Ari also took to comforting himself with food:

> Ari, twenty-one months, said he was hungry and sat down at the snack table. Mother said: "He is always the first at the table." Ari seemed very anxious and when the snacks were placed on the table took large handfuls and was the last to leave the table. His mum tried to limit his eating by moving the food away from Ari.

With mother unavailable for approaching and distancing behaviours, so crucial for the "practising" toddler (Mahler et al., 1975), it seems that Ari turned auto-erotically back to his own body for stimulation, as in his self-soothing symptoms, and filled his belly in the absence of more filling interactions with his mum. We leaders and the student observers noted how sad both mum and Ari made us feel.

Furman has written extensively about the phases of parenthood, how first the child is invested as a part of the parent's self, and then slowly the parents pass "bodily ownership" to the child. Though the narcissistic investment in the child—seeing him or her as a part of the self—is never fully replaced by the libidinal cathexis of seeing the child as a separate, loved person, the shift often represents a "precipice" for mothers more than for fathers. She writes: "Both parents include the child in their own mental self, but only the mother invests him also as a part of her bodily self, i.e., he is included in the boundaries of her body ego" (1996, p. 431). Furthermore, Furman writes, in giving up one area of control, for example, nursing, it is not uncommon for a mother to take control over a different area, such as sleep. She writes: "... spoonfeeding or rigid control of the types and amounts of food offered easily nullify the child's potential independence resulting from weaning; similarly, mother's ownership of nursing (what goes in) is often transferred to elimination (what comes out) ..." (1996, p. 434). As we would come to see, Ms B was terribly worried about what went inside Ari. Ari's solution to the confusion produced by his mother's enveloping presence alongside her yawning absences was to withdraw, holding himself together through his hair-sucking, ear rubbing, and overeating to create a second skin (Bick, 1968) where the relational patchwork of his first layer of skin had worn thin.

Rejection and collusion

As Ari approached two, there were many instances when play between mother and son would crumble before it ever got off the ground. Either Ari would walk away from mum because he did not want to be her "show pony" in reciting his colours, or Ms B would participate with Ari for a moment, and then turn to another mother or the leader for adult conversation. On the occasion of Ari's second birthday, mother's controlling interactions reached a high pitch with Ari as if serving to rid her mind of any hints of grief or worry as she took stock of what had undoubtedly felt a difficult year in their relational development:

> Bringing a raspberry cream cake, she bombarded him with questions after placing the birthday cake in front of him: "Whose birthday cake is this?" Ari answered his name and then Ms B asked, "How many candles do we have here, Ari?" Ari responded, "Two." Ms B pointed to the candle in a shape of a two, asking, "And which number is this?" "Number two," answered Ari. Ari stayed at the table a long time, completely at one with the cake as he ate it.

Observers felt they were watching mother administer an exam to her son. Ms B had asked me to take a photograph, yet I hesitated to show it to her as next to his jubilantly smiling Mum, Ari looked straight down at the cake. Though there were times when we felt upset with Ms B for her clumsy bids for Ari that left him withdrawn, it was equally upsetting and sad to realize how deeply mother wanted to be close to her son but did not know how.

It was therefore with great relief that we observed the delight between Ari and Ms B a few weeks after the birthday party when they played together with the Duplo:

> Ari and the assistant were playing with Duplo, putting little figures to bed. The assistant took a figure and asked if he could ride on a horse. Ari said "Yes," and taking the figure, tried to position it on the horse. Mother was standing nearby and offered to help the figure onto the horse. She took the horse and moved it along, humming a cowboy song. Ari first smiled and then laughed, and asked his mother to do it again. Ari then imitated what mother had done, and both clapped hands and laughed.

In this instance, Ari delighted in his mother's playfulness, and Ms B clearly enjoyed having her son join her, reducing her feelings of rejection. Yet, a few weeks later when Ari tried to place a large bull in a small doll-bed, mother laughed, saying, "Cows do not sleep in beds." Ari persisted in putting the large bull in the bed, but turned his body away and no longer involved mum in his game. We wondered if Ari's repetitive play of putting figures and animals to sleep made mother anxious, interfering with her ability to feel pride and delight in her growing son's imagination.

When Ari was twenty-six months old, Ms B came to me in the group to tell me she felt "lonely" when she played with Ari. With her husband working long hours, she felt her life very regimented: work, home to Ari, bed. I spoke to her about feeling empty, and possibly missing her husband both as spouse and co-parent. She denied this, and told me on the way out of the door that she would be missing next week's toddler group because of work. By telling us at the end, I felt dropped just as Ari must have felt at times when his mother's plans changed. The following week, brought by his nanny, Ari's "dropped" feelings came through in his play:

> Ari placed all the Duplo figures into the post office until no more [could] fit. They all faced the same direction. He pushed one last figure in and suddenly jerked his hand inside the building, crashing all the figures to the ground. The figures flew everywhere and his nanny looked startled. The assistant commented that it might have been very crowded in the building. Ari did not say anything, but sucked on his hair and pulled his left ear. Ari filled the post office again, then crashed the figures to the ground again.

Ari had stuffed the post office many times in the past, squeezing one more figure in until no more would fit. The assistant observed in herself that she had often felt the need to make space, opening doors when Ari played this game in the past. On this day, though, Ari and the assistant were more able to let the feelings be expressed through his play. Observing this scene, I felt spooked by how sombre Ari was as he watched the carnage. There was no excitement or pleasure in releasing his distress.

Mother reported the following week that she would have to miss three toddler groups due to work commitments. In the face of Ms B's busier schedule, we saw Ari rejecting his mother.

> Ari was playing with the Fisher Price house, placing all the figures around the table to eat. Mother stood over him asking, "What are they doing, Ari?" Ari did not answer. Mother asked again, so Ari said "Table." Mother asked Ari another question, who then stood up and walked away from his mother, clearly put off by the question. [26 months]

A few months on, Ms B revealed her ambivalence about having a second child. From their entry to the toddler group, she had said her husband wanted a second child while she did not feel ready and did not want to "give [one] to him" due to her anger that he worked such long hours. As we spoke, Ari played below:

> Ari said he had Mummy, Daddy and Ari figures, placing then all in one bed. First Mummy and Daddy faced one another with Ari facing the back of his mother. Next he turned the mother around to face Ari, so that father faced mother's back. Next Ari faced Daddy, while mother faced father's back.

Ari's play seemed to symbolize the lack of triangular relating that occurred in the family, and also reflected what had happened in our toddler group. We noticed how we had responded to the competition between mother and child for undivided attention by providing each with a special person, thereby protracting the distance between mother and child. Though our conscious motivation had been to provide and model attentive listening, playful interactions, and acceptance of both of them to help bring them together, we had unwittingly colluded in denying their grave difficulty being intimate with one another, and the concomitant difficulty of moving towards triangular and Oedipal relating, with all its agonies and ecstasies.

Rows on the path towards bodily and mental ownership

Ari was now thirty-two months, and as one of the more established pairs in the group, Ms B seemed more confident to note her grievance that the late mid-morning snack interfered with a "healthy" meal for Ari:

> The other toddlers were munching on raisins and bananas. Ms B brought out a large container of leftover pasta primavera that she had brought from home. Ari ate some apple and a few raisins. Ms B said sternly: "Ari, you make Mummy very upset if you don't finish your lunch first." Ari complied with a pained look and turned his face away before Ms B pushed the last of it into his mouth.

When I said Ari did not seem hungry for all that today, Ms B told me she wanted Ari to have a proper lunch before having "sweets" like raisins and bananas. Though I had tried to verbalize Ari's feelings about being asked to eat different foods from the others, I was also aware of mother's powerful feelings of anger about the sweet foods we offered. The prohibition on sweet flavours reminded us of how deprived and bitter Ms B was feeling inside. The assistant and I continued to be terribly concerned as to how to help their relationship in what was now their penultimate term, though there were many more hopeful moments such as these:

> Ari carried the big brown teddy to the garden. Once there, Ari grabbed mother's hand and led her to the swings. Ms B placed Ari in one of the swings and, at Ari's request, the bear in the other. Ari was smiling and making funny faces with his mum and the teddy. Another toddler noticed this and pulled his mum towards the swings. Ms B helped Ari and the teddy out to accommodate the other toddler, and Ari started to cry. The leader explained to the other toddler that Ari was playing with Teddy now but she [other toddler] could have a turn soon. Ari looked at the other toddler and then offered her the teddy. The leader and Ms B praised Ari for being such a good sharer and friend, and he then smiled with pride at his mum who gave him a hug.

It was touching to see how genuinely proud Mum was to see her son's concern for others, and more and more instances such as these nourished this mother's confidence in herself and in her son. Then again, it could be confusing for observers to see the inconsistency in Ms B's own developmental phases, one minute a proud mother, the next an angry and retaliatory sibling to her son. For example:

> It was time to leave. Ms B said, "We're going to Nan's, time to get your coat." Ari did not stop playing with the trains and did not look up when his mother repeated herself. She said it a third time, and Ari said "No!" Ms B's voice became louder and firmer, as she said they would come back next week, and Nan was waiting for them. Ari did not move. Mum said angrily, "Fine, you stay here, take your coat, I'm leaving." She threw the coat on Ari's head and went out the door. She later returned and forced the coat on him.

The following week, we had the opportunity to speak to Ms B about the incident. She admitted she did feel rejected when Ari did not follow her directions. I sympathized with how rejected she felt by her son, and reminded her of instances in which Ari found it easier to leave after he had had a good time with his mummy at the toddler group. Ms B's face looked as if a penny had dropped, as if she had never imagined she might have so much to offer her son. However, she still felt terribly threatened when Ari made different choices from her, as if Ms B had nothing good to offer unless his preferences confirmed her own:

> It was snack time, and as usual, Ari had water while the others had juice. Ari took sips of juice from the other children's cups, and his mother stopped him. I said it might be quite hard for Ari not to eat and drink what the others were drinking. Ms B said she wished we did not serve apple juice as it only rots the teeth and makes children want more and more sweet things. Taken aback by the strength of her disapproval of the juice, I asked the group what their feelings were about apple juice. One mother agreed that it was important that children drink water, but she didn't mind her daughter drinking juice here.

Ari ate his way through the conversation, before retreating to the Duplo toys. I followed him there, and watched as he put a family to bed. I commented that everyone in his family sleeps on their tummy after he had placed them so. He turned the figure of the Duplo boy onto his back as if to distinguish himself from the family. At least privately Ari could assert his own preferences—his own mind.

The following week at snack time, perhaps feeling more alone alongside Ari's increasing confidence at asserting himself, Ms B resumed where she had left off, arguing that apple juice was no different from sugary soda, it rotted the teeth. In our post-group discussion, the assistant leader and I were able to tease out how important it was for her to give Ari only good things on their special day, to make up for her sadness and guilt about not being with him the rest of the week. Ms B and I were eventually able to separate the drinks from how difficult it was to allow Ari to make his own choices, as if that rendered mum obsolete—psychical abandonment for Ms B. From that point, the assistant and I emphasized how much Ari enjoyed it when mum followed his lead, as that grew his sense of having his own self and mind. Ms B's fear of rejection decreased, too, when she felt his pleasure in having his separate ideas and wants validated by her.

Ms B gains confidence and Ari internalizes his mother

It had been agreed that Ari could stay until the end of the term after his third birthday. The new assistant and I reflected on how we had formerly "rescued" Ari and his mother from being together when it felt empty between them, reflecting that we too found the empty and lonely feeling between them unbearable. We resolved to help them through this by being vigilant about our feelings of needing to step in and rescue.

Ari had become a sociable, verbal, enthusiastic player with the leaders and other children. His preoccupation with sweets and stuffing himself continued, and mother had taken the assistant's words to heart that controlling all that passed through her son's lips would only create a preoccupation and not help him acknowledge his own bodily and psychic feelings. Ms B worked very hard to stop herself, though it was clearly still very upsetting for her to witness her son's tendency to overeat. Mother approached me to discuss why Ari, now thirty-seven months, overate. We discussed how Ari might be feeling quite hungry for something, and in not knowing what it was he was hungry for, ate to compensate. Mother asked if it was that he was hungry for her. I said: "You seem to think so." Mother felt guilty, and then spoke again about themes she had mentioned before, being solely in charge of the running of the household and the care for Ari, needing to support her overworked husband. I picked up her own feelings of depletion and emptiness and how hard it felt to give to her son when she feels she needs so much, too. I reminded her of many recent interactions in which both mother and son had played avidly, when she took Ari's zeal, and wondered what made that hard to sustain. Ms B said that she had always thought she was supposed to be teaching her son, and that the observers made her feel inhibited at the toddler group. Yet she visibly relaxed when we encouraged her to play as it was only she who had the didactic expectations.

Interestingly, what followed from this conversation and our efforts to encourage the two to play together more was quite remarkable. It was as if we had given mother permission to play and to be less self-conscious. As Ms B joined him more, Ari felt less a need to stuff himself at snack time. I had the feeling as I witnessed this change that there had in fact been many good interactions when Ari was a little baby, and they were now able to re-find one another. Rather than just allowing herself to let her hair down, as she had done when humming the cowboy tune aloud, she now appreciated their differences, which gave space for some separation between the two. The following observation took place at thirty-seven months:

> The assistant and Ari had played a game the previous week in which all the skittles were placed upright, and then kicked down. Ari had relished the game. The following week, Ari took his mum by the hand to the skittles. Ms B looked slightly uncomfortable, so the assistant came to say how important it was for children to play with messy and angry feelings in a fun way. Ari was busily turning them up and began to knock all the skittles over, then jumping up and down saying, "Come on, Mummy, let's do it again!" Ms B helped arrange the skittles again and this time joined her son in knocking them all down. This made Ari even more excited and they did it again. Though initially not sure, Ms B became infected by her son's obvious pleasure and began to giggle herself.

We were pleased the following week to see Ari lead his mother to the skittles basket and Ms B, with equal relish said: "I know what you want to do!"

The following observation, still at thirty-seven months, shows Ari not only looking for his mum but expecting her. There had been a time when the fact that they did not look for one another in our group made us feel so lonely that it activated our rescuing tendencies. They are again able to play with their aggression in the service of having fun with one another:

> Ari is walking around the room carrying a bowl full of red play-dough. He comes to the peg and hammer toy. He turns around to look for his mum. Once he has realized that Ms B is right behind him he points to the toy and says, "Look Mum," in excitement. Ms B smiles at Ari, then bends down to join in hammering the pegs with her son. Ari looks surprised when he sees the other hammer, then looks up and smiles in delight at his mother. They switch hammers and continue hammering.

Another change, so important for Ari, as it gave him more of a sense of himself, validating his own discoveries, was that Ms B became more flexible and interested in her son's ideas:

> Ms B and Ari put the wellies on the teddy, then stand, each taking one hand of the teddy. Ari suggests they take the bear for a walk. As they do, they pull the bear up in the air. As they approach the coats, Ari suggests they put a coat on the bear. Ms B looks at him and agrees. I was surprised. Ari and his mother begin to dress the teddy.

As Ari's two-year tenure in the group came to an end, we saw him actively seeking his mother, experiencing the excitement and curiosity that he used to lack. Ms B continued quizzing her son on occasions and Ari still loved to fill up his belly. But they were a partnership by the end, able to bear all the slings and arrows of that. Upon their arrival and the first one and a half years in the group, the empty and anxious feeling between them made us feel the need to step in to save them from the desolation. Despite the built-in time to think deeply about the parent–toddler couples we work with, we had acted on our feelings when we provided both mother and son with a special person. Later, by noting our feelings of needing to rescue them, we were able to establish ways to help Ari and his mother to find authentic feelings inside themselves, to come together and go apart without feeling they might never find their way back to one another. On their final day in the toddler group, of course there was sadness, but there was also true gratefulness in all of us for what we had gained.

References

Bick, E. (1968). The experience of skin in early object relationships. *International Journal of Psychoanalysis, 49*: 484–486.

Furman, E. (1982). Mothers have to be there to be left. *Psychoanalytic Study of the Child, 37*: 15–28.

Furman, E. (1989). Mothers, toddlers, and care. *In:* S. I. Greenspan & G. H. Pollock (Eds.), *Course of Life, Vol. 2: Early Childhood* (pp. 61–82). Madison, CT: International Universities Press.

Furman, E. (1992). *Toddlers and Their Mothers: A Study in Early Personality Development*. New York: International Universities Press.

Furman, E. (1996). On motherhood. *Journal of the American Psychoanalytic Association, 44S*: 429–447.

Greenacre, P. (1957). The childhood of the artist: libidinal phase development and giftedness. *Psychoanalytic Study of the Child, 12*: 47–72.

Mahler, M. S., Pine, F. & Bergmann, A. (1975). *The Psychological Birth of the Human Infant: Symbiosis and Individuation*. New York: Basic.

Winnicott, D. W. (1966). The child in the family group. In: C. Winnicott, R. Shepherd & M. David (Eds.), *Home is Where We Start From* (pp. 128–141). London: Penguin, 1986.

Zaphiriou Woods, M. (2000). Preventive work in a toddler group and nursery. *Journal of Child Psychotherapy, 26*: 206–233.

Zaphiriou Woods, M. & Pretorius, I. M. (Eds.) (2010). *Parents and Toddlers in Groups: a Psychoanalytic Developmental Approach*. London: Routledge.

Outreach

CHAPTER SIXTEEN

"Anna Freud in Africa"—Ububele in Alexandra township, Johannesburg

Hillary and Tony Hamburger

> *"The reward of the ending of apartheid will and must be measured by the happiness and welfare of our children".*
>
> —(Nelson Mandela)

The importance of the emotional world of the pre-school child

Ububele, an Nguni word, like *ubuntu*, encompasses more than its literal meaning, which is "kindness". It extends to include the idea of compassion and concern for others, a central ingredient of mental health. The root of the word is *amabele*, a breast that represents the nurturing mother and the early attachment relationship between the mother and her baby.

"Ububele" jumped out at us as a name for a mental health centre that we established on the border of Alexandra township, a dense black ghetto that still carries the scars of its apartheid past. Now ten years later, Ububele has established itself as an accredited training institute with local, national, and international connections. All our projects, with the exception of the "Working with Groups" training programme, are focused on the pre-school child (infancy to seven years old).

Every child is faced with developmental challenges that have to be negotiated. Even in optimal circumstances where there is the stability of a mother and father who are able to feed their children both physically and emotionally, there are constant developmental pitfalls to overcome if a child is to grow up with a secure sense of self. Many township children are faced with spirals of emotional suffering that arise out of poverty, unemployed parents, absent parents, overburdened single parents, physical and sexual abuse, and an HIV/AIDS epidemic that robs children of their vital primary relationships. It was in the hope of making some contribution to this critical state of affairs that Ububele was established.

The Ububele Nursery

Following a visit to the Anna Freud Nursery in London in 1999, we (both of us clinical psychologists and psychoanalytic psychotherapists) set up a nursery, tailored to meet the specific psychosocial needs of our children who came from the local township on our doorstep. While the well-equipped school follows a pre-school curriculum offering opportunity for creative play and active learning, the emotional development of each child is carefully monitored. Each week Hillary runs a seminar where the teachers bring the children that they feel need special attention for discussion. We follow the children inwards, into their psychic worlds, and outwards into their family and community life. To our delight we have become known in the township as "that place that talks about feelings", a literal translation from an African language.

The Umdlezane programme

A number of other projects soon took root. One that is closely tied to the Anna Freud Centre was developed with the ongoing support of Peter Fonagy, Mary Target, and particularly Tessa Baradon, who initiated and developed the Parent–Infant Project at the Anna Freud Centre and helped us establish a "sister" project at Ububele. We called our project the Ububele Umdlezane Parent Infant Project (UUPIP), which currently has an introductory training to offer.

Umdlezane refers to an indigenous practice during the post-partum period when the women in the family prioritize a mother's relationship with her baby. They take over the practical running of the homestead, freeing the mother to focus completely on her baby. It is not only the necessity of the mother-infant attachment that is crucial but also the quality of the attachment. Thus *umdlezane* appears to have many aspects in common with attachment theory.

The Umdlezane Project has a number of related programmes including a study group of practitioners working in the area, group and individual therapy for new mothers and their babies, and work discussion groups for nurses. Currently research and testing is being undertaken in mother-infant groups: this again is an adaptation of the AFC developed programme. Tessa Barradon leads this innovative research project in partnership with the University of the Witwatersrand, Ububele, and the Anna Freud Centre.

Another project stemming from the Anna Freud Centre is one for babies with teenage mothers. Training workshops run by Joan Raphael-Leff, for Ububele staff, Witwatersrand interns, and practitioners from Khanya Family Centre helped to increase understanding of this complex group, and to plan provisions for pregnant teenagers and group work with teen mothers, and/or young fathers in Alexandra, Katlehong, and Sharpeville. It was felt that the team's increased confidence is directly related to the extraordinarily warm and powerful training style.

The "Baby Mat" project

A so-called "Baby Mat" project now operates in three primary health care centres in Alexandra. A UUPIP trained psychologist and an auxiliary social worker/translator set up a floor mat in the corner of a busy post-natal clinic where mothers bring their babies to be weighed and inoculated. They are invited to bring any problem they might have with their babies to the Ububele psychologist on the baby mat. The short half-hour session is used to identify many emotional issues. The naming and the clarification of the problem appear to bring relief to the mother and the baby. We are often astonished by how much can be achieved in such a short intervention. More intensive individual help is offered when required at the Umdlezane Clinic at Ububele. The long-term goal of this and all programmes developed at Ububele is to find ways to disseminate them within South Africa.

Persona dolls

The Ububele Persona Doll project, designed as a therapeutic intervention for children between three and seven years, has become an integral part of the work in the nursery. The persona doll is a life-size rag doll that has a detailed personality and life history worked out by the practitioner during her training. This creates a "suspension of disbelief" phenomenon that allows the children to relate and communicate with a doll in a group setting, bypassing the practitioner as it were. In the nursery it is used by all our teachers to help the children become familiar with their emotional worlds. While this enhances emotional literacy when used by the teacher it can also be used as an effective therapeutic tool in the hands of a professional child therapist.

We believe that the persona doll is an aid to building emotional "muscle" so necessary for dealing with the vicissitudes of difficult lives. The following is an example of a persona doll session, which became overwhelming for the teacher who then brought in one of the psychologists to help in a follow-up session.

> The teacher's doll was named Lerato, she was four years old and she lived with her aunty in Alexandra township in 18th Avenue. Her mother lived in Kathlehong, a township on the East Rand. Lerato loved her aunty who had set up a small covered stand, outside her shack, a spaza shop, where she sold groceries. Lerato enjoyed helping in the little shop when she came home from school. They didn't work on Sundays when they both went to church where aunty sang in the church choir. Lerato was proud of her auntie who had a beautiful voice and knew many songs, which she would always sing at home.

These details about the life of Lerato facilitates the children's identification with her. The nursery children got to know Lerato well and looked forward to their weekly session with her. The doll, speaking "through" the teacher, brought different themes to encourage the children to talk about their own experiences. Not only difficult issues are brought (rivalry, prejudice, a new sibling, bullying, but everyday ones as well, such as a birthday party, a visit to a rural family, going to "big" school).

> On this particular day Lerato had brought an issue to the group about a boy who had hit her at school. One of the children pushed this topic aside as she urgently asked Lerato why she lived with her auntie and not with her mummy. (The teacher hadn't seen this as a problem,

> as it is common in South African townships for the biological parent not to be the primary caregiver.) Lerato explained that auntie did not have any children of her own while mummy already had Lerato's brother to look after. It was difficult for her to look after two children, as she wasn't well.
>
> One child wanted to know what was wrong with the mother. The teacher shrugged her shoulders. Lerato didn't know. And suddenly all hell broke loose. "I know what's wrong with her," shouted Tandiswe. "She has got AIDS and she is going to die," and with that she broke into uncontrollable sobs. That set the ball rolling. They all began to talk of relatives and neighbours who had died of AIDS and before long most of the children were weeping. The teacher was at a loss to know what to say as she attempted to calm and comfort them.

It was left to the psychologist to run a number of bereavement sessions in which she sought to bring the AIDS bogeyman out from under the bed so that they could deal with the reality of AIDS as an illness that could be treated. In addition she was able to help the children confront anxieties around abandonment, which underpinned fears of AIDS.

Play therapy

Often a child has to deal with trauma of such intensity that we think it requires individual attention in play therapy. Currently there is virtually no therapy available for children from most of South Africa's disadvantaged communities. Ububele relies on psychology interns who during the year of their internship are able to offer play therapy under supervision. Examples of particularly stressful cases are a boy whose dad is sent to prison for eighteen years for armed robbery and phones the child daily from prison; a four year old who has been raped by her sixteen-year-old cousin; a five year old, whose parents are mute but nevertheless subject him to their constant drinking and fighting.

A case history

Bongani was almost five when she arrived at Ububele at the beginning of 2010. Her great-aunt Maizie who brought her told us a heartbreaking story. Her sister, the child's grandmother, had extracted a promise from her before she died that she would look after Bongi when she was gone. There was no one else as Bongi's mother had died two years previously. Great-aunt told us that while she was honouring her promise to her sister she felt unable to take on another child at this stage in her life. She asked if we could direct her to a good orphanage. We saw our work as twofold: (1) to help Bongi deal with the trauma of her huge losses as well as adjust to her new impatient caregiver, and (2) to help Maizie parent Bongi.

We could understand Maizie's situation. She had brought up her own children who "were difficult and didn't help her now that they were grown up". She was a live-in domestic worker and Bongi was sharing her small room and bed with her. She was allocated to a counsellor who helped prepare the ground for a change in her attitude, which came suddenly half way through the year. Bongi overheard Maizie telling a friend that she was looking for an orphanage for her. Bongi became hysterical and cried all through the week until Maizie promised her that she would never do such a thing and added that she loved her. In this crisis Maizie discovered that she had become much more attached to Bongi than she had bargained for.

An intern (white) doing her master's degree in psychology took Bongi into weekly play therapy, under my (HH) supervision. At the beginning of our work at Ububele we had fretted at not being able to find enough black psychologists, as we believed that it was important for therapist and client to come from the same cultural background. We have since come to see that much can be done cross-culturally if the therapist is sensitive to the inner world of the child. Bongi's therapy showed us that neither race nor language necessarily hampered the process.

Over the course of the year the therapy went through a number of phases. In the first phase Bongi did not engage with her therapist. She would come into the play room, turn her back on the therapist, and settle down to playing with the family of dolls who she looked after with great intensity and diligence. She took one doll for a walk in the stroller while she strapped another onto her back: she filled the little pots with sand from the sandpit and then cooked her "food" on the stove: she bathed yet another doll and then put her to sleep while she rocked her in her arms. We understood her need to unconsciously communicate her experience of being the onlooker and outsider to a happy mother-child scenario: she omnipotently became the nurturing mother while the therapist became the envious, helpless, deprived observer.

For all that, she was so purposeful and contained in her play that after two months we decided that she was managing well enough for the therapy to end. (With our limited resources we needed the space for another child.) When her therapist told her that they would be stopping, Bongani's eyes widened in shock as she clasped her arms over her head and let out an animal-like howl.

The therapy continued. In the next stage she persisted with her doll play but now drew the therapist into the play, acknowledging her attachment to and need for her. This was followed by an aggressive phase in which she threw the dolls around and bashed strollers into the wall. And finally as the end of the year came closer and there was more talk about the end of her therapy and her going to primary school, this clever little girl found a solution to her problems. When her therapist commented on what a good mummy she was and how well she looked after her children, Bongi announced that she wanted a real baby and that she was going to get pregnant. When the therapist queried how she would do this she admitted that she didn't know how but that she would find a way.

Her behaviour in the classroom bore out her phantasy. She walked around with a small cushion under her dress and caused havoc one day when the teacher left the room for a short while. She took off her panties, lay down on the floor with open legs and invited the boys to "kiss my vagina". This necessitated some serious work with her shocked teacher who was all for having Bongi removed from the school. The following Friday our teacher's seminar was devoted to understanding Bongi's sexualized behaviour and once the teachers could understand that she was acting out her wish for a loved and loving person of her very own, they became warmly supportive of her.

Her November birthday was celebrated at the school with added enthusiasm. One of the teachers personally paid for a photographer, explaining that it was important for Bongi to be able to hold her good memories of her nursery in her hand. Bongi herself did not stop talking about the "best day" in her life and said to her teacher, "Everybody loves me so now I have to be good."

The poignancy of her statement did not blind us to the limitations of the help we were able to give Bongi during her year at Ububele. We nevertheless feel with some confidence that it will make a difference in the journey that lies ahead of her. In addition, Bongi's case leaves us with a conviction that much work can be done within seemingly bleak situations and limited human and financial resources.

The England of WWII in which Anna Freud developed her work with children in crisis resonates in our traumatized South African society. She truly finds a place in Africa as we go about our work at Ububele, mindful and appreciative of the support we receive from the Anna Freud Centre.

C. LATENCY

Clinical papers and outreach

Overview

CHAPTER SEVENTEEN

Overview of theoretical and clinical applications, and current developments

Anat Gedulter-Trieman

With the resolution of the Oedipus complex and with the establishment of the superego, the latency period is introduced. The latency period has received little attention in psychoanalytic circles. References in the literature are relatively scarce by comparison to the wealth of clinical and theoretical studies of early childhood and adolescence. This finding is intriguing considering that over many years of clinical activity at the Anna Freud Centre, the majority of those referred to the Centre were patients in the latency stage from five to ten years old.

Early on, Freud postulated the concept of the development of human sexuality with a period of sexual latency in the middle. This can be traced in the "Three Essays on Sexuality" (1905):

> There seems to be no doubt that germs of sexual impulses are already present in the new-born child and that these continue to develop for a time, but are then overtaken by a progressive process of suppression (p. 176).
>
> It is during this period of total or partial latency that are built up the mental forces which are later to impede the course of the sexual instinct and, like dams, restrict its flow ... this development is organically determined and fixed by heredity (p. 177).

Freud further elaborated in *Inhibitions, Symptoms and Anxiety* (1926): "The latency period ... is characterised by the dissolution of the Oedipus Complex, the creation or consolidation of the superego and the erection of ethical and aesthetic barriers in the ego." He described the reaction formation of morality, shame, and disgust built during the latency phase, referring to permanent changes in ego organization and object relations which will shape adolescent development and adult adjustment.

Extending this understanding, Anna Freud emphasized ego and superego development over and above changes in the functioning of the id (A. Freud, 1966c). Using a notion of a developmental continuum she referred to the widening scope of ego and superego during latency, from "egocentricity to companionship", from "play to work", and from a position of dependency to libidinal investment in people outside the family, impersonal ideals, and sublimated interests.

The process of gradual working through is seen as a fundamental feature of latency. Oedipal impulses are partly worked through and partly operative and defended against. Oedipal resolution is thus due both to fear and to loving and restorative impulses towards the parents. A resolution signifies an acceptance of the sexual and procreative parental relationship, and the renunciation of the child's sexual desires towards them. Re-working through at the beginning of latency occurs at a whole object level, as opposed to the part-object of earlier phases.

The relative relinquishing of incestuous wishes in the latency child concurs with advances in symbolization and sublimation. Curiosity is invested in intellectual functioning. Restorative impulses towards the parents are expressed by a growing capacity to learn and to engage in new activities (like sports and hobbies). The child widens his interest in other people and is preparing for exogamic object choice in adolescence.

Intellectually there is a sharper delineation between primary and secondary process thinking, between internal and external reality. This is reflected in more complex language development, such as the use of metaphors and in appreciating and making up jokes. The latency child is now capable of more abstract and complex symbolic functioning in his/her approach towards understanding of the world. Physical changes, with wider scope and intricacy of fine motor coordination, offer additional tools for mastering the environment and the growth of self-esteem.

Anna Freud noted a reorganization of defences which gives the latency period some degree of stability—sublimation, reaction formation, fantasy, regression, and repression are characteristic.

The rigidity of the (recently formed) superego is greater during the beginning of latency and devoted to censoring the remaining incestuous desires. In this early phase, tensions between the superego and the drives can result in heightened ambivalence which might be expressed in the child's alternation between strict obedience and rebellion often followed by self-reproach.

The child struggles to tolerate feelings of guilt and criticism from the outside, and his behaviour is not modified right away by either. In *The Ego and the Mechanisms of Defence* (1937) Anna Freud described what happens at this intermediate stage of superego development: "The attempt to internalize the criticism from the outside sometimes does not lead further than to identification with the aggressor, often supplemented by another defensive measure, namely the projection of guilt." Both defences in turn thrust the child into greater inner and outer conflicts.

Some young latency children, from about five to eight years old, might give the appearance of being in an emergency situation. As they are more conscious of their emotional distress they can show willingness to accept the analyst as a potential helper. Although they usually expect instant relief and often become disappointed and distrustful if this does not occur, they can become highly involved in the treatment.

Indeed, therapeutic chances seem to be better in early latency than at any other time due to the child's awareness of his/her suffering and the plasticity of the ego, being in defiance of both id and superego. The fluid state of the libido and the superego, being still open to modification, implies that the ego is not yet completely crippled by neurotic defences.

As the latent child develops, the ego is exposed to less severe conflicts—on the one hand, the sexual demands have become less exacting and, on the other, the superego has become less rigid. The ego now can devote itself to a greater extent to coping with reality. The average eight year old is ready to be influenced by the children around him and by adults other than his parents. As the child's perception of his parents' omnipotence subsides, changes in the ego's attitude to the superego occur. Identification transforms the child's relation with parents, preserving it and rendering it unconscious in comparison to the libidinal and hostile impulses that dominate the Oedipal drama.

Almost fifty years later, it is remarkable to see how influential Anna Freud's thinking on latency still is in our appreciation of the development and treatment of the latency child. The following four chapters will demonstrate in a fresh way, and with current relevance, clinical intervention done along the lines of Anna Freud's concepts.

Natalia Stafler's and Mark Carter's clinical papers portray a passage towards formation of a masculine/benign identification in boys of five, and seven and a half years respectively. The young patients' fragile egos seem flooded by their aggressive impulses, and by what are experienced by them as intolerable demands of the external world. The five year old retreats into omnipotent defences in order to avoid a reality where he feels helpless, like "a tiny insect that can be easily squashed". He refrains from contact with others. However, turning into the "murdered ant" leaves him overwhelmed and terrified. The omnipotence of the seven and ahalf year old has a more delinquent quality, but it becomes clear that this is a thin veneer, incapable of covering feelings of inadequacy, loneliness, and deprivation. Analysis proved to be crucial for the development of this boy, who could not afford to be "just a little boy" in the absence of a father figure to identify with and feel protected by. In those cases, as well as with Paddy Martin's six-and-a-half-year-old patient, one can see how the analyst is being used not only as a transference object but also as a *new* object and auxiliary ego. Paddy Martin's understanding of the aggressive and defiant outbursts of his patient, as driven by primitive anxiety concerning survival and integrity, helped keep the "gates and fences" firm enough to enable them to survive the constant attacks and to contain the patient's wild destructive feelings.

The crucial importance Anna Freud placed on working with the parent (or adult in charge) to support the therapeutic effort is manifested in all three of these clinical papers as well as in Pat Radford's chapter. In the latter, her description of her work as clinical consultant to a local primary school illustrates the value of supporting young children through work with teachers as well as parents.

* * *

In light of Anna Freud's invaluable contributions I would like to draw on my own clinical experience to explore some new challenges for today's latency child. The era of the internet, which enables rapid, almost unlimited modes of communication, is bound to create fundamental changes in individual psychic development, with potentially radical implications for the psychosocial realm. The accessibility of non-selective information sources and unfiltered audiovisual material exposes the latency child to an environment where not much remains latent.

Young children are commercialized and their toys are sexualized. The child is surrounded by explicitly sexual and aggressive stimuli.

The new objects made available for identification, as commonly portrayed by the media are beautiful, sexy, young, and glamorous. The centrality of visual perfection (with the aid of fictional means such as Photoshop) inevitably poses a great contrast to the child's image of himself and his parents, and presents an impossible act to follow. This can lead to difficulties in the formulation of his or her body image and extreme disillusionment with the parents and their ordinary appearance, resulting in undermining their authority.

Latency girls (and boys) can appear sexualized in their dress and demeanour, long before their body or mind reaches maturation. What starts as pseudo-maturation can escalate to a premature distortion in development.

Intense exposure and use of virtual reality might result in blurred boundaries between fantasy and reality, right and wrong. Such interference in ego and superego formation can be critical in this period, and may lead to poorly sublimated non-discriminatory expressions of sexuality and aggression.

As the latency child turns to his peer group, one wonders how the technological advances, mobile phones, email, Facebook and other new means of fast communication might affect the nature of object relations while these are being consolidated. The new phenomenon of "social networking" with its relentless remote communication, can pose a danger of leaving little room for the development of self-containment and tolerance of frustration. The risk of seeing the other as an extension of oneself, used for instant gratification, and as "switch-offable", can lead to a narcissistic and perverse psychopathology. The ever-growing need for harder core stimuli may dispose relationships to become transient, exploitative, and non-satisfying.

The rising new "epidemic" of ADHD diagnosis among school age children is leading us to greater awareness of the need for refined diagnostic tools. My clinical experience makes me wonder if what we at times perceive as "attention deficits" may represent the growing difficulty for the developing ego in coping with overwhelming external and internal stimuli. The bombardment can block development of the functions of the mind necessary for learning and the integration of psychic life.

Psychoanalysis by its nature provides a prompt alternative model of relations—steady, sustained, and meaningful, rather than erratic, instant, and virtual. This kind of therapeutic help can strengthen the emerging ego and superego formations and work through the anxiety and disturbance of the over-excitable latency child exposed to the incessant manic stimuli of modern life.

References

Freud, A. (1937). *The Ego and the Mechanisms of Defence.* London: Hogarth and the Institute of Psychoanalysis.

Freud, A. (1966). *Normality and Pathology in Childhood.* London: Hogarth.

Freud, S. (1905). Three essays on the theory of sexuality. *S. E., 7.* London: Hogarth.

Freud, S. (1924). The dissolution of the Oedipus complex. *S. E., 19.* London: Hogarth.

Freud, S. (1926). *Inhibitions, Symptoms and Anxiety. S. E., 20.* London: Hogarth.

Clinical

CHAPTER EIGHTEEN

"Finding the strength to say hello"—issues of male identification and separation/individuation in a two-year intensive psychotherapy

Natalia Stafler

Introduction

The story of Peter Parker, better known as Spiderman, is well known: an ordinary boy, an outsider, albeit very intelligent, struggles with his confidence and his ability to establish himself in social relations. By chance and through no means of his own, he is bitten by a genetically enhanced spider and acquires superpowers. Suddenly he is faced with the ongoing struggle between continuing his ordinary and lonely life and devoting his life to the higher good of saving humankind from evil perpetrators which would inevitably earn him the admiration of the common people, including his childhood sweetheart. In the end Peter Parker's confrontation with this dilemma facilitated a stronger belief in himself as Peter and not just as Spiderman and his ability to perform and relate to others in real life improves as a result.

Conversely, my little patient Kenny was faced with the dilemma of having to give up omnipotent superpowers, albeit imaginary, in order to allow himself to get in touch with the ordinary five-year-old boy inside him. He had to learn to relate to others in a genuine object related way whilst at the same time gaining a sense of self that enabled him venture into the "real world". His increasing ability to play allowed him to become creative and spontaneous without fully submerging himself in an imaginary world.

The therapy dealt with Kenny's narcissistic defences that guaranteed him a fantastical world of his own, albeit not object related. At the beginning of therapy his inability to tolerate any demands from the external world or accept frustrations was particularly striking. Narcissistic vulnerability obscured the degree of disturbance. At first it was difficult to ascertain the extent of Kenny's narcissistic disturbance and whether his underdeveloped and defective defence organization would lead, as Anna Freud describes, to an "irruption from the id rather than to compromise formation between id and ego" (1966b, p. 154). It was evident that Kenny has not yet reached the phallic-Oedipal phase with the formation of a superego to help him control inner forces of aggression and guilt. This led to an apparent struggle of modifying his identifications with the masculine, more aggressive aspects of his self which at first could only emerge in the form of sadistic fantasies.

I will describe the two-year journey with Kenny, initially in intensive four times weekly psychotherapy and subsequently twice weekly therapy, through different developmental stages, in and out of fantasy and into an Oedipal struggle which, however, is still ventured into with apprehension and frequent regressions. I will demonstrate Kenny's progress which, unaided by magic or genetically enhanced spiders, took place within the therapeutic relationship.

Referral and family background

Kenny was referred soon after his fifth birthday. Recent changes in the family's lives (separation from father and a subsequent move) had brought into focus long-standing difficulties. Kenny was described as a difficult baby with a sensitive disposition, crying inconsolably and finding it difficult to assert himself. At the time of referral he was reported to be shy and insecure, unable to stand up for himself and with a tendency to burst into tears, resulting in a number of temper tantrums per day. Prior to the referral he had developed a stammer and was still bed-wetting at night (wearing nappies). He was underachieving at school and was placed in a group of children with special needs, raising the parents' concerns that Kenny might have learning difficulties inherited from one of them. The parents did however contemplate the idea that his problems at school were of an emotional nature and interfered with his capacity to learn. School also reported an incident that involved soiling during the day.

Kenny is the older of two, his sibling being just under a year younger. The parents were in their early twenties when mother unexpectedly fell pregnant. Abortion was contemplated but instead they decided to get married and try to make the relationship work. The parents described being at a loss with the newborn baby, unsure how to care for him and overwhelmed by exhaustion and inexperience, struggling to bond with this "difficult" baby, feeling unable to be in touch with his feelings. Mother's own bleak history seemed to have increased her difficulties in relating to her newborn's dependency and neediness. She lost her own mother to a sudden death when still a young child and her father subsequently broke down, leaving her without any parental support. Mother recalled her first really positive memory of Kenny when he at two and a half asked her for a cuddle with his arms open wide.

In spite of a turbulent marriage and difficulties looking after their son, mother fell pregnant again shortly after Kenny was born. The birth of his brother coincided with Kenny's attempts to negotiate separation/individuation. Both children were exposed to parental arguments and fights as well as witnessing their parents under the influence of alcohol and drugs which at times escalated into perverse behaviour.

When Kenny was four years old the parents eventually separated after mother had met somebody else. She and the children moved in with her new partner, who was described as very sensitive, caring, and welcoming of the two boys. Mother also emphasized the importance and good relations of the new partner's extended family, highlighting the isolation that probably dominated their life prior to the new relationship.

In spite of the separation, contact with their biological father remained constant and the children spent time with him on a regular basis. This was ongoing throughout Kenny's therapy. His attendance was usually good and regular; however, it faltered after longer breaks.

Saying "Hello" or something like that

Meeting Kenny for the assessment

Even before I met Kenny, he and his brother had attracted some attention in the waiting room. As I came to greet him I could not fail to notice the similar looks of the children and mother, all parading an identical haircut, and identical hair colour and eyes. Kenny did not separate easily from mother, who seemed surprised by this. When I suggested that Kenny might want to show her the room we would be in, she asked if it was OK to leave her younger son behind in the waiting room, eliciting strong and immediate protest. This little incident offered a first insight into her struggle to ascertain her importance in the life of her two children as well as misinterpreting issues of rivalry, sameness, and differences between the two children.

Once in the room Kenny remained in the background whereas his younger sibling immediately ventured for the toys and seemed to try to take over the room, mother, and myself. When Kenny was ready to let mother go his brother tried to sneak out with some toys in his hands and did not give up his attempt to smuggle something out of the room even after being "found out".

Once alone in the room Kenny became active. He took the hand puppet and made it spew fire all around the room, voicing his aggressive, destructive, and damaging feelings as well as his pleasure in them.

Then the following took place:

> Kenny approached me with the puppet on his hand and made it stop in front of me. I formed my hand like a puppet and faced his. He laughed and started to open and close the puppet's mouth. I did the same with my fingers and for a few moments we were mirroring each other, looking at different sides of the room and back at each other. He then started to eat up my hand with his puppet. I reacted in surprise, wondering what was happening. Kenny replied that he was eating my puppet because there was "none".

The first moment of real contact, of my hand and his puppet saying hello, was ended by an act of oral incorporation, leaving none, eradicating the existence of my pretend-puppet. There was a sense that he could only allow the other to exist as part of Kenny, inside of him, without any identity or sense of a separate self.

This sequence was followed by a very sadistic and aggressive killing and murdering of the animals in the room, who could all magically be kissed alive again, just to be killed with even more pleasure. Whilst in fantasy Kenny seemed to be able to express his murderous thoughts without a trace of anxiety. When brought back to the here and now, Kenny hid away from me and seemed unsure how to relate and what to expect, voicing inappropriate requests like asking me to lift my shirt so he could see my body. I also noticed his rather piercing look, which felt as if he wanted to crawl inside me, and become one with me.

This feeling was borne out during the second assessment session, when Kenny expected me to know what was on his mind, becoming increasingly frustrated when I was unable to guess or understand him immediately, indicating our separateness. We got particularly stuck on Kenny trying to make me guess "Spiderman", which he initially tried to draw and subsequently explained to me with the help of the word "betick". My ignorance that this was Spiderman's action of shooting out the web from his hands was met with disbelief, confusion, and an apparent stronger need for us to merge, exemplified by Kenny's coming closer and closer with his face, repeating this word "betick" over and over again, as if like this he could make me understand.

After the assessment I was struck by the oddness in Kenny and in the quality of our engagement. Although I felt that Kenny showed some interest in the idea of making contact, this felt void and without substance, making me wonder about the narcissistic nature of his pathology. Sandler and Nagera (1963) discuss different forms of self-esteem regulation, suggesting that it is usually children with lowered narcissistic cathexis of the self that create daydreams in which they play a central or heroic role. I also understood the strangeness of his relating to me in relation to his poor sense of self, lack of theory of mind, and problem in asserting himself as a separate subject. His difficulties in making sense of affective states, anxiety, and feelings in general seemed to leave him vulnerable and depleted of coping strategies of external as well as internal dangers.

About monsters, murderers, and sleeping tigers

As therapy commenced and became established, Kenny worked hard to try to make sense of this new arrangement and the reasons for coming to therapy. Most striking was his struggle to relate to me and make use of me as an object. Kenny would either be fully engaged in playing out his sadistic fantasies in detail with the animals, cowboys, and soldiers; or at other times he would relate to me in a pseudo-adult way. During our second session, in the midst of a rather violent killing of the horses and the people, Kenny got up and said to me that he wanted to chat, making me sit opposite him on a chair. He then ventured into an account of his worries, of his fear of a troll who comes at night to kill his mother and brother, his fear of monsters that would appear suddenly from behind, emerging from the wall, wanting to either stab him or drag him back into the wall. Kenny seemed genuine in his plea for me to help him with these worries.

However, there was little sense of me helping him understand these, rather an expectation that I should be able to get rid of them, without his contribution. This was exemplified by his rather genuine questions whether he still needed to come back tomorrow, now that he had told me everything. When I questioned this idea he replied that he thought he could just leave all his worries here, or even better, lock them into one of the lockers. Although Kenny's account of his worries raised a number of questions in relation to his aggression and his fear of engulfment, I was mainly struck by the idea of being able to get rid of worries, of evacuating them through telling me about them. Later in treatment this very similar idea was represented by Kenny's frequent request to use the toilet, usually in sessions that dealt with his anger and frustrations.

It was very early in his therapy that I was faced with Kenny's inability to tolerate frustration and his flight into fantasy when faced with limitations and boundaries to his omnipotence. The notion of me as a separate being with a life extending outside the therapy room was met with nothingness, as if separateness simply did not exist. He would not acknowledge me in the waiting room or on the way to the therapy room. Our togetherness could only begin once in the room, as if contained within a safe womb, shielded from any external realities and any possibility of separation. Even within these boundaries Kenny managed to eliminate any notion of otherness or intrusion. His initial curiosity and exploration of the room and the locker came to a halt by only the fourth session. Having been curious about the other lockers present in the room as well as faced with the frustration of not being able to find out about their contents, Kenny abandoned his interest in his own locker and toys and no play material was used for almost four months.

There was a sense of Kenny's inability to bear restrictions and the accompanying frustration and anger about the presence of other children, maybe giving an indication of how he had experienced the birth of his younger brother. In the therapy room he pretended that the cause of his frustration (the lockers and the children) simply did not exist.

Instead of toys, Kenny and I had to use our bodies, enacting repeatedly sadistic fights and furious battles. There seemed to be little space for symbolization or separateness as I was made to enact the characters of his screenplay, without being allowed to bring in anything of my own. Interpretations or general variations on my part were not accepted. Kenny desperately needed to be in omnipotent control of our interactions and myself.

In the countertransference I found myself either increasingly bored or empathically engrossed with Kenny. I came to understand the boredom as stemming from my inability to assert myself as a separate being relating to Kenny, who seemed to use me as an extension of himself. I was allowed to play and be part of his fantasy as well as empathize with him; however, I was not to comment or assert myself in any way. At the same time there were moments during which I found myself enacting his fantasy play together with him, being interested and empathically involved, not only trying to understand what was going on but actually feeling his distress and pain.

> Kenny was lying on the floor and then pointed out a tiny insect, asking me if it was an ant. Unsure, he decided to call it "animal". He then tried to make it crawl onto his hand but the "animal" would not comply and crawled in the opposite direction instead. After trying a few more times he started to deliberately block the way and then started to touch it, at first tentatively and then more forcefully. I sensed that he was getting a bit frustrated and commented on how he wanted the insect/animal to crawl on his hand and do what he wanted to. In a whiney voice he said that he just wanted to hold it, he was not going to hurt it. I acknowledged this and wondered if maybe he did feel actually quite angry at the insect/animal for not wanting to be held. Kenny agreed and then flipped the "animal" around, making him lie on his back, helpless. I said that he was letting the insect/animal and me know what he thought about it not doing what he wanted. Now Kenny tried to flip it back, saying that he did not want to hurt it. He managed to turn it around and the insect/animal started to crawl again. Kenny seemed relieved and I talked about how worried he had got about having been able

> to hurt it. I was ignored while he turned the animal on its back again and then back around. He then suddenly got up, directing his attention to another part of the room. As I checked on the insect it was dead.

The horror of his capacity to kill this insect, which in both our minds had grown to be an animal, as well as the fact that he was able to kill it in my presence, was terrifying for Kenny and made both of us into murderers. I was overwhelmed with regret and guilt for allowing this to happen and found myself almost losing track of the fact that it was an ant that had died and not a human that had been killed. For the rest of the session and a number of sessions to come the room was filled with monsters and bugs, which could enter his body and control him from inside, showing his doubt at my ability to help him regain control over his aggressive impulses, wishes, and fantasies. There was a sense of Kenny feeling unsafe and unprotected in the room, resulting in fantastical, violent, and aggressive figures entering our room, which Kenny could fight, in the form of a super-hero.

It soon became clear that Kenny was convinced that the only way to fight and face these feelings was with omnipotent means and superpowers, providing an insight into the strength of his aggressive impulses. These overwhelming feelings of insecurity and lack of safety were thought about in relation to the parents' initial helplessness when Kenny was born, and their apparent difficulties to help him mediate his own murderousness while struggling to protect him from their own mutual aggression and the very mixed feelings they encountered towards their newborn son.

It also made me remember Kenny's inhibition during the first assessment session, when he allowed his brother to take over the room, remaining in the background until he was gone, and capable of giving way to his anger and aggression without the risk of really hurting or killing. I was therefore left wondering about the protective function of Kenny trying to keep me under his omnipotent control. As long as I was regarded an integral part of him I was protected from his rage and aggression and he was protected from the anxieties that this new relationship might cause him.

Kenny's struggle to modify his aggression was further exemplified by a repetitive game of sleeping tigers, where both of us needed to be careful not to wake them because otherwise something horrible would happen. The super-heroes were the only ones who could fight these tigers, and Kenny continued to be surprisingly absent in the sessions. It was a struggle to bring his five-year-old self, and instead Kenny came dressed up as a different super-hero for every session. He also persistently insisted on being one year older with every session, suggesting his difficulties of being just a five-year-old boy, with its limitations as well as pleasures and an ability to rely on the adult to help him modify his aggression.

This in turn made it difficult for him to use the male, aggressive part of himself, and he voiced concerns about looking like a girl and never being able to become as big and strong as his rather idealized father. Whenever Kenny seemed for a moment to be in touch with his five-year-old emotions they were accompanied by feelings of humiliation, shame, and sadness as well as a fragile sense of self, feeling misunderstood and isolated. To convey this he developed a nonsense language that made it impossible for us to communicate, in spite of being in such close proximity. In one session he told me the story of a little boy, whose name everybody had forgotten, including his mother.

Confusions

As my work with Kenny progressed I found myself feeling increasingly confused by this boy. There was a sense of our relating taking place on two levels. I was either made redundant as part of his fantasy play or else I found myself overly involved and empathic towards him, feeling his pain and sadness and a profound closeness in the room. I came to understand my role as serving as an extension to his omnipotence rather than a separate person with the ability to retain my own thoughts in the midst of overwhelming feelings.

I also became increasingly aware of the intensity of Kenny's struggle to move away from the oral and anal phase of functioning and allow himself to explore more age-appropriate pre-Oedipal and Oedipal concerns. In "real life" this was supported by his reluctance to give up the nappies at night-time, suggesting his regressive tendency as well as a worry of growing up into a "big boy". A rather strong libidinalization of his anality, conveyed in his fantasy play of indulging in his faeces and urine, suggested some perverse and rather disturbing tendencies in Kenny. In his "Three Essays on the Theory of Sexuality", Freud (1905) makes the link between the narcissistic object-choice and retention of the erotic significance of the anal zone. Kenny's overt investment in his body and its faeces suggests the use of his body as a means to gratification without the need for an object.

It was in relation to this that the first real frustration within the psychotherapeutic relationship took place and I finally decided to assert myself as a separate person unwilling to go along with his perverse fantasies. Kenny had come dressed up as yet another super-hero and we were playing "school", and I was reproached for making mistakes in my work. Kenny therefore decided it was time for a lunch break, which he used to indulge in "wee" and "poo", pretending to smear it all over his face in apparent delight. I meanwhile, was made to sit and eat my own lunch:

> Kenny then decided that I also had to eat his pretend "poo", threatening trouble if I refused to. I refused and instead talked about how much he wanted me to become an ally and part of this. He kept on insisting that I ate it, pretending to stuff it in my face, however remaining unsuccessful in making me pretend to eat. Slightly defeated at my refusal to go along and pretend to eat the faeces, he suggested that we should pretend I had eaten it but I refused to even pretend that I had. He insisted to just pretend. He increasingly felt more frustrated with me, telling me that I was not playing his game right, that I was destroying it all and that we could not play like this.

During this play there was no sense of inhibition or shame and everything was allowed and possible in "pretend" mode, giving way to perverse tendencies as well as a fixation in the anal phase. My refusal to play along, even in "pretend" mode, was felt to be destructive of the play at first, but it gave Kenny a certain sense of security in experiencing that his omnipotence was not real and that the extent of his powers over me was limited.

While the therapy room was invaded by this murderousness, aggression, and perversity his mother reported a marked improvement with Kenny: his tantrums had ceased, he was now settling in school, and fighting less with his brother. Having been faced with overwhelming aggression and murderousness throughout the term, I found myself slightly more hopeful that

Kenny's ability to bring his worries to the therapy room allowed him to develop outside and gain control of his impulses, without feeling too overwhelmed by them. There was a sense that my willingness to engage with him and to engage in his fantasies as well as to recognize and empathize with the pain and horror of his feelings might have helped him move out of his defensive omnipotence to explore other ways of relating.

Saying "Hello": our second attempt

Our first winter break from therapy was experienced as a real narcissistic blow to Kenny. There was a sense that the break reminded Kenny of the two of us being different and separate and he spent almost the entire first session back trying to eliminate these differences, wanting me to magically know what was happening inside his head. Although Kenny clearly had missed coming to his sessions I was left in doubt whether he had missed me as a separate person or just an extension to himself.

He returned for his sessions dressed as Spiderman, and there was a sense that on the one hand he was desperately trying to hide his more vulnerable side which actually did mind the break, whilst on the other hand allowing just these vulnerable aspects into the room for the first time. Kenny wanted to present as the invincible super-hero and spent a lot of time trying to reunite us, as if the break had never taken place. At the same time he offered me a glimpse of the vulnerable, lonely, and "not so clever" side of himself, asking me for help in remembering different characters of different movies as well as reporting his real struggle in making friends and participating in activities with them.

The lack of the acknowledgement of his locker also seemed to tie in with his sense of feeling little, vulnerable, and forgotten. It was only five months into his therapy that Kenny actually made an attempt to rediscover the toys in his locker. He was clearly pleased to see that everything was still in its place, kissing the play-dough for not having dried out, for remaining intact in spite of his denial and disregard for his locker. The joy was, however, short-lived since the rediscovery of his locker revealed his feelings of rivalry and jealousy about the existence of the other lockers. He appeared dressed as super-heroes, suggesting a retreat into omnipotent defences when faced with anger around separation. He was feeling disadvantaged in relation to sibling rivalry and the thought of other children taking up space in our room and possibly in my mind. In spite of this he persisted in asking for the key to his own locker, exploring its contents with apprehension as well as curiosity.

Now that Kenny had started to use the play material provided in his locker to express his dilemmas and conflicts, there was a sense of space having been created in the room, which could be used by both of us for thinking and understanding.

At the same time Kenny started to express some real interest in me (commenting for example on days I was wearing my glasses), attempting to renegotiate his relation to me as a different and separate object, with a mind capable of holding and remembering him. He would test me at the beginning of sessions if I remembered what we had done the previous session, obviously delighted when I was able to, in spite of him trying to trick me. It was only within this more object related relationship that a full treatment alliance was established, and Kenny worked hard together with me to try to make sense of his now symbolic play, conveying the depth of his muddles and confusions as well as a progressive pull towards understanding. I was surprised and impressed with the rather insightful and clever boy, who seemed able to make use of his creativity and to feel pride in his achievements, in addition to increasing insight.

Through his play Kenny was now able to convey his internal world and struggle to me, spending an extensive amount of time trying to make sense of his external family situation and his real muddle about which baby belonged to whom and how anybody could have two fathers. Consciously he seemed very clear in this regard. He told me how his mother had been married to his father, when one time she went shopping, where she met the new partner. They saw each other, fell in love and Mum then left Dad. After this account he asked me whether I now understood how he had come to have two dads. This story conveyed Kenny's deep sense of being replaceable. People could be disposed of the moment something or somebody else makes an appearance. This was very much understood also in relation to the appearance of his brother and Kenny's own concern about being replaceable.

Through the use of displacement (onto the tigers) Kenny tentatively started to explore his murderous feelings towards his brother. His play centred around a deep concern about babies, a wish to dispose of them as well as a worry of the babies being taken away:

> Kenny started playing with the snappy crocodile and told me that he was on the tiger's team and helped steal everybody else's babies. As he was playing he mistakenly called me by his brother's name. He looked at me and smiled, telling me that he had just called me that name. I took the giraffe and made her wonder if maybe Kenny had been thinking about his brother just when talking about the snappy crocodile who made babies go away. He made the crocodile answer to the giraffe that she was "clever" before looking at me and saying that he did not really want his brother to go away. I commented on his worry that thinking and wanting something might make it happen for real. Kenny replied that he thought I would be saying something like this, before taking the giraffe from me, saying that now he would be the "clever one".

Although omnipotent fantasies still tended to invade Kenny's thinking, he seemed more able to step out of them. Also, Kenny's new-found ability to actually experience remorse, shame, and conflict around his aggressive fantasies was understood as a progressive step in integrating and relating to his objects as a whole. There was a sense of both of us now being able to retain an observer function, capable of reflecting and thinking as opposed to acting.

Transference

During and throughout the second term of therapy Kenny developed a very positive and loving transference to me that made being with him enjoyable and fun. I found myself looking forward to our sessions, and Kenny openly expressed his trust and love towards me while continuing to explore and think about this new-found relationship. During one session, approaching the break, Kenny insisted on leaving the room with his toys outside his locker. I commented on his apparent difficulties in believing that I could still think about him, even if we did not see each other and even if his toys were not left scattered all over the room. Kenny looked at me and smiled shyly. I commented on his look, and he said that this would be like "love".

His very positive transference in turn made it even more difficult for Kenny to acknowledge and contemplate the idea of having to share me with other children. Once, after seeing me with another patient, a boy slightly older than him, I found myself vigorously trying to make Kenny accept my interpretations about his emerging anger and jealousy. Kenny, however, ignored my comments and all attempts to interpret to such an extent that I found myself wondering whether he had actually seen me with the other boy or whether my own anxieties and feelings of guilt had got the better of me:

> Kenny engaged in solitary play, leaving me out, ignoring me. I watched him play on his own, and feeling increasingly confused, remained in the background. After a considerable amount of time without talking (apart from Kenny's noises as he made the figures fight and kill each other), I commented on Kenny playing as if I was not there. Kenny looked at me and said: "Like with the boy in the waiting room." Now I was even more confused (had he seen me or not?), and Kenny explained that he pretended I was not here like he pretended that the boy in the waiting room was not there.

I was struck by Kenny's own insight into his defences, increasingly convinced that his omnipotence and denial were used defensively rather than indicative of a more profound narcissistic pathology. At the same time there was fragility around these defences and an almost immediate retreat into either fantastical omnipotence or messy and anal modes of coping when faced with frustration and anxiety.

Kenny now expressed a growing curiosity about differences between boys and girls, which increasingly gave way to his struggle to identify with a male object, complicated by a deep-rooted confusion about the sexes and adult relationships. Kenny seemed to hold on to the notion of the phallic mother and openly expressed his wish to be a girl, envying her ability to have babies. I observed that when he was brought to the clinic by his highly idealized father, Kenny was able to express his aggression in a more role-appropriate way, skipping stairs and taking risks instead of being the good, well-behaved little boy. In relation to me he tried to find out if I could like and support him as a boy, or if I preferred Barbie over Spiderman.

As Kenny continued to explore this field, and moved tentatively into a more Oedipal state of relating, he was able to present his worries around masturbation, and castration anxiety, as well as strong feeling of guilt for having "sexy" thoughts. During one play he made the crocodile bite off the elephant's tail and, holding it in his hands, he said that without the tail the elephant was not a real elephant, he needed his tail for fighting. This was followed by vigorous attempts to stick the tail back on as well as Kenny's fantasies of intercourse as a rather aggressive act, involving the elephant spraying water onto the giraffe. His confusion about the genitals was striking as Kenny was trying to figure out whether the elephant's tail was used for fighting or rather defecating. Infantile sexual ideas around intercourse were predominant in the material of this now six-year-old boy. They highlighted his deep struggle and made me wonder about the extent of his confusion about the sexes, as well as what he might have witnessed as a child in relation to his parents' sexual relationship.

With the long summer break approaching, themes around sibling rivalry and Oedipal issues faded into the background, and Kenny became openly concerned about the break and the loss of his sessions and new-found space. His feelings of rejection were conveyed on anal, pre-Oedipal as well as Oedipal levels, depending on the strength of his accompanying anger. The angrier he was the more regressed and messier his expressions (making the cars defecate all over my room, encircling me so that I was unable to leave). As opposed to the previous, shorter break, Kenny now seemed able to convey his difficulty, sadness, and dilemmas around his feelings of rejection, and was surprisingly open about his attachment to me, almost confessing his love and need for me. At the same time he found ways of expressing his ambivalence, which was strongly felt in the countertransference and my own sense of disengaging prematurely, maybe like him, to avoid the actual separation. In relation to this he showed an increasing interest in the calendar, wanting us to continue it "for ever", marking the date we would be back with a smiley face and a smiley man, exemplifying that now he could actually trust me to be back, happy to see him, in spite of the long break.

When it was time to say goodbye before the summer Kenny, still in the room, waved and said "Bye," adding that now he had said it. In the waiting room Mum encouraged him to say "Bye" again and told him to give me a hug. Instead, Kenny picked up a big teddy bear who he hugged with affection. In spite of his mother's suggestion, Kenny was able to make use of his new-found assertiveness, and capacity for transitional objects and space, leaving me convinced that he would be able to hold on to the sessions as well as to the belief that I, too, would be able to hold on to him in my mind. The worry of either of us drying out (like he imagined the play-dough would), seemed to have been overcome by his positive feelings. We had finally managed to find each other, as separate beings.

When saying "Hello" is not so easy after all

After the summer break mother failed to bring Kenny back to his sessions or to make any contact. Returning a phone call she conveyed her impression that Kenny was doing really well, that she did not have any further concerns, and that she thought it was not necessary to bring him back to therapy. It seemed that lack of contact with the clinic during the break had brought back for mother feelings of abandonment, associated with the loss of her mother as a child and a need for self-sufficiency. Eventually she came to understand that terminating Kenny's therapy was not in his favour.

The beginning of therapy was therefore delayed and mother struggled to bring him regularly. This left both Kenny and myself in the dark about when we would meet again, having sporadic meetings and usually not seeing each other more than twice a week. It was not until the middle of the term that we contracted for Kenny to continue his therapy, however with the prospect of reducing session frequency.

The material in the sessions was dominated by Kenny's sense of disappointment with me. He experienced the difficult start as proof that I had not been able to remember and hold on to him and that I did indeed prefer other children over him. Furthermore, the break might have elicited feelings related to the separation from his father and the subsequent move. Especially in the beginning he was concerned about who else had been in the room and who had taken over his time with me.

However, unlike in the beginning of therapy, Kenny did not retreat into omnipotent fantasies, taking on the role of super-heroes, but instead seemed to be defending himself against the painful feelings by pretending not to register or hear me (he would start the session by putting his head down the corner of the couch, reminding me very much of an ostrich who does not want to see and does not want to hear). There was a sense of the rather manic denial being replaced by a more subtle and depressive mood, serving to suppress the angry and aggressive feelings towards me and Mum for jeopardizing his therapy.

As he continued to struggle with themes around aggression, there was a sense that Kenny had to re-explore if he still had the permission to allow himself to show me these feelings. They were usually displaced onto the tigers, with Kenny disowning them by pretending not to be in the room. The tigers came to represent the most frightening part of his self, while he, Kenny, pretended to have no recollection at all.

Through his play he seemed to try to find out if it was indeed his anger and murderousness that has caused the break between us as well as the impending reduction in sessions. The fact that the sessions did not start as planned might have been experienced by Kenny as a confirmation of the omnipotence of the aggressive and angry feelings he had for me for taking a break in the first place. The regressive pull became especially apparent in the similarity of his play to the early days of therapy; his fantasies dominated by sadistic torture and killing, as well as his refusal to use any of the toys, preferring us to enact with our bodies instead. I came to understand the fragility of Kenny's apparent rapid progress and the strength of the regressive pulls, wondering about the stability of the progress he had made over the past year and his mother's ability to support it.

The sessions were now filled with games of hide-and-seek, clearly conveying Kenny's need to find and be found, to claim and be claimed in the midst of the reduction of his sessions. It took almost the entire term for Kenny to come to terms with this reduction, repeatedly expressing his wish for things to go back to how they used to be. Similar to the first break from therapy, the sudden reduction was felt like a narcissistic blow and exemplified Kenny's ongoing difficulties with accepting boundaries and frustrations. Kenny drew a picture of Spiderman in the inside of his locker, writing "Spiderman to the rescue", conveying his wish for omnipotent powers, however now not claiming to have them inside him, and acknowledging the painful reality as well as his helplessness.

Kenny's difficulties in owning up to his aggression was further emphasized by his belief that his mother would not approve of him if he were to exhibit any aggressive behaviour. There was a clear sense of Kenny's struggle to express his masculine identifications without losing his mother's approval and love. The material continued to convey a strong worry about issues relating to gender and Kenny's attempts to identify with the aggressive male. He was struggling to be in touch with his phallic narcissism, conveying his difficulties with respect to the process of identification and the acquisition of sexual identity (see Edgcumbe & Burgner, 1975). In relation to this, somatic ways of coping with his fear emerged (repeatedly needing the toilet), as well as a tendency to allow aggression into the room only in a regressed, anal way (through passing wind), exemplifying his wish to rid himself of these feelings.

In parallel to this, Kenny showed an increased need to be in control of the beginning and ending of the therapy sessions. He was dealing with the loss of the sessions by taking charge and feeling big and in control and at the same time experimenting with the extent of his own aggression and assertiveness. Anxieties re-emerged with the approach of the second winter break; however, Kenny was able to bring them into the relationship and to allow these worries to be examined, experiencing his anger as well as attachment in a seemingly more age-appropriate way.

I am who I am and if you don't like it just leave the room

Kenny returned from the break without any of the dreaded complications. There was a sense that the smooth return to therapy allowed for Kenny to rediscover a space to explore and think about his worries, rather than trying to expel them and get rid of them. The material in the sessions was dominated by Kenny trying to assert himself as a phallic boy and to explore Oedipal material in a playful and creative way.

In relation to me, Kenny became increasingly more daring, trying to push boundaries and test limits, while still carefully monitoring my reactions, as if testing whether I was supportive of this new development or did not approve of it. The windows in the room, which initially represented a closed womb, were now opened and Kenny would throw out toys or try to lean out himself as if ready to break out. It was during this time that I was informed that with the help of his mother he managed to let go of night-time nappies successfully.

We spent a number of sessions playing made-up board games with strict rules, which only Kenny was allowed to adjust in his favour. While noticing the increasing engagement with latency age activities, I understood this as an attempt to take control in light of rules he feels that adults make without consulting him (i.e. missing/reducing sessions). He conveyed a strong wish to be grown up. However, his wish for power now seemed to be age-appropriate and reality-oriented as opposed to the previous confinement to his own fantastical world. His favourite play figure became the phallic and powerful lion while I was left to use messy play-dough man. During play Kenny chatted a lot to me, for the first time allowing me to be part of his life outside the therapy room. On one occasion Kenny told me with pride about having fought with his brother and how, after having been reprimanded by mother, he suggested to her to just leave the room if she did not like it.

For the first time, Kenny seemed to take pleasure in asserting himself as a phallic boy, whilst also conveying his struggle of having to give up more infantile ways of coping to make way for six-year-old Kenny, who was becoming increasingly aware of his abilities and limitations. He now used the sessions to try to understand his sense of feeling held back and his worries about the nature of his changing relationship with his mother. On the one hand he clearly wanted to break out and "fly away", and on the other hand he felt uncertainty about the stability of their changing relationship. After having observed a pigeon outside our window and watching it fly away, the following took place:

> Kenny took the phone and started to tie the cable around his leg, telling me that he was making feathers. With the phone dangling from his leg he started to run around the room, explaining that these were his feathers and he was flying. I commented on the paradox of flying while at the same time being tied up, and that maybe he was letting me know something about not being able to just fly away and grow up because something was holding him back. He ignored me but as he was "flying" around the room he took more and more furniture

> with him (by entangling it with the cord), commenting on what he was doing. I said that the burden seemed to become bigger and bigger and he now was banging the phone on the floor as he continued to run around the room. I continued to comment on his uncertainties of being allowed to grow up until eventually Kenny asked for my help to untangle him.

Kenny clearly conveyed his wish and need for my help to untangle him, not only from the merged relationship with his mother, but also to receive my permission to untangle himself from the rather idyllic relationship we had been finding ourselves in. He came back one session, asking me for a chess game. I found myself contemplating during and after the session whether I ought to provide him with this game, the first thing Kenny had ever asked for, worrying about the idea of having to spend a number of sessions playing chess. My own dilemma was solved by Kenny's suggestion of making a chess game ourselves. However, I was left thinking about my own difficulties in letting Kenny go and allowing him to develop age-appropriate activities, asserting himself as the six-year-old boy he was, with the inevitable distance and possible boredom this would bring between us. This gave me an insight into Mum's possible struggle of allowing Kenny to separate from her.

Whilst in therapy Kenny continued to struggle with issues of gender identification, separation, and aggression, at home he retreated to wearing and wetting his nappies at night. This regression showed the extent of his difficulties in separating, growing up, and expressing his aggression overtly, rather than hidden away in his nappies. It also made me wonder yet again about the role of aggression within this mother-child dyad. The choice of symptom seemed to be the preferred and more accepted way of expressing aggression for Kenny as well as mother. Rosenfeld (1968) emphasized the unconscious ambivalence which manifests itself in withdrawal of cathexis from the child and can play a crucial role in toilet training and tolerance of age-adequate aggressive behaviour in children. Franco de Masi (1999) further noted the effect of a mother's inability and unconscious unwillingness to allow her child to emerge from symbiosis and to help him acquire an independent identity.

Just before our second summer break the battle of power and control entered the therapy room in a different form. Kenny, now openly able to express his curiosity and interest in me, soon came to understand that this was mutual and that I was just as interested in him as he was in me. With much enjoyment he discovered his ability to withhold information and used this new-found capacity with pleasure, letting me know what it felt like not to know, to be curious and left with the fantasies as well as the frustration. In spite of this I came to learn that Kenny was making very good progress in school as well as achievements in his after-school club, and that he was voted by the other children to become the class representative for next year. Kenny described the number of responsibilities he would have, but most and foremost he was able to convey his relief and joy in having been chosen for being Kenny, without needing help from Spiderman. This recognition allowed him to continue exploring his muddles about Oedipal issues as well as gender identification without feeling ashamed or afraid of not knowing. Kenny left for the summer break feeling secure as to his space in my mind and in my room, certain that I would be there to greet him after the break.

After the summer Kenny only came for five more sessions. The struggle of the past year to return Kenny to his sessions was repeated. The beginning of therapy was simply forgotten—in spite of my name featuring in the diary—and followed by a number of cancellations.

Mother related to me that she has been accepted for a much sought, but demanding training course which meant her having to renegotiate and reschedule daily activities. During a number of phone conversations we agreed to change the session times to accommodate her new schedule. A few minutes before the first scheduled session mother phoned and asked the receptionist to pass me the message that the time was not suitable after all. This was the last time I heard from her and Kenny. Any attempts to contact her remained unanswered.

In the countertransference, I found myself feeling increasingly angry and sad about this sudden, and in my opinion too early, termination of Kenny's therapy. I came to think about the sudden and painful loss I was made to experience as representing the depth of the difficulties between Kenny and his mother around separation and individuation. It seemed that it might have been too painful to allow Kenny not only to grow up, but to make meaningful relationships of his own accord, which mother was not part of. Although we had finally managed to say "Hello", unfortunately there was no opportunity for "Goodbye".

Conclusion

In this paper I attempted to demonstrate Kenny's experience and the therapeutic process within our relationship. In particular I focused on his narcissistic defences and use of aggression, as well as his ability to form relationships, and as Winnicott (1969) suggests, acquired a capacity to "use" the object. In spite of apparent progress in many areas I am very aware of the regressive tendency that remained with Kenny, leaving me with questions about the extent of his narcissistic difficulties, as well as concerns for the development of more perverse solutions that do not require the object for libidinal gratification. Anna Freud (1966b) distinguishes between regressions in favour of development, and permanent regressions during which drive energies remain deflected from their age-adequate aims, and ego as well as superego functions remain impaired, damaging any further progressive development. Given Kenny's progressive pull towards development, separation, and masculine identifications, I was left hoping that he would continue to overcome the regressive tendencies and build upon the work we have been doing during our two year journey.

The transference was used not only to make sense of Kenny's experiences but also to gain a better understanding of the dynamics within the mother-child relationship. My own at times rather hesitant and protective manner towards Kenny made me wonder about both Mum's feelings about Kenny, and Kenny's relation to his mother and his constant awareness of her weaknesses, limitations, and ambivalent and mixed feelings towards him. This was exemplified during our last session, when after yet another exploration about his confusion around sexuality, Kenny turned away from me and said that he would like to come back again four times a week. At this point I understood this as his need for more time and wish for space to explore this important subject that was exciting and worrying at the same time. Given that this was the last time I saw Kenny I am left wondering about how well attuned he was to mother's difficulties in sustaining therapy. His final declaration of his attachment to me can be either understood as a plea for the continuation of therapy or as his way of ensuring he be remembered by me with affection and warmth.

Those of us familiar with the story of Peter Parker are aware that he has not yet found a solution to his dilemma and is still caught up between his real life and the life of Spiderman.

After two years of therapy and maybe especially because of the abrupt ending, I am left wondering about Kenny's ability to find a way to cope as Kenny or if eventually he will have to resort to a super-hero's omnipotent ways of coping.

References

De Masi, F. (2003). *The Sadomasochistic Perversion: the Entity and the Theories*. London: Karnac.

Edgcumbe, R. & Burgner, M. (1975). The phallic-narcissistic phase—a differentiation between preoedipal and Oedipal aspects of phallic development. *Psychoanalytic Study of the Child*, *30*: 161–180.

Freud, A. (1966). *Normality and Pathology in Childhood*. London: Karnac.

Freud, S. (1905). Three essays on the theory of sexuality. *S. E.*, *7*: 125–245. London: Hogarth.

Rosenfeld, S. (1968). Choice of symptom: notes on a case of retention. In: *Beyond the Infantile Neurosis*. London: Goodwin Press.

Sandler, J. & Nagera, H. (1963). Aspects of the metapsychology of fantasy. *Psychoanalytic Study of the Child*, *18*: 159–194.

Winnicott, D. W. (1969). The use of an object. *International Journal of Psychoanalysis*, *50*: 711–716.

CHAPTER NINETEEN

"With great power comes great responsibility"—a new object experience and finding space to be a boy: analysis of a six year old

Paddy Martin

Introduction

Anna Freud, in her book *Normality and Pathology in Childhood* (1965c), outlined the importance of conceptualizing child development in terms of Developmental Lines along which the ordinary child progresses at varying and not necessarily always corresponding rates. Some of the more important lines conceptualized were "progression from dependency" to self-reliance and adult object relationships, from "early suckling" to mature feeding and the attainment of control of bodily functions; alongside the physical paths were important developments in terms of moving from "self-centred" to more reflective and socially minded behaviour. While described in separate terms, these lines of development are of course entwined and reflect each other and it might be said that play and behaviour in the therapeutic setting become the tools by which disturbance or difficulties in development may be addressed.

In this chapter charting the progress of a six-and-a-half-year-old boy described as having an "attachment disorder", I focus on the importance of mixed developmental work and therapy in helping him move back onto a line of development, aspects of which had become fixated and regressive in tendency, impairing many aspects of his biological, emotional, and cognitive development.

Working with Samuel was extremely demanding but also rewarding, and I was often struck by his ability to evoke a fondness in others despite his very difficult behaviour, illustrating that the "indiscriminate" behaviour of the child with attachment disorder, while pathological, is nevertheless a strategy. From the beginning of treatment, it was clear that Samuel's emotional and social difficulties and developmental delay constellated around a particular vulnerability in his attachment insecurity and poorly articulated object relational world. He lacked a sophisticated and emotional grasp of the object world both internally and externally.

He frequently displayed aggressive and defiant behaviour linked to a deeply primitive anxiety about his survival and integrity. Samuel's behaviour was a noisy insistence of his fight for survival, for a space to be in the context of being an unwanted and sometimes unloved baby.

The task of therapy was to address the developmental deficits, and to achieve this by promoting and reflecting upon an authentic relationship as it formed between therapist and child, allowing Samuel to develop some sense of safety in his object world through the mitigating experience of a developing relationship. None of this was achieved by technique alone and perhaps the most important aspect of the work with Samuel was the genuine nature of attachment and bond that formed between us.

Technically, I found myself treading a fine line between open and important interpretation of Samuel's anxieties, and working more in the mode of *developmental therapy*, as described by Anne Hurry et al. (1998), providing something of a holding environment for Samuel in which he was able gradually to integrate his feelings and develop a more sophisticated way of object relating.

So this chapter really describes a process of developmental therapy to help a child move *into* latency, developing ordinary and healthy psychic structures and defences such as symbolization, repression, identification, and inhibition.

Background information

My involvement with Samuel began after he had already been in therapy for some time, as a result of his then current therapist's (necessary) departure. Samuel was originally referred because there were concerns that he was significantly adult focused, and unable to initiate interactions with children. He had difficulties understanding boundaries, displayed angry behaviour such as hitting adults and being verbally abusive, particularly to his father; and he could be very destructive at home. His parents were very concerned by his behaviour and felt at a complete loss to know how to manage him.

Samuel was diagnosed by a consultant psychiatrist as having a marked attachment disorder illustrated by his frequently running away from his parents in the street and inappropriately approaching strangers, asking them to take him home with them. He had ended up at police stations, much to the embarrassment of his parents when they had to collect him; he seemed to enjoy his parents humiliation in this.

Samuel's speech could be very indistinct and hard to understand. He was behind in his school studies, delayed in reading and writing. When I first met Samuel there had been some considerable improvement reported in his symptoms, particularly at school as a result of a year and a half of once weekly psychotherapy with his therapist and ongoing regular work with a speech and language therapist. This progress was apparent not least in Samuel's ability at times to label affects and understand the symbolic aspects of his play, but he was still striking in his presentation as a poorly integrated, affectively dysregulated boy, who was indiscriminate and exaggerated in both bodily and verbal relating to adults, significant or otherwise.

Samuel came from a middle class family. Mr and Mrs P had already been married for sixteen years and Samuel was not a planned child. Mother had two adult daughters by a previous marriage. The parents' feelings about the unexpected pregnancy were deeply ambivalent, particularly for the mother. Samuel was born six weeks prematurely and spent some time in the special care baby unit. Mrs P was very depressed at this time and found it difficult to bond with Samuel.

When he was ten months old Samuel's mother, already struggling, decided that she would combine her task as a mother with work, by running a nursery from home. She thought this would "help" with looking after Samuel and was surprised that it made matters worse; Samuel could not stand the presence of other babies at home and he would stay in his room for long periods. If he did come out, he would be very quiet and withdrawn.

Consequently, there were significant factors in Samuel's early development both in constitutional and environmental terms that interacted in a complex way. While his mother's post-natal depression, difficulty bonding, and ambivalent feelings towards the pregnancy were clearly significant factors blighting the facilitating environment, his constitutional development will have been affected by his prematurity of birth. Equally, being born premature and kept in an incubator in a special care unit for the first few weeks of his life would have interfered with his parents' ability to form a bond, to hold their child, however mixed their feelings may have been.

It seems that right from the beginning of his life, Samuel's experience of holding and handling, of being in the mind of the other was severely disrupted. Such disruptions can be seen as contributing to cumulative and early relational trauma (Baradon, 2010) and will be experienced somatically, impacting upon regulatory mechanisms, expressed and re-expressed through implicit rather than explicit memory. Samuel, while having gained some insight from his therapy to date in understanding his feelings, was nevertheless unable to contain and manage affects at a bodily level, and his unpredictable, challenging, and risky behaviour when his security felt threatened was dominated by an over-activation of the bodily stress mechanisms. His impulsive behaviour and taking action when anxious seemed linked to unprocessed activation of the limbic system, a literal fight or flight response that stamped its hallmark on a troubled and disorganized attachment.

At age six, when I began work with him, Samuel was still frequently running off from his parents and proving difficult to control. Developmentally, he was delayed in his speech, toileting, and sleeping, returning most nights to his parents' bed. He had great difficulty relating to peers, often shying away, and school reported him as very quiet and responsive, but preferring adult direction. The transition from one therapist to another had led to some serious regression as Samuel was faced with this loss. It appeared that more was needed and this was a good opportunity to increase the sessions to twice weekly. In terms of the physical and developmental aspects of this particular therapy, the increase in sessions made a great difference to the overall experience of the therapeutic environment for Samuel.

First meeting

In their book *Techniques in Child Psychoanalysis* (1980), Sandler and colleagues talk about the issues around managing a change of therapist, which however difficult can be a valuable experience for the child and in terms of learning about his or her own particular object relationships. As they say, "A successful changeover requires that the child establish a treatment relationship with the new therapist *and recognizes* as well, that he is relating to a different person from the previous therapist." In this case, the transition became all the more meaningful as Samuel's previous therapist was female and he was now embarking on a therapeutic relationship with a male therapist.

While there was a transition of therapist, the parent worker remained constant, and this greatly helped to protect the therapy. While Samuel's therapist met with him for the last time, just prior to a holiday break, I met with his mother before we all met together to facilitate the changeover. I was due to begin seeing Samuel on his own after this break.

As I listened to Samuel's mother, I got a strong sense of her embarrassment and frustration with him. She began with a warning tone saying, "I don't know how much you know about him ...", before going on to describe how difficult he was to handle; saying she was at a loss to understand him. She could not stand all the noise and aggression; he was so unlike the rest of their family. It was as if Samuel was an alien body to her. She spoke of her mixed feelings when he ran off, part of her wanting to just let him go. She often felt ashamed with him outdoors and would give in to his demands to keep him quiet. Her husband, she said, was more easy-going but too lenient and allowed Samuel to act terribly towards him; she told me, "He uses words no six year old should use." She observed that Samuel had been a lot worse recently, without reflecting on the impact of this transition.

When Samuel and his therapist joined us, he was all energy. He burst into the room, making an immediate impression on me as he seemed to lurch around the room haphazardly. He was a slightly overweight boy but also big and he seemed to fill the room; he spoke in a loud, cheerful voice. His smile was engaging and I immediately liked him despite his rather brash manner. At times his speech was quite indistinct. He had an inappropriate, over-friendly manner; he wanted to sit right next to me and told me I was handsome and how *much* he liked me. He approached first his old therapist, then me, bringing his face right up, so that our foreheads were touching, his eyes right next to mine. It felt uncomfortable but I tolerated it and said that I thought he was trying to see right inside me, to see what I was like and if I was like her.

In this first encounter, I was made a "good", liked therapist, and the fact that he was meeting me in relation to losing his current therapist was ignored, except when I directly referred to his comparing us: Samuel's response being to collapse briefly but theatrically to the floor. In terms of how the change of therapist could reveal Samuel's way of object relating, here was evidence of the disturbed attachment, apparently showing no anxiety in being handed over to an unfamiliar object. His response to me was indiscriminate and idealizing and showed just how lacking was Samuel's sense of a secure base.

As he brought his face up close to mine, in this first meeting, I wondered about this communication. I found myself thinking about Samuel's need to see into me as perhaps a distortion of the gaze between mother and baby; how he lacked this experience, subsequently finding it difficult to regulate the distance between us, physically and emotionally. It was clear that his mother was deeply uncomfortable with this intrusive gaze. I think my ability to tolerate it sent an important message that I could accept Samuel in all his parts without wishing for him to "run off". This was something he tested to the full in the early sessions, often trying, sometimes successfully, to run out of the room; he was surprised, but not distressed the first time I refused to let him do so and by my continuing to keep him in the room.

Regression and disintegration against un-integration

The sense of getting the distance right continued in the early sessions, as Samuel tried to keep all his good and bad feelings split apart, which was played out in terms of the transition from one therapist to another. His idealization of me was unrealistic and equally, he showed no grief or rage in relation to his previous therapist, completely denying the significance of the loss of this relationship and with it any dependency. However, his play was all about transition and comparison as he chose between his old and new toy boxes, and played with two toy farmers pointing out how they were the same, and how they were different.

Extract from the first session:

> He tells me that he likes me as he goes over to the door and puts the crocodile and bear down on the floor by the door. I say he wants very much for us to like each other and to keep his crocodile and bear feelings by the door, and he says, "Yes." I comment on how it is quite hard to come here today. In some ways it is like before, but I am a different person and he does not know what I will be like. He takes the two identical farmers (one has a walking stick) and sets them up opposite each other. He points out to me how one has a walking stick and needs it because he has difficulty walking. The other is okay and does not need it. He takes the farm hand and says that this is the "big boy". I say that this is very similar, he's got two farmers to look after the animals and they are almost the same but not quite. I say, "And then there's the big boy with them." He nods and agrees and I wonder if he feels like he would want to be a big boy sometimes and have both these farmers as his friends. I come and sit next to him at the desk and he looks at me and then away and I sense he is awkward. He asks me if I will turn off the light now. I do so wondering if it felt to him like I was too close. [Session 1]

An important part of the early work with Samuel was around managing this change, helping him to recognize his feelings of loss, however painful, in terms of his therapist, and to relate to me as a different therapist with whom he was continuing the work. His over-stated and immediate liking of me, it seemed, was an attempt to deny any such loss. Sandler (1990) notes a complicated link between separation anxiety and reactions to the change of therapist. Samuel, while professing nothing but good and positive feelings towards me, would act in ways that showed his level of anger and rage at this latest "abandonment" by his old therapist, easily stirred up whenever I was *not* perfect, and enacted in our constant separations each session. This was a developmentally fragile area for Samuel, whose difficulties with early bonding had been exacerbated by maternal depression and a separation at ten months, as his mother began her nursery full of strange babies. This no doubt impacted upon the normal phase of stranger anxiety. In relation to this, Samuel made clear his intense dislike of the baby doll I had put in his new box; he would try to destroy it before ejecting it from the box and placing it out of sight. I saw this not only as an attack on the babies his mother had chosen to take care of, rather than devoting herself to him, but also an attempt to cast out his own baby feelings of vulnerability, shame, and rage.

While Samuel's idealized attachment to me felt uncomfortable at times, it was apparent that he really was trying to make a connection to me as a wanted good object with no bad, rejecting feelings; he would try to take my hand to the room; and when my hand was not forthcoming, he would bump into something, shouting "Ow!", accusing me of being unfriendly, uncaring. I articulated this contrast between an idealized therapist and an uncaring one; how important it felt that I show him in very concrete ways that I like him, and how this linked to the question whether his previous therapist had really liked him and if so, why she had thrown him out, got rid of the "baby" Samuel.

Samuel's ability to hold himself together when anxious was precarious, and invariably my interpretations of these anxieties would send Samuel into a rage, attacking both me and the room, often becoming gleeful as he tested out how much I could bear him, how much he could embarrass me. But in play, he showed his need for help with containing his aggression; gates and fences were needed to keep the wild bear and crocodile separate from the other animals, gates and fences that continually got broken. The two almost identical farmers were needed to help him manage this task. Samuel appeared to recognize the level of his denied dependency and showed me his awareness of the power of this object relationship, as if referring to the more vulnerable feelings he had in relation to me and his need for my strength—he quoted Spiderman, warning me, *"with great power comes great responsibility"*.

Samuel would become extremely anxious if I was not active in the room, and needed to keep us both busy, often attacking my thinking by shouting or singing repetitive pounding soundtracks that were tuneless and grating. I was struck by how irritating and aggressive these attacks felt, more so in fact than his also frequent physical attacks on me, the room, or the box and its contents.

Samuel indicated a dangerous and fragile attachment to a primary object that he did not feel adequately held by. He was furious each time I let him know we were near the end of the session. He played a violent story using the family dolls and a huge plastic plane that he had acquired from the waiting room at the beginning of his first therapy. The plane was filled with the family together going on holiday, but it kept crashing heavily against the walls, the family inside falling out and dying, getting attacked by wild animals, dinosaurs, and monsters. His feelings often escalated until by the end of the session he had completely destroyed everything in the room, thrown over the box and its contents, scattered them, and turned over all the furniture. This wilful disintegration seemed to be a necessary defence against the more terrifying threat of un-integration.

What appeared to be most important to Samuel at this early point in the therapy was the idea that he was held in mind by me. The crashing plane was trying to hold all the family together and keep them safe, but became completely buffeted by angry and destructive monsters; the plane seemed to reflect his internal state. Sometimes the family was destroyed and sometimes it would just manage to land safely. Significantly, it was play carried over from his previous therapist, and linked to the change of therapist; while Samuel was forced to give up one toy box for another, the plane represented a bridge across both old and new. It belonged to neither, and symbolized, I thought, himself in the therapy: an awareness of an overall, ongoing process that precariously strived to help him hold his internal objects together over all the breaks and changes.

In these first sessions, each time I acted differently to his previous therapist, Samuel would be surprised and would invariably push against this unexpected difference, this reminder that I was not her. Through this, we were able to get at his painful feelings of loss. One day, while in the consulting room, Samuel became furious with me for not letting him go to the waiting room to bring in extra toys from there. He tried to push his way past me and was clearly surprised when I stood by the door and told him we were staying in the room. I spoke about how much he was missing his old therapist, how he wanted his old toy box too and he agreed. I commented on how hard it was not to have both and reminded him how last week he had chosen some things from his old box to keep in the new one. He asked me if I had done that and I said that I had and he thanked me. I spoke about how we had been able to keep some of the old toys that reminded him of his old therapist and put them together. He was delighted, exploring the new box and told me, "I'm proud of you." He now felt that he had "loads" of toys. I said that perhaps he was "proud" of me for not forgetting his old toy box completely and keeping something from his old therapist. He agreed, no longer trying to leave the room, and then he asked me if I knew his old therapist, did I ever see her. I reminded him of when we first met all together and I said that now he was letting me know that he really missed her and wondered if she was still around.

Samuel's play for the rest of this session was around exploring the relationship between us and how I differed to his previous therapist; what kind of "farmer" would *I* be, was I able to contain all the animals; was I able to withstand Samuel's own wild animal feelings and still provide something good afterwards in a benevolent way:

> He goes to the box to get all the animals out and sets them up on the table and he asks me to help him. They are all set up in the same direction and are going somewhere. The farmer with the stick is put on one side and he is there to "look after the animals and protect them". Then he takes out the female farmer and says that "he is the one who feeds them". I reflect this statement back to him and how the one farmer looks after and protects while the other has to feed them. He puts play-dough down at the end as "food" and water and tells me that all the animals are good, none of them are nasty. I comment on how they all must be good. But then he puts a fence down one side to keep them together and he has to repair it with sellotape. I comment on how he needs all the animals to be good right now and has repaired the fence to keep them in their place. He talks about how the crocodile is not bad but is very hungry and I wonder if being a very hungry crocodile can lead to bad things happening and feels quite dangerous. [Session 2]

In this early session, Samuel related to the two roles of the farmers, reflecting, in his mind, a sense of how different therapists could give him different things and how this in turn reflected, I thought, parental roles of mothering and fathering. He looked for both these roles in me now, sometimes equating me to the "Daddy" family doll (called Paddy) that needed to be very strong with the little boy, and at other times to the mother. He was concerned that his aggression could be very destructive, making him both dangerous and unlovable. On one occasion, after running out of the room, he played with the calf feeding from the mummy cow and asked me, "Does it hurt the cow when the calf feeds?"

Often, Samuel's feelings of anger or frustration would become too much and he would "act out" directly, smashing the toy plane around the room, throwing items across the room before attempting to rush out of it. I interpreted many of his feelings of anger and loss in terms of the loss of his previous therapist. The frequent running out of the room seemed to combine a need to "escape" intolerable anxiety as well as a wish to "check" that his mother (or father) would still be in the waiting room for him, that he had not destroyed them. It also seemed to be an attempt to find his former therapist. My interpretations were helpful only in the context of physically, sometimes, holding on to Samuel, keeping him contained. Gradually he related to me as a different therapist and allowed himself to acknowledge his loss.

Containment—transition and transitional space

As mentioned, an element of Samuel's aggressive play and running away was his need to "test" me, and I felt it was important to keep hold of Samuel and whenever possible keep him in the room. Despite a sometimes fierce attack, there was clearly relief in this for Samuel, in establishing the boundaries of a setting that contained him without becoming punitive. I felt that Samuel was discovering just what kind of an object I was, that would hold on to him however aggressively or angrily he behaved. I remembered his first looking into my eyes, as if trying to see inside, wondering perhaps what my capacity was to be with and tolerate him.

Klein's concept of the paranoid-schizoid position is helpful when thinking about the use of splitting and projection, as Samuel did when he became overwhelmed by anxiety. When not a disappointing object, I became idealized as the "good" therapist, but when that idealization was frustrated, he became furious and hateful towards me. This hate and rage would become unbearable and was then projected out so that I became for Samuel a potentially terrifying monster, a hulk with fierce red eyes. What was helpful to him was my refusal to play into the projective identification, of *not* "actualizing" this monster (Sandler, 1993), and thereby presenting myself as a different developmental object.

It was important to receive and tolerate all Samuel's projections and thereby take the role of the "container" (Bion, 1962). Samuel found it difficult to bear his own feelings, and at times of high anxiety, thought would stop and action take over, and I thought about how this reflected a baby, a bodily ego that simply had not learned the capacity to think; a baby ejecting raw, unprocessed feelings outwards. My role was not just to withstand these feelings and attacks, but to help Samuel in making sense of them, to act as a receiver of all the raw unprocessed affective mess, and give it *back* in a form that could now be tolerated.

These were pre-Oedipal elements that needed working through for Samuel, before he could move on developmentally. Later phallic strivings, with and against the object, felt far too dangerous without a sense of the object's ability to survive his attacks. He had to learn repeatedly to *use* the object (Winnicott, 1971b) and to see it survive his destruction of it; this was a task that Samuel carried out with some dedication towards me.

Over time, this "containment" gradually facilitated for Samuel a move from fragmentation to integration, which was remarkable and linked to his growing sense of a whole integrated object-therapist, whom he now became concerned about. His wish to repair signalled a move into the depressive position. His ability to do this was detectable from the start of our work together and suggested how much work had already been done with Samuel, so perhaps it is important to recognize that there had been much regression in Samuel in response to the loss of his old therapist. Addressing this transition and loss enabled him to begin moving developmentally and emotionally forward.

One day, Samuel had run out of the room to get a bottle of water, following a comment by me linking my inactivity to his anxiety in relating to a depressed object. Samuel showed me in the next session the importance of helping him to preserve the good object:

> When I go to pick him up, he makes me wait a bit and then comes to follow. He has a toy car in his hand and I tell him that that stays here in the waiting room. He tosses it to the floor and follows me. He goes straight to the box and puts up the "Stay out, beware" sign from the previous session, onto the wall and I comment on his retaking ownership of the room from Friday and wanting perhaps to keep out any bad feelings. He is pleased and amazed to find his water bottle in the box, from Friday. He drinks deeply and thanks me, telling me he is "proud" of me. I reflect on his surprise that I kept the bottle. [Session 7]

This bottle from now on became an important symbolic link for Samuel during this difficult period when he often needed to run out of the room. He would leave his bottle each time, and over time I would refill it. At first, I wondered why I did this, having been so firm about other boundaries, but it seemed important for him; he made a point of drinking from it each session, and its survival intact and his ability then to take in the water from the bottle seemed to represent what was going on between us. Samuel's attachment to me was growing now, in a way that felt more genuine and reciprocal. Despite his angry behaviour, I looked forward to our sessions. But, as his attachment grew, so did Samuel's outbursts around breaks and frustrations. My cancelling a Friday session had a profound impact on Samuel. Initially, he tried as hard as he could to keep me the "good" object before becoming unable to contain his anger and aggression; the bottle and its contents now became poisonous and attacking. He began by attempting to sellotape me to the door of the room, to stick the door shut and to make sure he and I both stayed in the room. I reflected on his wish that we could both stay here until Friday, and his anger that I was going to be away. He told me he wanted me to stay there "forever". When I had to let him know we were coming to the end of the session, he became angry and agitated and tried to attack me with scissors and to tie me up. I took up the angry feelings and confirmed we would see each other again on Monday, but he refused to leave the room and as I began to pack away some toys, he filled his mouth with water from the bottle and spat it at me, showing his oral fury and frustration, repeating this until the bottle was empty and the floor now drenched. It felt impossible for Samuel to keep anything good inside.

Over the next few weeks, I continued to interpret Samuel's anxieties and feelings of rage, but in the context of a therapist who can see him as bad and angry sometimes, and yet bear him and want to see him again. Correspondingly, he began to show a capacity to take more symbolic control of his feelings, at first in quite concrete ways, such as bolting the door. He acted out less and wanted to leave the room less often, instead claiming the space, creating "No entry" signs and "Samuel and Paddy" signs, leaving behind his marks or drawings on the walls, or a mess in the room, demanding I leave it until next time—I would take this up, emphasizing my ability to hold him safe in my mind.

This was a difficult phase in the therapy, addressing Samuel's sense of loss in the context of becoming attached, and it was particularly important that Samuel felt there could be a containing space for all his feelings. He was often challenging of boundaries but there was clearly relief when they were maintained. It helped Samuel to realize that his object could hold a "wholesome" view of him in all his parts, good and bad, without splitting off and projecting the negative aspects.

However, as we neared the long summer break, Samuel's anxiety became greater than he could bear, expressed in angry and destructive outbursts beneath which lay feelings of great deprivation and neediness. My interpretation at this level had a significant impact on Samuel when, just before the break, I spoke of his angry feelings towards me in terms of his *fear* that I might go away and not want see him again:

> No one survives, and I pick up on his fear that somehow, the angry plane has destroyed everyone, the woman, the man and the little monster … He continues to bash the man with the plane for a while and gets quite intense—the man is me and he is the plane. The man flies in my direction and I take hold of him and put my hand around him. Samuel demands it back and I say that maybe I need to think about protecting this man and keeping him safe and Samuel now tells me with irritation, "It's not you, it's just a toy." I say, "But it's what you would like to do to a therapist who goes away." He smiles and holds the plane over his head as if to hit me directly with it. I hold his gaze and he stops … He now wants to know if I am angry at him for breaking the plane. I talk about how worried he is that I am angry at him … He nods and I say, "It seems that there is a lot of worry in Samuel today about me getting angry at him and him getting angry at me." He listens and I say, "And I think then you go away … and spend a lot of time worrying about it and what will happen next time when you come back." He nods to this. I say, "Will I be angry at you? Will I even want to see you?" He nods and says, "Just because I'm angry at you, you're still my friend." I say that I think this is very important to him, that being angry does not mean that we cannot be friends. He agrees, looks at me with his rather dreamy, appraising look and smiles. I say, "Maybe that's part of what you really worry about … that it all gets so messy at the end sometimes and that I might be so angry at you that I would not want to be your friend any more." I talk about how important it is then that I can still look after the man, the woman, and even the monster no matter how angry he is, and he says, "Yes, because you can be angry at someone and still be friends." [Session 18]

As we got closer to the summer break—Samuel then became very good; he seemed desperate not to spoil things in my mind so that I would want him back. It felt important to try to get hold of all the feelings but although Samuel was able to acknowledge some of them, he remained terribly worried about showing his anger now. This led to us making a "book" about our sessions and us, saying goodbye and hello and, most importantly of all, thinking about each other over the break. Samuel was pleased to "tell our story" and to hold on to it. At first, he wanted only smiley pictures of him in the book which I linked to his need to be good; I took up the fear of my having a "shouty" Samuel in mind over the break and then not wanting to see him. Through the book, I introduced the idea that I could have all aspects of Samuel in my mind without the good ones being destroyed. Samuel expressed his fantasies that we could be together on holiday; he drew maps of where we lived and all the important places he went so that everything was all "connected up"—so I would always be able to find him.

In our final session before the break, Samuel brought me three "letters" he had written (one for each week we would miss). Inside each letter were simple pictures of a smiling Samuel; he acknowledged his fear that I would forget him over the break and he wrote that in his book.

> He now wants to do a drawing to add to the book … He tells me it is important that I take it home and at the end of the session he reminds me of it, saying, "That one you must take home." I tell him that I will, that I will keep it with the letters he gave me. On this picture he draws Samuel and then gets me to write, "If you forget me Paddy, don't worry. Because this is a boy who you are going to remember—S". I say how really very worried he is that I might forget him and then just not be there after the holidays to meet him. He nods and we go through the last part of the book. [Session 20]

Identification with the new object

Samuel had moved on to a more integrated object world where aggression and loss did not feel so terrifying, did not threaten him or his objects with complete annihilation, and this freed him to move forward developmentally, to become more concerned with phallic and Oedipal concerns and strivings. He began to display this both positively and negatively as he showed both competitiveness against, and identification with, me.

When Samuel returned after the break, he was initially quiet and subdued; he examined me very carefully and decided I looked different, my hair was different and he tried to push it back into its old shape. When I picked up on his worry that I was still the same Paddy, he frankly acknowledged this and told me he had missed me, and when I spoke of his wondering what I had been doing all this time, while I was not with Samuel, he then told me he had lost the book; he had been worried about telling me this. I took up his fear that I would be angry at him, and not want to see him, linked to his own anger at me over the break and his worry that he had not been able to keep the symbolic link between us alive. Samuel's relief was palpable as he now decided we would make a new book. He wanted to make a reparation.

Over the next few sessions, Samuel's new book, replacing the old book, became an important project—this book would be much longer and Samuel would take more and more paper, covering each sheet with lines for writing our story on. He made it clear that he was thinking about how long *we* would have together, and the old book being replaced by the new book also represented the change from one therapist to another, and inevitable endings.

Surviving the first break had a significant effect upon Samuel; he seemed to have internalized the loss of his first therapist, and the transference to me deepened as he now trusted me, for the time being, to stay. He added my name to his old folder that he had kept, and one day he came to the room showing me proudly how he had brought back the family doll of me that he had taken away in secret. I reflected on his sense that a person *can* go away and come back.

Samuel's struggle with integrating the "good" and the "bad" elements of himself now moved into the symbolic realm—into repetitive drawings and energetic games or stories where good and evil characters battled it out. At times, in the play, Samuel projected bad aspects of himself onto me, now feeling safe enough to make me bad.

As Samuel played out his ongoing battles, I saw signs of more phallic development, sometimes in rivalry and sometimes in a wish to identify with me as a masculine object from whom he could get different things. Interestingly, Samuel's father had begun to take a firmer and more assertive approach with him and this had clearly helped Samuel in feeling more contained, more owned by his father. But it also aroused difficulties in his Oedipal strivings with his father that were further complicated by his relationship with his much older sister, who would taunt Samuel, stirring up powerful feelings of anger and hatred while making him feel small and vulnerable.

He told me of his humiliation that his sister had beaten him in a fight, his difficulty in being, by far, the smallest and weakest in his family yet wanting to identify himself as a strong boy who could become a strong man. Samuel showed a wish to identify with a therapist, who had shown that he could tolerate and be firm with Samuel's aggression and yet be on his side. He wanted help to make sense of these terribly destructive feelings stirred up by feeling so small and helpless, and unable to protect himself; projecting his aggression outwards only left him feeling surrounded by monsters. He related more and more scenes and stories from films that revealed this difficulty.

> "Aragorn was really angry with the monsters," Samuel said. "Gandalf told Aragorn he is outnumbered by thousands of monsters that are not on his side. Aragorn said he would take his soldiers. Gandalf said the horses were restless, the horses were scared. Gandalf said, "I will give you a powerful sharp sword. This is a great one." "Thank you," said Aragorn—"but I hope it is even more powerful and magic. … " As we write the story, I reflect to Samuel on Aragorn being angry at the monsters, a bit like how Samuel gets angry and how he wants very much to fight them, but also, I say, like the horses, he feels a bit scared. He wishes he could be more powerful like Aragorn and fight off these monsters; wishes he could have fought off his sister. Samuel nods to these comments, then continues the story. "Legolas told the dwarf, we will take good care of you. The dwarf went to talk to his friend Aragorn. They started wanting to have the ring and wanting to fight these monsters." [Session 32]

His positive identification with me meant that Samuel was working hard now at trying to contain his angry feelings in the transference. He needed help integrating the negative and positive aspects of his relationship with me. Following his seventh birthday, Samuel *was* able to express his disappointment that I had not gone to his birthday party, and his equal distress at missing his session immediately beforehand; he then cast me in the role of a more complex character, who was both good and bad, but ultimately and importantly helped Samuel, and redeemed himself. This character was then needed to save a helpless little Hobbit with a broken arm.

Samuel's own arm had been hurt in his fight with his sister and seemed to represent his castration anxiety. His identification with me as a strong object was less idealized, but aspiring, and there were indications that fights and disagreements could be repaired sometimes, with help from another, without always ending in disaster. This seemed to indicate Samuel's gradual process of internalization and integration of good and bad elements linked to a more completely mourned object, a wish for reparation and trust in his object relations. His parents now reported considerable improvement in Samuel's behaviour. In our sessions Samuel stayed willingly in the room, and this was mirrored in the external world and his no longer running away. He was learning to sleep on his own, and his interest in learning and writing leapt forward. Samuel's speech became clearer and more distinct and he became interested in his own achievements, seeking approval. School reported great improvement in reading and writing and that Samuel was more able to tolerate frustration and show a desire to master tasks instead.

Remembering—a whole object

At the end of October, after half-term, the department I worked in moved to a new location within the same setting. This raised a lot of anxiety for Samuel and his fear of losing his therapist came back to the fore. We spent lots of time drawing maps of the department and how to find it, how to get from the old one to the new one. Samuel found various ways of symbolizing his anxieties about the half-term break and the move, and was able to use these effectively to help him manage this period. There was some return of his old symptoms but in the main Samuel was able to speak of his fear that he would be forgotten about, his conflict about growing up however much he wanted to be bigger, because he knew that it also meant changes and the end of things, living with his family, coming to therapy. Symbolically, he said goodbye to the old room and began a story of Paddy and Samuel, that he told me firmly was "to be continued ..."; we would finish it when we next met, in the new room.

When Samuel came for his first session in the new premises, I bumped into him with his mother coming into the area and Samuel shouted "Just in time!" He had become extremely anxious. Apparently forgetting the move, his mother had taken him to the old department and found no one there and they became disoriented trying to find their way here. In the new waiting area Samuel quickly explored the space and became friendly with all the new people there. He was excited by the new room, which was bigger and better with extra things, a white board, a sink. He told me, "I am really proud of you!" He again idealized the new and denied the loss of the old. His way of managing uncertainty and anxiety was to quickly appropriate this new environment.

In fact, he soon expressed other feelings; he became very aware now of all the other people that came to this department and his jealousy of my spending time with other children was apparent—he would lock the door to keep himself from running out but also to keep them out. He wished to be the "only" child in my mind and despite his initial delight in the new things in the room, he was troubled by these "shared" resources. He took out all the pencils he considered "not his" from the shared pot.

At the same time, he tried to maintain a good Samuel in my mind, for fear that I would not want to hold on to him, and this linked to another event going on: his mother going on holiday with his two older sisters and Samuel's terrible feelings of loss and abandonment. It was his fear that it was his behaviour that made him unlovable, and he linked his feelings directly to the loss of his first therapist:

> There is more and more fighting in the pictures and his character (Frodo) shouts, "It's not safe here." And I reflect on his not feeling safe, and he talks about his sisters saying to him that they "do not love him any more". I reflect how hard this is and how worried he must be and he tells me about "once" (last Christmas) when his mother said to him that she was "fed up" with him and did not want to live with him any more. I reflect on how hurtful it was and how he was worried he would be left. We talk about his finding it hard to know that his mother loves him when she says she is "fed up" with him, and he agrees; and we touch upon his own angry feelings and how frightening for him it is when he feels angry and his fear is that that will make people leave him. He tells me that he misses H (his previous therapist), and I identify her with the "lady of light" who "looks after" Frodo. He tells me that he misses her a lot but not as much as he will miss me when we finish, but that won't be for a long time. I reflect on his sense of loss and how perhaps he worries that I might get angry at him and "fed up" with him and not want to see him any more … We talk about his fear that H will forget him and he is able to say that he does not think she will forget him completely and that perhaps she misses him sometimes too. [Session 39]

It was clear that Samuel's process of mourning his lost therapist had helped him think about other losses, and to be less fearful that he was the unloved baby. While his mother was away, he got the important job of looking after the plants with his father, symbolically able to hold on to and nurture a relationship. He told me after their return of how he was both crying and screaming with joy to see them again.

As we came up to Christmas, Samuel again tried very hard to be good and expressed in many ways his need for a strong, auxiliary therapist; partly this seemed to relate to his difficulties and fights at home, particularly with his one sister, and his need to explore more fully his confusion around masculinity and being the smallest in the family. In his stories, people became monsters and this reflected the way his mother and sisters changed in his mind when they became angry, overlaid by his own projected angry and hateful feelings. He was again preoccupied with my appearance, that I might change if he became angry with me; he felt these changes in a concrete way, telling me I looked like a monster, or a werewolf; and in turn he identified himself at these times as a horrible, Gollum-like Samuel that I would abandon.

The Christmas break raised a lot of anxiety and anger for Samuel; we needed another book and another calendar but none of it felt like enough. I took up the significance that it was after the Christmas break that his first therapist had started talking of finishing and how this coincided with his mother's being so "fed up" with him over that Christmas, as he reported it, that she "did not want to live with" him any more.

We talked about how we would finish one day, but not at Easter, and I compared this to his learning to sleep on his own—at first he was frightened but now he liked it; he had an easier attachment that allowed him to be more independent. In Samuel's mind, the link between us finishing one day and his being good or bad became less of an issue. He was more open about his feelings of loss when we would finish, but seemed to know now that it was not about whether or not he was a good and lovable child. He noticeably became more and more tolerant of his own mistakes in the sessions, keen to show me all the things he could do and laughing when he sometimes got things wrong.

Mourning, loss, and integration

When Samuel returned after the break, he seemed a little nervous and serious—he had something to tell me; his teacher had spoken really nastily to him. It seemed this teacher had been angry at Samuel and I wondered if he thought I might be angry at him. He wondered if I ever got angry and then he told me sadly how he had not finished the Christmas card for me; he insisted he never got angry at me. I reflected on how it seemed like neither of us was to be angry and yet how hard it felt for him to miss his last session here before the break and his worry that I might have been very angry at him for not coming.

Samuel began to regress in some of his play, reintroducing the crashing, broken plane with the fragile family inside. A difficult period followed, where Samuel, referring to the tsunami disaster that had happened over the holidays, was flooded with anxiety that he could not contain. It all seemed to focus around finishing and leaving; Samuel would find it difficult to end sessions and would demand that I hug him, angry when I did not, and my interpretations around the Christmas break just did not feel right.

At the beginning of a session in February, Samuel ran into a different room to our own before running out again. I was soon following him down the corridors of the hospital in which I worked, in a way that reminded me of our early sessions. As I interpreted his need to know once again that I would not let him go, he insisted I write him a story about "Samuel the Scientist". I spoke about Samuel the scientist who conducted an experiment to see what "P" would do—would he hold on to Samuel or let him go. Samuel then "marked" my work, and told me it was good. I wondered if he had been thinking about finishing again: perhaps he had heard that someone was leaving (the parent worker was). He shushed me and then told me that *he* was going to be moving away; he was going to go a long way away and he would not ever see me again. He told me how sad he was about this.

Unfortunately, it turned out that this was true; his parents were planning to move. This move was planned for the summer; it meant that we would be finishing sooner perhaps than originally planned but there was time to manage this ending. Although for their own reasons they had found it very difficult to let me and the parent worker know, Samuel's parents were regretful and mindful of the impact this would have on him.

In the end, working on this ending was helpful to Samuel, and it was a sign of his improvement overall that he was able to do so. He showed a lot of thoughtfulness in this, appropriately sad and reflective. He used drawings and stories to symbolize his wish to keep a connection between us; he drew a new house and a path leading to it. I talked about his worry that we will lose each other, that I would forget him and he might forget me. He wanted to know if we were "really good friends" and told me how much he would miss me. He said he would never forget me, then added to the drawing a "cookhouse" and a cook, and told me "there is lots of good food". My having helped him, he told me how "fantastic" the picture was, giving me all the credit, and I reminded him that this was something we had worked on together.

Now Samuel seemed much more contained and integrated in an age-appropriate way, possessing a repertoire of communications to express his affective state of mind, without becoming so easily overwhelmed. But he was still worried that his anger could be so great that he would destroy me and all the good work we had done.

Instead of turning to the dark side, Samuel became reborn as Luke, who survives after the death of his mentor and keeps his voice alive inside. Our final session was appropriately sad and Samuel expressed his difficulty and ambivalence about leaving: he had made a card to say goodbye but then forgotten to bring it. He wanted to take something away, wanted to take everything, but in the end he took his folder of drawings, leaving me some, and the old broken plane that had been there from the beginning and with both therapists. Despite some very mixed feelings, he knew we would remember each other.

Discussion

Samuel was first referred with what was termed a severe attachment disorder, and Bowlby warns that attachment patterns tend to persist. But whilst old established negative "internal working models" of expectation and behaviour can persist, new internal working models that are less pathological and serve the individual well can be established through new relational experiences. These more benign internal working models mitigate older patterns and ultimately allow for better emotional and physical regulation. Impulsive and uncontained behaviour lessens as affects feel more manageable and can be better articulated, and represented, mentally and verbally. Attachment theory is helpful in drawing our attention to the biological imperative that is the need for security and safety, and how this impacts upon development at all levels—particularly when this biological need was inadequately met. The failure to find a "secure base", a solid receptive and reflective whole object, impacts upon emotional, social, and cognitive development as bodily and mental regulatory processes are disrupted. There is dysregulation at all levels and lack of an integrated core sense of self. Feelings and perceptions become overwhelming. The attachment disordered child can be characterized as the child that feels his/her primary caregiver is both a source of safety and protection, and of threat and danger.

As such, from the very start of his life, Samuel's difficulties were rooted in early developmental relational trauma and needed a correspondingly developmental approach. When I came to thinking about writing this chapter and the way the work had proceeded, I found myself thinking about the difficult balance between interpretative work and more developmental work—a concept that was well captured by Bion's (1962) notion of "containment", which assumes an active process between two minds, where the role of the container is to both tolerate and contain the projections of the other, and through the process of reverie to metabolize, and *make sense* of these projections and the feelings elicited by them, and *give them back* in a modified form that can now be tolerated. In particular, acting as a sort of "container" for Samuel, tolerating his behaviour, as well as interpreting, felt crucial. We were developing a language for his feelings and his experiences that he could take back in and use.

Importantly, having internalized one therapist, through the loss Samuel was able to use me differently, to begin to work through his identifications as a boy, enabling him to make sense of and structure his aggression which felt particularly dangerous.

I want to equate this to *Anne Hurry's* (1998) writings on the use of the analyst as a new developmental object. Sandler and Sandler (1998) have emphasized the importance of role responsiveness and working in the "here-and-now", which Anne Hurry sees as part of a growing interest in the interaction between child and analyst, as it represents the situation between child and parent. The idea is that the analyst can become a developmental object by providing a safe, holding environment where the child can then experience a different way of relating with the object. In this way, the analyst in the "here-and-now" is not just "re-constructing" the past psychic life, but is *constructing* new formulations: a new object relationship in the experiential realm, interplaying over time with a different object experience and thereby modifying the already established fantasy object relationships of the more deeply unconscious non-experiential realm.

Samuel's aggressive behaviour and play, acting out furious battles between good and evil, were repulsive for his parents who found it difficult to tolerate this level of violence and consequently were unable to help Samuel regulate and organize his affects so that they remained overwhelming for him too. He seemed locked in a struggle for survival and needed someone to join him in his fantasy world, his inner world, full of unprocessed feeling, to help him make sense of it, a sort of alpha-functioning.

This kind of work can and does go hand in hand with interpretation, particularly in interpreting the affective states, the anxieties behind the defences. But the work is equally focused on a way of being with the patient that the patient grows to know, an innate, new forming of internal working models. This links closely with Stern's (1987) ideas of how a "core sense of self" is constructed and how it can be skewed by early experiences. The repeated process of therapy with another can over time gradually build up new "schemas-of-being", and through these, modification of a "schema-of-being-with" another—much in the same way, I would assert, that Sandler's experiential realm can impact on the unconscious non-experiential realm of object relations.

In conclusion, Samuel experienced first a female and then a male therapist and it seemed there had been a certain overarching progress, through the two therapies and managing the transition. During his time with his first therapist, the parent worker was seen as highly significant in helping Samuel's mother in becoming more genuinely attached to him. Likewise, as I began to work with Samuel, his father became a more assertive presence, setting firmer boundaries around him. This is not to say that the maternal and paternal functioning in the therapists or the parents was strictly gender based; indeed, at times it was apparent that Samuel needed a maternal-type functioning that his father was more able to give—he told me movingly of his father's holding him in his arms after a nightmare and singing him gently back to sleep. But the overall experience for Samuel in therapy was one of developmental emotional growth by a revisiting of his very early object relations, which allowed him to re-attach himself in his family. Working through the loss of his first, and then second therapist, helped Samuel to mourn properly the loss of the object and thereby internalize something integrated and good for himself that he could take to further and to new object relationships.

References

Baradon, T. (Ed.) (2010). *Relational Trauma in Infancy: Psychoanalytic, Attachment and Neuropsychological Contributions to Parent–Infant Psychotherapy*. Hove, UK: Routledge.

Bion, W. R. (1962). *Learning from Experience*. London: Tavistock.

Hurry, A. (1998). *Psychoanalysis and Developmental Therapy*. Madison, CT: International Universities Press.

Sandler, J. (1993). On communication from patient to analyst: not everything is projective identification. *International Journal of Psychoanalysis, 74*: 1097–1107.

Sandler, J. (1996). Comments on the psychodynamics of interaction. *Psychoanalytic Inquiry, 16*: 88–95.

Sandler, J., Kennedy, H. & Tyson, R. L. (1980). *The Technique of Child Analysis*. Cambridge, MA: Harvard University Press.

Sandler, J. & Sandler, A. -M. (1998). *Internal Objects Revisited*. Madison, CT: International Universities Press.

Winnicott, D. W. (1949). Mind and its relation to the psyche-soma. In: *Through Paediatrics to Psychanalysis*. London: Tavistock, 1958.

Winnicott, D. W. (1962). Ego integration in child development. In: *The Maturational Processes in the Facilitating Environment*. London: Hogarth and the Institute of Psychoanalysis, 1965.

CHAPTER TWENTY

"The robot, the gangster, and the schoolboy"—intensive psychoanalytic psychotherapy with Luis, a latency boy in search of a father[1]

Mark Carter

Introduction

Luis, a deprived and neglected eight-year-old boy, was developmentally delayed emotionally and cognitively. He showed the destructive trend of an "antisocial tendency" (Winnicott, 1956) and was on his way to becoming an "explosive delinquent" (Wilson, 1999). Stealing, the other main trend of this inclination, was part of Luis's therapeutic material but was not one of his referral symptoms. Luis's household included a variable number of delinquent men and as the therapy progressed he showed me his emerging identification with being a gang member. Drawing together thinking from a range of writers and psychoanalysts, Canham (2002) understands the "gang mentality" as being antisocial, anti-parents, anti-life and anti-thinking, offering the individual a way of freeing themselves from consciously experiencing their vulnerabilities, dependence, anxieties, and terrors, via projection in pathological group processes.

While at the same time, Luis's search for a father figure was based on ideas of a person who seemed good, consistent, and boundaried, and so he remained open to a new figure to identify with. When the first holiday in the four times per week psychoanalytic psychotherapy shattered Luis's somewhat idealized good father transference, his rage became the predominant theme of the work. The containment of this anger in the therapy allowed Luis's vulnerability, which he had protected with a "robot" stance as he called it, to be seen and understood. Realizing that his therapist would not retaliate or humiliate him, Luis then found himself in conflict between his gangster identity on the one hand and being a small boy who was able to have "ideas" and "make things" on the other. Surmounting this crisis and identifying more firmly

[1]I am very grateful to Debbie Bellman for her supervision of this work.

with his therapist enabled him to establish a schoolboy identity with enough internal resilience to maintain this development successfully.

Luis and his family

Luis had serious aggressive outbursts that had been a worrying aspect of his behaviour since nursery school, and had led to his permanent exclusion from his primary school. Before his exclusion he had been frequently losing his temper violently and attacking pupils, staff, furniture, and equipment. The restraining policy used at school was found not to be suitable; rather he needed to be soothed after an outburst. He was also restless and had poor concentration. At the time that I met him (aged eight) he was considered to have low to average academic ability and cognitive capacity, and he could not read or write (which he found hard to cope with). He was also receiving four hours of home tuition a week and had been out of school for a few months.

Luis lived with his siblings (boys aged eleven and four, and a girl aged two) in his grandmother's house. Grandmother was Spanish in origin and still had strong family links to her home country despite living in London for many years and raising her family in this city. Various, mainly male, members of the extended family and family friends would come from Spain and stay in the house, to such an extent that it was very difficult to keep track of who was living there at any one time, although there were usually quite a few of them and some stayed for a long time. To Luis all these men seemed to be subsumed under the label "uncles". These men sometimes behaved in a delinquent manner and one or two of them had spent time in prison. When Luis was with one or other of these men he would assume a tough silent demeanour and slight swagger. The very first thing that Luis told me in the first assessment session was that he was the strongest in his local gang of friends and that he wanted to do boxing to get even stronger. He later gave the impression that his "uncles" looked out for him.

For the first three years of his life Luis lived with his mother and father. He and his siblings were then removed from this environment, having suffered emotional and physical abuse. They were placed in the care of the maternal grandmother, who appeared to be the main provider of care and affection for Luis. Luis's father subsequently left his mother and, following a period in prison, had no further contact with the boy. Luis's brothers and sister had different and also absent fathers. Luis's mother had regular contact with her children, although she did not live with them. About one year before the work in the clinic began, mother had been diagnosed with chronic fatigue syndrome (or myalgic encephalomyelitis). According to grandmother, Luis and his mother had always quarrelled a great deal. The first time that his mother brought Luis to a session was one month into the work. I noticed that she looked thin and unwell. In the waiting room mother gave the impression of being very emotionally cut-off and lacking in energy and was hard to engage in conversation. I noticed that Luis seemed not to be relating at all to his passive mother and it seemed difficult for him to acknowledge that he was with her. Luis had brought a remote control robot with him and he played with it for the whole of his remaining session time. I thought this reflected something about how he had to be with his mother, hardened and without feeling, with little interest invested in him. The session felt overwhelmingly sad to me and Luis used this image of a robot to allude to himself on many other occasions.

Grandmother was a tall woman with an elaborate jet-black hairstyle, who would arrive for sessions in an old large stately looking but rusty car. She was involved in the support of Luis's therapy mainly through regular review meetings, as ongoing parent work was hard to maintain. However, a very helpful social worker was involved with this family and I frequently linked up with him. Social services were giving grandmother a great deal of support as she had a lot to cope with and seemed over-stretched at the centre of this household. The household seemed to be in perpetual turmoil because of the frequent variation in the number of occupants and their unsettling activities, and basic care and organization was hard to maintain. The children often appeared to have to look after themselves and each other, and reliability in bringing Luis to and from sessions on time was often an issue. Grandmother was able to engage in the thinking around therapy to an extent and she had a sense of humour and was caring, although at times she also came across as being a little emotionally distant.

The first term of treatment

Maternal transference—care and neglect

Luis was slim, with black curly hair that was sometimes cropped very short, and he had a neglected, unkempt look about him. His speech was slow and he stumbled or stuttered over some words. He was often unclear when talking, not only because of his difficulty with pronunciation, but also because of the confused content of what he was saying. He appeared sad and a little distant, rarely making eye contact. In the initial assessment sessions he seemed painfully withdrawn and he looked frightened. I found myself wanting to give him more time, perhaps responding to his experience of not having enough.

In the first few weeks of the therapy Luis would respond to any moment of emotional contact between us with a big smile where he seemed like a much younger child. He found the most basic skills such as drawing, or cutting out, extremely difficult, if he attempted them at all. His tolerance of his lack of skills was very low. He also brought elements of his own self-care, abandonment, and neglect in the stories he told at the beginning of the work; telling me, for example, how he had to look after an injured boy in the park while the boy's parents were away for three years. There was something good and caring that came across in these stories, although mothers were represented as punitive, absent, and castrating. He also brought some intense material about his anxieties and how unsafe he felt. Using his younger brother as a displacement figure, he talked about being scared of the dark and having bad dreams. He recounted how his mother told him stories about monsters, witches, and vampires. Typically, Luis then denied that vampires were "scary" because they did not exist any more as they came before dinosaurs were "invented".

In the countertransference Luis evoked strong maternal feelings, not only in terms of wanting to provide physical care, but also in terms of wanting to keep all the aspects of his life, particularly his anxieties, in mind, so that he would experience someone thinking about him in that way. I was then responding to the sense of physical, emotional, and mental deprivation and lack of containment in a child who was still able to evoke a positive emotional response in adults. This early material seems indicative of Luis's strong ambivalence in maternal object representations, which was to become more apparent as the therapy proceeded.

The missing man

The following vignette comes from the first therapy session:

> Luis took out a toy man from his box and then placed a plastic toy net over the man on the table. He said a few words describing this and I acknowledged that the man was "trapped". He then stuck the four corners of the small net down with plasticine, and said that the man was "stuck". His face then brightened and he went on to tell me about a computer game that he had at home, but the batteries were finished so he has to use his "imagination" if he still wants to play it. He stumbled over the word "imagination" and I clarified it. He went on to describe that when he is on his own at home, when his friends are not around, he uses his imagination to think of a "wrestler" which he "'tends" (his word for "pretends") to fight on his bed. I acknowledged this and he described fighting the pillows on his bed as well, pretending that they are men and beating them. His descriptions moved on to include cars, speedboats, guns and going into buildings and shooting "baddies". It took me a few minutes to realize that he was talking about another computer game.

Luis's wish to have an attachment relationship to a paternal figure was evident. He seems unsure how to keep such a figure in his life. In the absence of a father, or batteries, or friends, he uses fantasy. These absences give an impression of Luis's loneliness, his wish for a father to fix things or to provide, but also a father with whom to work out his phallic-narcissistic concerns. In this session Luis also made a "very very strong robot", as he called it, out of plasticine. He added that the robot was made by a "doctor", who was also a robot, but one who made robots. This is perhaps referring to a fantasy that maybe I—in the figure of a doctor—may actually turn out to be the maker, or the "making-better man", that he is looking for.

The work continually vacillated between the maternal and paternal transference as Luis was deprived in both spheres. In relation to his mother, and perhaps others in his environment, Luis adopted an emotionless strong robot stance. He thought a father would make him into a stronger robot rather than the weak one that he felt now, thereby utilizing phallic-narcissistic concerns to strengthen this defensive position.

In this first term he represented himself as invulnerable, with others being the injured, broken, or frightened ones. He was often a "James Bond" type with a special weapon and thus he would often resort to omnipotent fantasies to cover up his feelings of lack, vulnerability, and powerlessness. The theme of who I was, and so who he could be in relation to me, ran throughout the therapy, well beyond his initial anxieties about starting. It seems then that not only did he take a defensive stance in this first term, but he tried to be what he thought I would like, in the hope that I would like him and he would get his needs met.

Defences and the emergence of aggression

Luis went to great lengths to keep any expression of aggression out of the room, or at least away from me, at the beginning of the work. He employed the defences of denial, avoidance, splitting, and projection (A. Freud, 1937), and also controlled the activity in the room so that our relationship remained smooth, and he could protect his wish to view me as a good father. He spent the majority of his session time involved in a repetitive aggressive game, where he seemed closed-off from me, leaving me out and casting me in the role of a passive observer. These games involved a toy that he seemed identified with in a phallic way, sometimes a horse or sometimes a small fast and tough car, fighting and winning against lots of enemies.

Luis often took a long time in his play to arm the protagonists with increasingly more powerful weapons; sometimes they did not even get to battle because the time was taken up with preparation. It felt like it was important for him to be prepared and to arrive with his defences in place. These battle games can also partly be understood as an aggressive coming together, in which Luis is trying to work out how he can be in the room with me and both of us survive when he has these angry feelings.

After the first few weeks Luis then began to test me to see how I would respond to his aggression. On one occasion, when we met after a missed session, he began to play cars in such a way that a car would accidentally hit my foot and he would giggle. I mentioned that the cars were trying to get me and tried to elicit a response from him about why they were doing this. He did not answer, but in the next session the following occurred:

> Luis returned to exactly where he left off and said that he was going to "get" my shoes. I had set my shoe as the boundary for his "getting" me, but Luis found this increasingly difficult. He began to build fences and traps around my shoes in order to stop the cars from hitting them. These defences grew more and more elaborate, pushing the cars further away from me. Eventually Luis put plasticine around the car tyres to stop them from moving. After I took up this stopping of the tyres, he freed the cars' wheels and brought in many other toys to attack my feet, although the fences still held.
>
> In the following session he returned to testing me with the cars, allowing his boisterous feelings to emerge until his car hit my knee. He looked at me with great uncertainty, and I verbalized what had happened and that he was wondering what I thought or what I was going to do. He started to build fences against the car as he had done before. I asked him why he thought the car needed to be stopped? He said that he did not know. I wondered if it was because he felt it was a wild little car that needed to be controlled. He did not reply but he started to play with the two cars in an increasingly violent manner with big smashes and crashes. I made comments about him showing me some angry feelings and I linked this to the previously missed session, to which he simply replied "Yes".

The aggression in Luis, that was to emerge more fully in the second term of treatment, was suggestive of what Anna Freud referred to as a "lack of steady love relationships in early childhood", which disrupts the "normal fusion between the erotic and destructive urges" and so "aggression manifests itself as pure, independent destructiveness" (A. Freud, 1948b, p. 48).

Winnicott (1956) describes two trends in the "antisocial tendency", where the genuinely deprived child looks for the wider environment for management. He conveys how stealing is the trend to look "for something, somewhere", and destructiveness is the child "seeking that amount of environmental stability which will stand the strain resulting from impulsive behaviour". Stealing was sometimes in Luis's material although he never actually stole.

Rage and destructiveness, however, was a predominant theme. According to Winnicott, the wider environment gives a new opportunity for ego relatedness in a child such as Luis who has perceived that it was an environmental failure in ego support that has led to his sense of being deprived.

The Christmas holiday shatters the "good father" fantasy

When I told Luis about the first holiday in the work he brought the following story:

> He arranged a tidy doll's house with two brothers and two sisters in separate bedrooms upstairs, with Mum and Dad downstairs watching TV. He went on to tell me that the windows were open at night because his "uncles" wanted to let in the fresh air. Luis mentioned that creatures might come in, particularly bats and vampire bats, and he described hearing the wind at night. I acknowledged that this might sound "scary". He added that people had smashed windows in his house. Again I acknowledged his fears. He said: "It was lucky that Andrés (one of the "uncles") was there with his friends and that they had baseball bats." I replied: "Perhaps this makes you feel a bit protected, but that maybe angry people with baseball bats can also seem scary." Luis added, "… and my Grandma wasn't there." I mentioned his sense that at other times she protected him in the house. I also added: "Perhaps—like in the doll's house here—you would like a daddy in the house to protect you." He said a thoughtful "Yeah", and then talked in an unclear way about there being four different daddies, and that daddies had made babies with mummy. I wondered where he thought his daddy was? He replied: "He was a long way away, but he comes back when it is snowing where he lives." I said: "There were some comings and goings that seem difficult for you, just like here."

This story was a typical mix of fantasy and reality, beginning with his fantasy of a safe and conventional family but his fear quickly transforms this image. The real unsettling nature of the house was clear from external sources, and also the approaching holiday felt like abandonment for Luis, repeating the initial loss of his father. He had wanted me to protect him from his external and internal fears and yet he felt I was leaving him with his "uncles" and an absent grandmother or maternal figure, as he perceived it. The "uncles" toughness that Luis seemed to identify with actually left him feeling frightened, unprotected from violence and danger.

In the weeks before the holiday Luis went through many attempts to keep me. One poignant example of this was when he brought into his session a little battered plastic toy saxophone and serenaded me. He was unable to do more than tunelessly squeaking, but this made it all the more moving as an attempt to impress me in order that I would not leave him. He wanted to be a good boy for a good father. For most of the penultimate session before the break Luis sat in silence, showing me his control, and punishing me with his silence. But there was also a sense of despair and rage—he had done everything in his power but there was still going to be a holiday that he felt helpless to prevent. It became very difficult for him to maintain his idealized fantasy of me as the good father. I was now to become the abandoning, depriving, and bad father who left him.

The second term of treatment

Rage at the beginning of term

Luis's anger towards me started to build up towards the end of the first session back after the holiday. He threw a paper rocket at me and then pushed the table against my legs. He then trapped me with chairs, turned the light off, and tried to scare me with vampire stories. I was being vividly shown how frightened, powerless, abandoned, and "in the dark" he had felt. Luis found many more ways to express his rage directly, as well as his fear of it. His destructiveness against the room began with him attacking the desk with a ruler, and his verbal abuse began when he used an empty sellotape roll as a pretend mouth through which he could say "rude" words. In later sessions he sang a song with lyrics that repeatedly berated "crappy uncles". He also brought a story full of rage of how he and his friends were going to get everyone out of this building and then destroy it and the police would help them.

> Luis brought material concerned with me stealing from him, and said all my stickers were "girl's stickers". When I interpreted his feelings of castration he brought up an interesting description of me as wearing a "mask" before Christmas when I was a "goodie", and then after Christmas I took off the mask to reveal myself as actually being a "baddie". He then wanted to make a phone call to the police for them to come and arrest me. The police story continued with Luis taking control and sitting in my chair, I was a thief in his house and he called the police to put me in prison. At one point Luis made the comment that his uncle Andrés must like prison because he does "naughty" things and gets put back in there.

The holiday had shattered his idealization of me as the good father, and left Luis feeling rage at the humiliation of not being able to hold on to a father and being left feeling abandoned and castrated. Inhibitions of his rage and destructiveness could now be discarded when he wanted, as there was no longer a sense of him being a good boy for a good father. The use of the police showed how he felt that I did something very wrong, but their confused role was indicative of his unstructured superego. Luis was looking for a non-delinquent attachment figure that stayed with him, and his "uncles" had not been what he wanted. My mask had been cast aside to reveal a baddie who was no better than all the other men in his life. With this confusion over who is good and who is bad, Luis elected to play it safe and assumed a position of the toughest, or a robot without feelings. This time, he wanted to be in charge of when the police came and took people away, turning passive into active (A. Freud, 1937). Maybe he also feared that I, like some of people in his life, would be sent away to prison, and believed that it was only a matter of time before I too would go, but at the same time wanting me to go, to punish me.

Rage becomes less dangerous

The negative transference had now opened up and so I could become subject to his extreme rages, although at times he would still try to keep things smooth in the room. His behaviour included throwing things around (sometimes at me), messing up the room or kicking things, and verbally abusing me. However, in time Luis discovered that his rage was not met with retaliation, but rather had been acknowledged, and he learnt that it was acceptable to be angry and his anger could be understood. Furthermore, our relationship had survived his anger and I had returned from the break. Interestingly, the freeing up of Luis's rage in the room entailed a greater willingness in him to risk exposing the issue of his competence and feelings of inadequacy with me. Encountering a non-retaliatory object meant that his anger when he failed could be tolerated in the room and also gave him hope that I would be a non-humiliating object as well.

This was the beginning of him being able to be 'just' a little boy. He initiated the two of us making paper aeroplanes and was very proud of his achievements, which I encouraged. He was still incredibly fragile, however, and the slightest difficulty resulted in the partially made planes being torn up. He also started to come up with more ideas about things he wanted to make, even drawing plans for us to use in the construction. He began to be able to ask for help, which hitherto had been impossible for him because this involved an admission that he could not do something, thereby denting his omnipotence. As well as reflecting on how awful it felt for Luis to find doing things so difficult, I tried to mirror him in order for him to develop some self-observation during his efforts. I could now link some of his difficulties to those he had experienced at school, as the rage he experienced when he could not complete a task was probably a factor in his outbursts at school. He was also finally able to show me one of his biggest humiliations—writing—in a game of hangman that he initiated.

From then on Luis often used shared activity as a way of being in the room with me, and I was beginning to be established in Luis's mind as a man who facilitated his competence and did not humiliate him, and was fair and consistent and always returned after I left. I was safe for him to identify with. But this conflicted with his fears about unreliability, lack of safety, and unavailability, and so his defensive tough guy, or robot stance, would often reappear. Luis's fear of abandonment, for example, was brought to the fore again with my announcement of the next half-term break, and he showed his rage in the sessions in similar ways as before. However, he now also expressed his feelings through two drawings. The first drawing showed his destructive rage and his omnipotent defence, as he defended his town and its people and the king and queen and their home from the helicopters dropping bombs. Later he drew the clinic with a happy sun, preserving it for when he got back, and he also drew smiling faces in his name written above the building.

My time away from him at half-term left him feeling rejected and not in control, small and humiliated. On his return he drew volcanoes, symbolically depicting his volcanic feelings that threatened to erupt and actually did erupt in some of the sessions. It seemed as if he got into the vicious circle of his angry projections making me a frightening person, which he then responded to by strengthening his defences and becoming full of rage, and then I appeared even more frightening. He seemed to respond better at these moments when I said something more soothing, such as sympathizing with how awful it felt to be so angry, or how awful it felt for him to feel so small. My countertransference response to Luis's rage in this part of the work was more maternal and containing. Luis's raging attacks and my survival of them over time helped Luis in developing greater integration between love and hate (Winnicott, 1956, pp. 206–207).

Meeting the gangster

It was becoming clearer that the phallic component to Luis's material was a defence against feeling small, rather than a more secure attainment of that developmental phase. After we were able to survive and move beyond his angry response to half-term, he revealed some of his preoccupations in a session which had started with him measuring his height outside the room:

> Firstly he played his enclosed fighting aggressive games with cars. I was a spectator until I said: "Perhaps with these goodies and baddies fighting, it is as if they are not sure if they can be in the same room together." In response Luis stopped his fighting play and put the cars into a garage. I called the garage a "safe place", which prompted Luis to arm the cars with big weapons. I said: "The cars want to be big and strong. Maybe this was like you telling me how tall you felt at the beginning of the session today". Luis then said: "The cars are like robots." I replied: "We have talked about robots before—that they are big and strong, but have no feelings." Luis said: "That's because they have no hearts." I replied: "Right, so they don't have any feelings—good or bad—poor robots!" Luis then said: "Robots break easily." I replied: "It seems like you feel that robots are fragile as well?" He then made a little plasticine man and immediately squashed it. "So the poor little man has been crushed," I said. He took the plasticine that had been the man and turned it into a hammer on the end of a pencil, which he then used to crush another plasticine man that he had just made.

Luis responded better to simple step by step comments, allowing him to move at his own pace and preserving the empathic contact between the two of us. This approach was often more effective than elaborate interpretations. Luis seemed to be showing me how difficult it was for him to be in the room with me and that he has to feel big and tough to protect himself. The transference was revealing how Luis had been made to feel humiliated about the smallness of being a child. When he is being tough, or developing a defensive armour, he loses touch with his feelings. He cannot allow himself to feel because otherwise he is left with feelings of vulnerability that he cannot tolerate. He feels angry at having such vulnerable feelings and so he squashes or crushes them, in order to feel safer. He cannot tolerate these vulnerable feelings because his environment has not been available enough or tolerant enough of these feelings and in some ways it has partly been crushing him as well. In his play he seems to be showing me how the crushing of vulnerability can be passed from one person to another.

This vignette also seems to include the anxiety that this is a precarious internal position to be in, as even robots are fragile. In the work that followed I began to try to empathize with these feelings by interpreting how being small felt like the worst thing in the world for him, and that being big felt like the best thing. Luis started to shift more rapidly as he increasingly believed that I would not humiliate him, so he could lower his defences and his robot stance more and be a vulnerable child with a protecting and caring adult. He started to include me in his fighting aggressive play. He also introduced a new game where we had to throw plasticine balls at targets. This was the beginnings of competition, although it was clear that he still had to be the winner. He then really began to show me his prowess in this game, showing off his jumping and throwing—a more genuine phallic-narcissism. It became clear that the purpose of

Luis's robot position was not to defend against all feeling but specifically against the feeling of smallness and humiliation and also his early longings that he seemed to perceive as "wimpish". Furthermore, in one session Luis even told me that "small people are important", which was a significant step on his way to being a young schoolboy.

As noted, Luis had possibly been heading towards becoming what Wilson (1999) has termed an "explosive delinquent". This is a delinquent that functions at a higher level of organization than other types of delinquents, but has "periodic outbursts of violence and revengeful preoccupations". This is because this young person is highly sensitive to perceived rejection or humiliation. The causes of this are complex but can reside in an accumulation of narcissistic injuries in response to the mother's extreme ambivalence. This begins in the early mother-infant relationship and is characterized by mother's sudden and unpredictable swings from over-involvement to withdrawal of affection, or even hostility. These injuries engender a deep sense of hurt and anger, which Kohut (1972) describes as constituting "narcissistic rage". The child then uses compensatory grandiose or idealizing fantasies to defend against this intolerable vulnerability (Wilson, 1999, p. 320). After Luis made his statement about the importance of small people, he made a brief comment about him being a gangster. In the following session he acted out his omnipotent gangster fantasy:

> Luis had arrived wearing a T-shirt with some rub-on tattoos displayed on his arm. He was smiling and he shyly turned away from me on his seat and then turned back to me holding up a very small crooked rusty penknife. "Ah, a knife," I said. He held the knife up in a powerful posed manner. "Now you feel like a big man," I said. "I'm a gangster," Luis replied. This led Luis into a brief description of him being the leader of a gang of gangsters. He had taught them all their fighting moves. He boasted that his gang had first twenty, then thirty, and finally forty members, and they had at least ten fights a day and always won. As he talked he brandished his knife a little and I said: "Holding the knife makes you feel strong here with me and in control." "Shut up!" said Luis. I replied: "You want to control what I say, too."

Getting in touch with his vulnerability and "smallness" in the sessions with me was then fraught for Luis, because of his internal fragility and with the un-protecting, humiliating, and neglectful aspects of his environment. The compensations in grandiosity and omnipotence are clear for him, as is the defensive value in identifying with his aggressors (A. Freud, 1937). Being a member of a gang has a "lure" according to Canham (2002, p. 114) because it "promises a life without any of the pains that recognising difference, dependency, the inevitability of death and vulnerability entails". Canham also states how "ganging" is used as a solution to the pains involved in having ambivalent feelings. It might be described as a kind of manic defence where "dependence on the object, and all this implies, is utterly repudiated" (2002, p. 116). How much Luis was part of the gang in reality I was never sure; he did use fantasy a great deal, but his environment also contained figures with innate potential for Luis's identifications of this kind to be cultivated, rather than limited.

I felt that Luis was now strong enough for me to analyse what he was telling me, even though it exposed his vulnerability and made him angry. At this point I felt that him bringing a knife into the session was an enactment of his wish for phallic power in the room and so a symbol in fantasy, rather than a wish to harm me physically.

Luis seemed to want to know what I thought of these freely and passionately expressed ideas about himself that he was now bringing. A little later in the same session:

> It was not long before Luis returned to talking about being a gangster. I connected being a gangster with wearing tattoos, and Luis seemed pleased by this. He continued that he was the leader of the gang of all his "mates", and that I could join the gang if I guessed the password. I said: "Perhaps you are interested in what I think about being a gangster and would I want to be one?" "Shut up," Luis replied.

Luis is here seeking my affirmation of his feelings and identifications, which would solve the conflictual feelings he was beginning to experience. His wish for my affirmation shows his strong positive transference that is confounded by his identifications, am I part of his gang? Where do I fit into his ideas of male figures? How do we fit together? Typically, he tries to keep hold of the knowledge and the power, as he is the one who knows the password that could exclude or include me.

A little further on in the session:

> Luis brought up the subject of stealing again and talked about the police coming to take me away. But the police then became baddies and when I questioned this he said that he hated the police. I said: "Maybe sometimes it felt difficult to know who was a goodie and who was a baddie in the people around you." Luis replied: "No, 'cos I have a computer to tell me." Luis added: "I'm James Bond and he kills goodies." "I thought that James Bond *was* a goodie," I replied. "He is," said Luis. I said: "Well it seems like it is difficult for you to tell who is a goodie and who is a baddie—and that includes me—am I a goodie or a baddie?"

Again we see Luis's confusion over good and bad, right and wrong, and the roles of people around him. He is still not sure if I will turn out to be a baddie, and my not embracing his gangster identity arouses fears that I will reject him—touching on his feelings of deprivation and abandonment, and so the idea of "stealing" appears in the material. He defends against confusion and vulnerability by returning to his defensive toughness, becoming a James Bond who has all the answers and the equipment and is neither good nor bad. This is indicative of the instability in Luis's representational world (Sandler, 1962).

The following excerpt, a little later on in the session, shows how his feelings of vulnerability lead him to try to make me feel scared and vulnerable, so I could understand how he feels:

> Luis angrily continued to threaten me and said that he was going to stab and kill me. I said that perhaps part of him did not want to hurt me and was a little worried about these angry stabbing feelings. Luis replied: "No. All of me wants to stab you." He then listed the parts of my body that he was going to stab, which included my arm, eye, and elbow, adding with more emphasis that he was going to stab me in the "head", "heart", and "willy". I said: "The head is

> where we think, the heart is where we feel, and the willy ..." "Is what we piss through?" Luis interrupted me to say. "Yes, it does mean that ..." Luis then quickly added: "I'm a boy."

Luis's frustrations are mounting and his "gang mentality" is shown in the threatened attack on the non-gang attributes of thinking, feeling, and authentic potency (Canham, 2002). My having acknowledged his attack, however, allows Luis to tentatively assert his masculinity that had been so castrated in his environment, as he is able to say that he is "a boy". Luis is briefly connecting with a more real identification, which has been a developing aspect of the therapy. But a few minutes later his anger had returned and the session then reached its climax, as shown in this next vignette:

> His threatening behaviour prompted him to get up and start strutting around full of rage and he continued to threaten me. I made a comment about him feeling angry and wanting to be a tough gangster who does not have worries. Luis then started to sing his "crappy uncles" song. I said: "Perhaps it feels like your uncles are bad to you sometimes and it might feel really difficult to live with these bigger men." "Shut up!" Luis said, and I felt like this had connected with him. His anger escalated and he threatened me by swiping his knife down through the air, although still at some distance away from me. I acknowledged his strong desire to hurt me.

In the midst of his rage he hears my comments about his defensive identity and responds with an association to one of the main sources of his feelings of smallness—the big "uncles" that he lives with. My sympathetic acknowledgement of his difficulties brings his rage to a climax because his vulnerability is exposed, and yet it also indicates the difference between his uncles (as he perceives them) and me. After this point his rage gradually decreased, until:

> He lent on the desk looking out of the window and his stomach rumbled very loudly. He tried to say that the noise was me a couple of times. When I wondered what he felt or thought about his tummy rumbling, he said angrily to the window that he did not get breakfast this morning. I said: "How awful it felt not to be given what you need, perhaps it felt like you were not important enough to be given breakfast this morning." He made an angry noise, and I said: "Yes, it makes you very angry." He then started angrily kicking the walls of the room and pieces of cardboard.

Luis feels able to express his rage without fear of retaliation or punishment and feels that I will listen to his hurt feelings. The needs of a little boy are heard. He then rages against the room rather than his therapist.

This gangster figure almost seemed to burst into the sessions, vividly coming to life and showing Luis's tendency to over-invest in his fantasies with the potential to act them out. A further comment on the process in the therapy would be how the internal "gang" structure strongly seeks to preserve itself (Canham, 2002) and is here reacting dramatically to this therapeutic process that had now begun to threaten it. I have suggested that the fusion of Luis's libidinal and destructive impulses had been compromised in his development. Underlying the "gang mentality" there can be a way of resolving this struggle between these two opposing impulses by attempting to get rid of the dependent self and thereby love and concern for the object, and identifying with a destructive narcissistic part of the self, which also feeds into a sense of superiority and self-admiration (Canham, 2002).

Vacillations

In the session that followed the above extracts, Luis not only wanted to repair the damage that he feared he had caused, but he also expressed his new-found identification with me. He decided to make things, and he also began to talk about having "ideas" for the first time. He made a "stereo" out of some cardboard and he then had the idea of making a book, but he did not begin this yet. He did, however, begin to make a "mirror" out of cardboard. He drew his face and wanted me to look in the mirror and see his face instead of mine, which he thought was a "good trick". He then wanted me to draw my face next to his in the mirror. In the following session he wanted to make this drawing of us appear old, like a historical document, so he put holes around the edge and coloured it in to make it look faded and stained. It seemed then that Luis was wishing for him and me to have a shared history together. This material suggested how "the self is built up in relation to the other and to the other's view of the self, and shared experience of positive affect is essential to the development of the sense of a separate and authentic self" (Hurry, 1998, p. 38). Material around this time was also indicative of the shift to "group" thinking and behaviour, as Canham describes, away from the "gang mentality" and "where individual members can explore themselves through each other's experience of being with them" (Canham, 2002, p. 125).

However, a couple of sessions later his new fragile identification with me was shaken with the release of his "uncle" Andrés from prison, and another holiday at the end of this second term was approaching:

> Luis arrived for his session with a large prestigious looking toy boat in nearly new condition. He then told me a long story about having lots of money and lots of large toys. When the coming holiday was mentioned he began to play with the dolls. In this play I was preserved in ice. After I mentioned him wanting to keep me safe during the holiday and safe also from his hot feelings, he started to do a rap. The lyrics of the rap included the line: "I am what you say I am." I mentioned that perhaps he wanted to be like me sometimes, and he told me that this was his music that he plays on his stereo. I asked if it was gangster music. He said: "Yeah, I'm a gangster," and with his bravado building he continued, "You could be one but you don't want to be." He then got angry when I noted his interest in what I thought about him being a gangster. I then said: "I also know you as a boy who has lots of ideas and makes things."

As was often the case with Luis, he attempts to impress me with stories of all his toys and money as if he hopes to buy me or impress me enough to prevent the anticipated rejection of the Easter break. He is showing me all that he has, all his wealth, denying his experience of loss and deprivation. When his angry feelings are acknowledged, he then brings rap lyrics that seem to indicate that he is also trying to be who I want in order to keep me; although the lyrics may also suggest that he feels that my acceptance of him is on my terms. My not joining him in his gangster activities may be experienced as disapproval of him. Things are further complicated by the return of Andrés from prison. Knowing that he will be left with his "uncles" during the holiday, Luis will then have to be tough again, identifying with his "uncles" in order to feel liked and accepted. He fears that his new identity and little boy feelings may well be lost and so it will be even harder to secure me to him. I am drawn into reassuring him of his new identity.

The vacillations in Luis's material can be usefully linked to the idea that "new models of self-with-others built up in treatment … do not obliterate old models. They are built up alongside the old: the potential for activation of the old remains, particularly under conditions of stress" (Hurry, 1998, p. 51).

Approximately one week before the Easter break Luis showed me how he wanted to castrate me by making a large cardboard image of a man who he was violently kicking in the "willy", as he put it. Later he tried to glue this image to the carpet, perhaps showing his wish to stick me in one place. In the following session the rage continued with the kicking and ripping-up of the cardboard, but then he abruptly stopped as if he decided that he had had enough of that, and he announced that we were going to make "books". He sat on the floor, inviting me to join him, and we discussed what the books were going to be about. Luis said that his story was going to be about "a boy who was about to move house. He lived in the city and was going to live at the seaside." Luis told me that the problem that he had with making this book was that he actually could not write, although he could write his name. He was clearly feeling much safer with me so he could tell me about one of the things that he found so humiliating, and as we got to work he was able to ask for my help with the writing. In addition to the boy in the story going to a new place, Luis also decided to "spring-clean" his therapy box of toys and materials, suggesting that perhaps a new chapter in his therapy had begun. In the context of the coming break he seemed to be trying to keep me close by identification.

He had always been looking for a way to keep me and now he seemed to have found something as the boy who could sit down alongside me and think of stories and make books with me. Luis's choice of making books has further meaning for him in terms of repairing the humiliation of his exclusion from school, as he understood it, as well as his problems with literacy. He was allowing me to know about his vulnerabilities without fear that I too would reject him.

The summer term

At the beginning of the following term, Luis's grandmother reported that he was more verbally angry at home rather than physically, and he was able to say why he was angry, which he had not been able to do before. The social worker agreed with this and added that he could have a proper conversation with Luis for the first time, and that Luis actually initiated conversation with him, asking him questions, for example. He also noted how he had attended a play-scheme over Easter with eight other children that he did not know and there had been no problems. All these changes were reflected in the atmosphere of the therapy where Luis was relating to me in a generally more alive way and often seemed happier. He was still angry at times but was able to use language to express this a lot more.

Luis was still fragile, and my interpretations could now aim at supporting his growing sense of phallic potency, including, for example, suggesting that it seemed as if sometimes he could forget that one day he will grow up and be a big man. Luis was identifying with good super-hero characters now, and he was pursuing more sublimated avenues for his aggression, such as a marbles fighting game.

Luis had been accepted at a school for children with his educational needs, to start after the approaching holiday. His anxieties about this began to come through in the sessions, and he would often resort to his familiar omnipotent stance to ward them off. He also became anxious about losing me when he went to his new school. In one session where this anxiety had been present Luis started to grow angry. I mentioned how he was trying hard not to be angry and that he was wondering if I would accept him when he was angry. He then calmed down and quietly said with his head bowed that he had been "kicked out" from his last school. We were then able to talk about the feelings this had aroused and his worry that it might happen again.

In one session he noticed some evidence that another child had been in the room. This made him angrily resort to his omnipotent stance, and he also attacked me and the therapy by saying "Thinking is gay". Luis went into a long description of how he understood the world. He said that he was a "cool person", and explained to me that a cool person is a "gangster", and everyone else—including me—was normal and not cool, and normal people were in fact idiots. I picked up on his division of types by saying: "Why can't you be a big boy who can think and feel and write stories and also be cool?"

Luis was generally more contained now, relying less on his old rigid defences or his more manic defences, and his new identifications were more durable and his representational world more stable. This was particularly evident with the book-making, where he wanted me to make a book alongside him while he continued making his. The story in his book developed so that the mother and boy went into a removal van and travelled to their new home, and when they arrived they went into the house to look for their rooms. Luis also invented the story for my book entitled: "A boy and his mother's first Christmas", which followed this mother and child through from the preparations for Christmas, to Father Christmas coming down the chimney to leave presents, and finishing with Christmas lunch.

The last year

As part of my liaison with Luis's new school I drew up a timetable for his integration that slowly increased the length of time that he spent there each week, to ensure that he did not become overwhelmed, and so minimizing the risk of his behaviour breaking down.

By the first therapy session back after the summer holiday, Luis had just started at his new school. I was deeply moved when I entered the waiting room to see Luis sitting upright with his brand new school uniform on, holding up a book as if reading it. He seemed to be looking for my approval and was clearly very proud of himself. There was some strain for Luis as he started his new school because he was trying very hard to "get it right". At first he did not want to speak about his school in his sessions, but after a while he began to tell me how well he was doing—nearly top of his class in some subjects—and he brought some of his work to show me. This success was verified by grandmother, who added that there had only been one moment of mild oppositional behaviour from Luis at school.

Following a successful first term in his new school, we agreed to reduce to twice weekly psychotherapy sessions for a further two terms, enabling Luis to attend his school full-time. Due to external factors, it was agreed that therapy would then finish at the end of the second year.

One significant change in the material over this last year was that his desperate need to win, when we were playing competitive games, was decreasing, and he would actually get cross with me if he thought that I was letting him win. The countertransference had swung more to the paternal aspect and Luis felt safe enough to bring competitive Oedipal feelings, sublimating his aggression in this play.

Discussion

This paper attempts to illustrate the intricate links between the impact of early deprivation, abuse, and loss, and the current family context where elements of neglect, deprivation, and humiliation continue and lastly, how this has implications for a child's developing attitudes towards society and functioning in the wider social environment. The process over time of the psychoanalytic psychotherapeutic intervention introduced into this child's life has also been described, and its effects for the child on these interconnected levels.

The antisocial tendency, as Winnicott (1956) describes it, implies hope, because the child feels deprived of something good that they once had and they are taking their protest out on the environment where they feel that their problem originated. Despite feeling the narcissistic injury of maternal ambivalence, loss, and abandonment and also the later humiliation in his environment, Luis had not yet given up. He had also internalized some understanding that adults would help him, and could be good and boundaried (despite being unclear about where such boundaries lay). Wilson (1999) notes that some children have an inherent temperament that is more resilient than others, although in this case I would also suggest that any positive early experience with parental figures was built upon in the positive aspects of his important relationship with his grandmother. Following the loss of his father when he was three years old he had held onto a rather idealized father figure in his mind, which was expressed in his initial idealized transference towards me. The strong transference was then built on Luis's ideas, expectations, and longings that he already had about relationships, and he was able to elicit a strong countertransference indicative of his needs, and effective in getting them met. Despite all he had had to contend with in his life, he still had hope and was willing to risk forming relationships with a new adult and to allow them to become a new developmental object (Hurry, 1998).

It is difficult to evaluate how internal resilience and hope is maintained in individual childhoods where there have been adverse circumstances, although Hurry (1998) helpfully describes how internalized models of self-other relationships can be various and differentiated, and how "even a single secure/understanding relationship may 'save' a child" (p. 46).

The early material was shaped by Luis's deprivation, loss, and humiliation and the defences used to manage this, including his idealization of me as the 'all good' father he had been looking for. This idealization was then shattered with the repetition of the early loss of his father by the first holiday in the work. My return from this holiday gave him the opportunity to repeatedly attack without fear of retaliation in the safe context of the therapeutic setting, expressing the deep-set and long-held rage with its explosive character that his familial and social external environment had found difficult to manage. I became an object that could survive his anger and think with him about it, facilitating greater integration. This often required robustness and patience alongside following him sensitively to support his needs and avoid humiliating him. He was able to develop a greater capacity for thinking and could then think more about his reality rather than relying on fantasies. He acquired a more viable coherent sense of himself, feeling more competent, recognizing his value, and tolerating his vulnerabilities. These developments allowed him to rely less on his primitive rigid defences, and he seemed to become less anxious.

The strength of his transference, and the attraction for him of the use he could make of the therapy for his own development, gained enough momentum in the process of the work to challenge the "lure" of the gangster identification (Canham, 2002). His forward development itself in the therapy was undermining the defensive value of the "internal gang" structure (Canham, 2002) for him. Moving away from the "robot" and the "gangster" allowed him into a more thoughtful, creative, life embracing place, where being a schoolboy was acceptable and sustainable. Canham's (2002) view of the hold of the death instinct in a "gang mentality" is a chilling suggestion for Luis's future, casting the gradual shift in his identifications in a serious light.

Further significance of the benefit of the work for Luis is shown in Woods's (1996) description of how antisocial behaviour that defends against loss, paradoxically often brings further loss. For Luis, his raging outbursts had ruined much for him, leading to the loss of school life and peers (thus confirming the rejection and loss he feared), and so initially he worked hard to keep this rage away from me. As Woods (1996) also describes, society can repeat the cycle of deprivation for the delinquent, and thereby confirm the sense of rejection and justify further attacks. Luis had been withdrawn from school after it was no longer possible to manage his aggressive behaviour; minor criminality had been an aspect of his family context; and so, along with his internal disposition, he had significant factors in his life that favoured his development of delinquent behaviour. However, therapy had placed Luis on a path that meant he did not receive another rejection from his new school, thus breaking the potential cycle of social deprivation.

Luis's grandmother pushed the local education department for him to be sent to an appropriate school for his needs, and she will continue to support him and safeguard his interests. Another positive sign for the future was that he had been able to make a positive identification with the male headmaster of his new school.

This paper argues for early intervention with children like Luis, before the formation of a delinquent character, which, as Wilson (1999) notes, is very difficult to work with therapeutically, particularly once the individual has reached adolescence. At this developmental stage a young person can find engaging in psychotherapy very difficult, and adaptations of therapeutic technique and other innovations in treatment can be necessary when working with the characteristics of this stage of life (Baruch, 2001).

Antisocial behaviour has long been a social concern, and more recently gang membership has been very high on the social and political agenda. (For example, see the website of the

London Criminal Justice Board on gang and group offending: http://lcjb.cjsonline.gov.uk/London/4068.html). In their caseloads most local services and agencies have children and young people with these behaviours, or with potential to be drawn in this direction, and can struggle to make a significant positive impact with some of them. This chapter illustrates how deeply entrenched and powerful are the psychological, familial, and social dynamics involved in some of these kinds of situations, and how detailed and long-term work can be beneficial, with a necessary emphasis on early intervention. It seems reasonable to suggest that if this work is undertaken the long-term costs to society may be reduced, as well as potentially improving the future outcomes for individuals and their families.

References

Baruch, G. (Ed.) (2001). *Community-Based Psychotherapy with Young People*. Hove, UK: Brunner-Routledge.

Canham, H. (2002). Group and gang states of mind. *Journal of Child Psychotherapy, 28*(2): 113–127.

Freud, A. (1937). *The Ego and the Mechanisms of Defence*. London: Karnac, 1993.

Freud, A. (1949). Notes on aggression. In: *Selected Writings* (pp. 37–48). New York: Penguin, 1998.

Hurry, A. (Ed.) (1998). *Psychoanalysis and Developmental Therapy*. London: Karnac.

Kohut, H. (1972). Thoughts on narcissism and narcissistic rage. *Psychoanalytic Study of the Child, 27*: 360–400.

Sandler, J. (1962). The representational world. In: *From Safety to Superego*. London: Karnac.

Wilson, P. (1999). Delinquency. In: *The Handbook of Child and Adolescent Psychotherapy* (pp. 311–327). London: Routledge.

Winnicott, D. W. (1956). The antisocial tendency. In: *Through Paediatrics to Psycho-Analysis*. London: Karnac, 1987.

Winnicott, D. W. (1960). The theory of the parent–infant relationship. In: *The Maturational Processes and the Facilitating Environment*. London: Karnac, 2003.

Winnicott, D. W. (1963). Psychotherapy of character disorders. In: *The Maturational Processes and the Facilitating Environment*. London: Karnac, 2003.

Winnicott, D. W. (1965). *The Maturational Processes and the Facilitating Environment*. London: Karnac, 2003.

Woods, J. (1996). Handling violence in child group therapy. *Group Analysis, 29*: 1.

Outreach

CHAPTER TWENTY ONE

Child psychoanalysis in schools—an Anna Freudian tradition

Pat Radford

Introduction

In her 1954 paper "Psychoanalysis and Education", Anna Freud reflects on the impact of misconceptions regarding the findings of child psychoanalytic clinical research on the lay public. She writes: "Little of this work has reached the lay public of parents and educators, except the misunderstood notion that since the causation of neurosis dates back to the first year of life, it is the behaviour of the mother which proves decisive for the child mental health or illness ..." (p. 320). She goes on to explore all the internal and external factors and dynamics which influence the early emergence of neurotic symptomatology in her characteristically clear and systematic style, highlighting the need to move away from a "mother-blaming" culture.

Interestingly enough, even today those of us working in schools and tending to the needs of young children and their families still find many of the misconceptions and obstacles encountered by Miss Freud and colleagues when trying to engage with school personnel and parents. The nature of our task is further complicated by countless parenting guides and specialized teaching manuals and curriculums available to parents and teachers. However, at the end of the day we encounter the same basic challenge: that of translating our understanding of the internal world of the child and how it is shaped by its interaction with the external world of peers, family, and teachers in order to promote a collaborative and mindful partnership. Fifty years on we continue to seek the same goal of inviting parents and teachers to reflect on the developmental and relational journeys children embark upon when they enter the school setting.

Anna Freud began her own career as a teacher and although some of the ideas expressed in her writings, such as those in her paper "Answers to Teachers" (1952), are representative of a different era, the core of her contributions (which constituted pivotal components of the training at the Hampstead Clinic in London) remain as valuable today, and very useful to the child psychotherapist working in schools. These include detailed observation of children in the context of their peers, and in interactions with significant adults; and use of clear theoretical frameworks such as the "Developmental Lines".

Anna Freud's legacy lives on in the development of specialized services in schools such as the Primary Years Prevention Programme created in 2008 at the now, Anna Freud Centre in London, with the purpose of early detection of emotional difficulties in children aged three to seven. A successful collaboration with five local schools resulted in services to children and families who otherwise would most likely not access their local mental health services. Anna Freud's influence is also evident in early education centres in the United States such as the Hanna Perkins School in Shaker Heights, Ohio and the Allen Creek Preschool in Ann Arbor, Michigan, where the legacy of developmental psychoanalysis has continued to guide the evolution of innovative ways of serving the emotional needs of young children and their parents.

As evident in many of the contributions to this book, the Anna Freud Centre has undergone many changes other than its name since Anna Freud's passing. However, in the midst of all these changes, a small project at a local primary school managed to survive and hopefully inspire and inform new generations of Anna Freudians working in schools. Not only did this project (which came to an end in 2009) serve the needs of children, parents, and school personnel for more than a decade, but it provided the opportunity for graduate students and clinical trainees to practie Anna Freud's detailed observational methods and to apply concepts such as the developmental lines to their unfolding understanding of the nursery child. The rest of this chapter is a narrative description of the history and structure of one such project, as developed twelve years ago at the AFC. It highlights the continuity and strength of Anna Freud's legacy of innovative applied psychoanalysis.

A child psychotherapist working in a school

In 1998 Sheila Sansbury, head teacher of Robinsfield Infant and Nursery School in north London, approached the Anna Freud Centre with a request for assistance from a member of the Centre in advancing the development of early learning in her school. Robinsfield had a socially and culturally mixed school population, with very varied degrees of emotional, intellectual, and linguistic development. The head teacher had had experience of the emotional care and psychological thinking provided in the Hampstead Nursery, which her own son had attended aged three. She was therefore asking for a similarly qualified Anna Freud therapist to help in the development of her nursery and infant school. The Anna Freud Centre asked me if I would undertake the task, with a roving commission to do whatever seemed relevant to the needs of staff, children, and parents/carers as appropriate in the varied situations outlined by the head teacher. For more than a decade I attended the school once or twice a week to offer what help I, a trained child psychotherapist, could give to the emotional life of this exceptional school.

My morning's work began in the hall reception area where the head teacher greeted the parents and children on their arrival, and thus I became a familiar figure to the adults. A brief discussion with Sheila would fill me in on any problems in which I might be of assistance, such as a staff member's concern about a pupil's puzzling behaviour; a parent worried about her child and requesting a private talk with me; spending time with teaching assistant staff to explain more of my approach to behavioural problems in particular children, etc.

I was free to undertake whichever request seemed most urgent and accessible. However, I would inevitably start with a visit to the excellent nursery school of about forty to sixty children, where the value of intervention in any possible worries at the earliest stages of a child's education was much appreciated. The nursery head teacher would direct my observation to a child whose behaviour was of concern to the staff. Using my therapeutic understanding to assess the levels of anxiety which might be overwhelming a particular child, I would discuss my observations with the nursery staff to consider the most appropriate help.

Parents were often present in the nursery and would either approach me directly or through the nursery head teacher with anxieties about their child. I offered a private confidential interview if this was appropriate, always trying to follow up my concerns about the whole problem. Parents with an intimate worry often found it easier to approach me as I was not a direct member of the educational establishment. I was, however, available to help support staff when care and protection issues arose, and I might have had concerns myself after being in touch with a child and his/her parents. Eventually, as more parents requested talks with me, the head teacher suggested that, with a colleague, I institute fortnightly one and a half hour parent groups. We decided these should be open to parents of children of any age and any cultural, ethnic, or social affiliations. This proved to be one of the most useful interventions. Although I would sometimes introduce a topic (e.g., feeding, sleeping problems, etc.), the parents spontaneously brought their own problems for fascinating discussions. The common sense approach of parents with children at different levels of development enhanced the skills of less experienced carers. My colleague and I acted as mentors, particularly if some abstruse psychological theory intervened or if an archaic problem reappeared in the adult as the child's difficulties were explored. The open door approach of these meetings allowed shy or anxious members to listen without feeling any pressure for active participation. Frequently, however, at the end of the meeting someone would request a private meeting. Each group meeting was truly a learning experience for most of us about the emotional depths of even the youngest toddler. Our awareness was amplified by the many and varied ways in which carers' own experiences, old and current, influenced their parenting.

I would also visit classes at the request of concerned teachers, for helpful understanding of a particular child's difficult behaviour which was disturbing the class work: perhaps an autistic little boy, an angry depressed girl, an explosive, aggressive boy. Having stayed in the class observing by whatever method seemed appropriate, I would discuss with the head and the specific class teacher possible helpful interventions. When a child clearly had profound emotional and psychological problems, because of my connection with the Anna Freud Centre I would, after discussion with the parents and head teacher, refer the family for psychological assessment and possible more intensive and long-term treatment at the Centre. Some parents were financially unable to accept such therapeutic help, but the school found a sponsor and once weekly psychotherapy for a year was made available for five young children who otherwise would never have been able to obtain psychotherapeutic support of this nature. This was so helpful that further funding was obtained for an extension of this project, partly because appreciation of each case's successful treatment influenced many other parents' approaches to their own worries and possible help.

Walking down the corridor I would often be stopped by a parent I did not know whose "friend" had suggested she speak to me about her problem. Even more so, children would stop me to report some worry or even some success. I felt very rewarded and grateful for the opportunity I had to work at this school, always supported and inspired by the head teacher and all her staff and by the Anna Freud Centre.

In sum, the psychological expertise I was able to give to the school furthered the well-being of much of the school community and aided it in its difficult tasks. Many times, the head teacher shared with me that having access to a child psychotherapist enriched the whole school and freed staff to focus on the task of teaching, at the same time as increasing their awareness of developmental and emotional issues presented by young children. The Anna Freud Centre has been able to continue work in schools through the efforts of younger graduates such as Norka Malberg, Tobby Etterly, and Natalia Stafler. It is wonderful that they perpetuate this endeavour which is so much in line with Anna Freud's work in her nursery school and at the heart of our tradition.

References

Freud, A. (1952). Answering teachers' questions. In: *The Writings of Anna Freud, Vol. IV* (pp. 560–568). New York: International Universities Press.

Freud, A. (1954). Psychoanalysis and education. In: *The Writings of Anna Freud, Vol. IV* (pp. 317–326). New York: International Universities Press.

D. ADOLESCENCE

Clinical papers and outreach beyond the consulting room

Overview

CHAPTER TWENTY TWO

Overview of transitions, clinical application, current developments

Luis Rodríguez de la Sierra

Since her death, Anna Freud seemed fated to disappear from the minds of many psychoanalysts to the point of denying her importance, and almost her existence, even in places where indisputably she reigned for many years during her life. Taking into account her prolific and important contribution to psychoanalysis, that phenomenon is not only incomprehensible but terribly unjust. Recently something interesting has started happening: a slow but certain come-back in the UK and elsewhere, including France and the USA—countries where she was once well known and had become an almost complete stranger.

Her work today is as relevant as it was while she was alive as it provides us with original and useful ways to understand not only the behaviour and psychopathology of children but that of adults as well. Her great and invaluable direct experience with children fed her understanding of human development, and that coloured the many insights and ideas which she brought to her contributions to psychoanalysis. The elegance and deceptive clarity of her formulations remain unsurpassed, but her later theoretical ideas lacked the illustrative clinical material of earlier papers. Her thinking is not always easy to unravel without recourse to the observational experience and clinical work on which it was based.

This book is one of several attempts to restore Anna Freud and her ideas to their rightful place. Florian Houssier's last book, *Anna Freud et son école: Créativité et controverses* (2010), tries to do the same in France. Hopefully more will follow.

Anna Freud was a very modest woman who never tried to steal the limelight. Indeed, at times, she undervalued the importance of some of her own contributions to the theory and practice of psychoanalysis. The best example of this is her reluctance, while she was alive, to give their rightful place to her innovations in technique for working with children suffering from developmental deficiencies—techniques she named "developmental help". These originated from her developmental theories and, unlike her modest approach, nowadays many child psychotherapists from all persuasions consider them as comprising part of the "proper" child and adult psychoanalytic repertoire.

The concept of her "Developmental Lines" is one of her great contributions to the understanding of human nature from a psychoanalytic perspective. It has applications to adults and Marie Zaphiriou Woods (2003) has written an excellent and illuminating paper on the developmental approach in the psychoanalysis of adults.

Anna Freud, like all analysts who accept the dualism of the drives, and give sexuality an essentially organizing and disorganizing function, refused to amalgamate adolescents with children and adults. Like Freud, she insisted that the upsurge of drive energy which occurs with puberty presented us with an imbalance between the id and the ego, debilitating the latter. To her this meant that the adolescent had little toleration of frustration, and sought immediate satisfaction instead of sublimatory substitutes. The anxiety connected with the weakening of the ego causes the defences to become even more rigid. By so stating she gave quite a special and specific place to adolescent psychopathology. Her position was very different from that of Winnicott (1961, p. 79):

> There exists one real cure for adolescence, and only one … [It] belongs to the passage of time and to the gradual maturational processes; these together do in the end result in the emergence of the adult person. This process cannot be hurried or slowed up, though indeed can be broken into and destroyed, or it can wither up from within, in psychiatric illness.

As to Melanie Klein's views on the subject, apart from one short paper on puberty (1922), and the chapter where she expresses her views on "The technique of analysis in puberty" (1932), she says nothing afterwards. I assume that relates to the importance she attributed to destructive aggression as an expression of the death instinct from birth, which deflected attention from the libidinal drive and its fate during the sexual maturation that is so central to the process of puberty and adolescence.

Some psychoanalysts maintained that treatment was not only possible, but very necessary. Jeanne Lampl-de Groot, the Dutch psychoanalyst, thought that the reluctance to analyse adolescents was due to the fact that the period of adolescence had not been properly psychoanalysed in the course of the analyses of many adults, psychoanalytic candidates included.

Adolescence, as we know, is a turbulent period of time in life. Young people experience hormonal and physical changes that affect their moods and emotions. Very few psychoanalysts nowadays doubt that psychoanalysis can help them resolve the new and confusing feelings with which they contend. Anna Freud was the first to describe adolescence, and the study of adolescent moods has remained one of the most promising means of approaching our topic. Since her comment has attained such fame in psychoanalytic literature, I would like to quote it in full:

> Young people who pass through the kind of ascetic phase which I have in mind seem to fear the quantity rather than the quality of their instincts. They mistrust enjoyment in general and so their safest policy appears to be simply to counter more urgent desires with more stringent prohibitions. Every time the instinct says, "I will", the ego retorts, "Thou shalt not", much after

> the manner of strict parents in the early training of little children. This adolescent mistrust of instinct has a dangerous tendency to spread; it may begin with instinctual wishes proper and extend to the most ordinary physical needs. We have all met young people who severely renounced any impulses which savoured of sexuality and who avoided the society of those of their own age, declined to join in any entertainment and, in true puritanical fashion, refused to have anything to do with the theatre, music or dancing. We can understand that there is a connection between the foregoing of pretty and attractive clothes and the prohibition of sexuality. But we begin to be disquieted when the renunciation is extended to things which are harmless and necessary, as, for instance, when a young person denies himself the most ordinary protection against cold, mortifies the flesh in every possible way and exposes his health to unnecessary risks, when he not only gives up particular kinds of oral enjoyments, but "on principle" reduces his daily food to a minimum, when, from having enjoyed long nights of sound sleep, he forces himself to get up early, when he is reluctant to laugh or smile or when, in extreme cases, he defers defecation and urination as long as possible, on the grounds that one ought not immediately to give way to all one's physical needs (1936, pp. 166–169).

Anna Freud goes on to say that this repudiation of instinct differs radically from ordinary repression in that no loophole is left for substitutive gratification. Instead of compromise-formations (corresponding to neurotic symptoms) and the usual process of displacement, regression, and turning against the self, we find almost invariably a swing-over from asceticism to instinctual excess, the adolescent suddenly indulging in everything which he had previously held to be prohibited (1936, p. 170).

In 1958, twenty years after she had first written about it, she returned to the subject. Her paper on adolescence is now a classic and unsurpassed study of adolescent psychology. In 1966 she returned once again, and for the last time, to the subject, and wrote one of her lesser known papers on the theme, "Adolescence as a developmental disturbance". In this paper she completes, with the deceptive simplicity which characterized her, what she had started in 1936 and continued in 1958. It is a paper that deserves re-evaluation and diffusion among those interested in the subject. At the risk of repeating myself I would like to point out that in this paper she not only advocates that psychoanalysis can help adolescents resolve their problems, but insightfully talks about the confusion those developmental problems provoke in the young person and also in those around him, hence the title of the paper. She explicitly alerts us to what normally takes place during that developmental phase, and how important it is for the adults to take it into account before making unreasonable demands on the young person whose energy and interest are occupied with what is happening to them at that time, rather than with what the adult world and society in general expect from them. Norka Malberg, in her rich and very interesting paper, "When silence and tears speak: psychotherapy with an adolescent girl" (this volume), returns to this rarely cited paper of Anna Freud's in her closing remarks, and we have to thank her for that.

While Anna Freud was always very interested in the psychoanalytic understanding of adolescents and followed closely the work of her fellow students (Aichhorn, Bernfeld, Erikson, Hoffer), she was reluctant to engage in their treatment herself, and this continued to be the case at the Hampstead Clinic for many years. However, after meeting Moses Laufer, one of her students with a very keen interest in the world of adolescents, she supported and encouraged him to continue doing so. Because of their association, Anna Freud actively worked towards the creation of what was to become Laufer's central psychoanalytic interest and it was thus that the Young People's Consultation Centre was eventually born in the period between 1961 and 1962. Anna Freud's enthusiasm for Laufer's work was such that in the course of the following two years his Centre became an extension of the Hampstead Clinic for the treatment of adolescents and for the training of those wishing to work with them. (In 1965 Laufer modified and expanded Anna Freud's "Diagnostic Profile", specifically for the assessment of adolescent disturbances.)

In her 1958 paper, Anna Freud starts with an historical review of the existing psychoanalytic literature on adolescence, then gives a very good, clear, and insightful description of adolescence, and concludes by defending the possibility and necessity of offering young people psychoanalytic treatment. Shortly before her death, the number of adolescents seen at the Centre seemed to increase and in later years it multiplied even more, to the point that a fair number among the staff, including myself, were frequently treating and assessing adolescents.

Anna Freud not only encouraged us to work with these patients but, as Brafman (2000) rightly points out, with their parents. In her 1958 paper she states: "... it may be [the adolescent's] parents who need help and guidance so as to be able to bear with him. There are few situations in life which are more difficult to cope with than the adolescent son or daughter during their attempts to liberate themselves" (pp. 225–278).

Many of Anna Freud's ideas are still valid when thinking of this group of patients, and her emphasis on how crucial is the making of a relationship *before* analytic interpretative work begins is absolutely true in our work with youngsters. It certainly has played a very important role in my own work with young people suffering from alcoholism and drug addiction. In this volume, Doris Venguer's paper, "Female adolescence and the uses of the body", on the psychoanalytic treatment of an adolescent girl, Michaela, is another excellent example of the present day use of Anna Freud's ideas; and the same can be said about Helen Ritzema's description of William, an adolescent boy opting for the delinquent solution, in her clinical paper, "The terrorist and the boffin". These two chapters differ in many ways but, like Norka Malberg's, they bear the imprint of Anna Freud's teachings and ideas. All these papers show an integration of Anna Freud's contemporary clinical ideas and concepts which strengthen the developmental approach characteristic of child psychotherapists trained in this tradition. Finally, Joan Raphael-Leff's work is an excellent example of such integration and the impact that Anna Freud's tradition of training and research has had on the psychoanalytic community and beyond. Her course targeting mental health workers working with teenage parents encapsulates the essence of Anna Freud's vision of educating professionals in allied fields through the use of the psychoanalytic lens.

Nowadays, the concern about adolescence has increased even further and we witness many psychoanalytic events organized around this subject both in the psychoanalytic milieu and outside it. In this context, we should always remember Anna Freud's original interest in, and hearty support for this cause.

References

Brafman, A. (2000). Working with adolescents: a pragmatic view. In: I. Wise (Ed.), *Adolescence*. London: The Institute of Psychoanalysis.

Freud, A. (1936). *The Ego and the Mechanisms of Defence*. London: Hogarth, 1942.

Freud, A. (1958). Adolescence. *Psychoanalytic Study of the Child, 8*: 225–278.

Freud, A. (1966). Adolescence as a developmental disturbance. In: *The Writings of Anna Freud: Problems of Psychoanalytic Training, Diagnosis, and the Technique of Therapy, Vol. VIII* (pp. 39–47). New York: International Universities Press.

Houssier, F. (2010). *Anna Freud et son école: Créativité et controverses*. Paris: Éditions Campagne.

Klein, M. (1922). Inhibitions and difficulties at puberty. In: *The Writings of Melanie Klein, Vol. 1. Love, Guilt and Other Works, 1921–1945* (pp. 54–58). New York: Delacorte Press/Seymour Lawrence.

Klein, M. (1932). The technique of psychoanalysis in puberty. In: *The Psycho-Analysis of Children*. London: Hogarth.

Laufer, M. (1965). Assessment of adolescent disturbances—the application of Anna Freud's diagnostic profile. *Psychoanalytic Study of the Child, 20*: 99–123.

Rodríguez de la Sierra, L. (2000). Working with the addict. In: I. Wise (Ed.), *Adolescence* (pp. 72–88). London: The Institute of Psychoanalysis.

Winnicott, D. W. (1961). Adolescence: struggling through the doldrums. In: *The Family and Individual Development* (pp. 79–87). London: Tavistock.

Zaphiriou Woods, M. (2003). Developmental considerations in an adult analysis. In: V. Green (Ed.), *Emotional Development in Psychoanalysis: Attachment Theory and Neuroscience* (pp. 209–225). Padstow, UK: T. J. International.

Clinical

CHAPTER TWENTY THREE

"Desperately seeking a mother"—female adolescence and the uses of the body[1]

Doris Venguer

It seems to be generally accepted that a strong fixation to the mother, dating not only from the Oedipal but from the pre-Oedipal attachment to her, renders adolescence especially difficult. [...] lack of a mother fixation, far from making adolescence easier, constitutes a real danger to the whole inner coherence of the personality during that period. In these cases adolescence is preceded frequently by a frantic search for a mother image; the internal possession and cathexis of such an image seems to be essential for the ensuing normal process of detaching libido from it for transfer to new objects, i.e., to sexual partners.

—(Anna Freud, 1958, p. 152).

Twenty-five years ago, during my training at the Anna Freud Centre, my analyst used a phrase that has remained with me throughout the psychotherapeutic and analytic work with my own patients, as well as in my own personal life as a daughter and a mother. Paraphrasing Margaret Mahler (1971) she said: "We are all trying to work out the optimal distance between ourselves and our parents."

Achieving this "optimal distance", as we know, is a recurrent process that begins very early. We each start life connected to our mother, gradually "emerging" through the physical and emotional relationship with our caregivers in our cultural environment; and progressively building our identity, while being immersed in a constant exchange of subjective interactions.

[1] I would like to thank Marianne Parsons for her insightful comments on this case.

Stepping away: adolescence

In psychoanalytic thinking, adolescence represents a key stage of the development through which the young person achieves further individuation by negotiating emotional distance and detachment from the internalized parental objects (Blos, 1967). During this particular developmental phase of negotiating optimal distance, the dramatic oscillation between closeness and separation reflects the internal reorganization of the individual's psychic reality. The adolescent is faced with the crucible of biological, psychological, and cultural pressures while her caring objects are going through a transformation themselves. In this chapter I will present details from the analysis of an adolescent that conveys these dilemmas.

In order to understand the restructuring processes that are taking place during the adolescent upheaval, we cannot ignore the role of the external influences that have shaped the young person's personality. Separation and identity formation, as Erikson pointed out, do not begin or end in adolescence: "It is a lifelong development largely unconscious to the individual and to his society. Its roots go back all the way to the first self-recognition: in the baby's earliest exchange of smiles there is something of a self-realization coupled with a mutual recognition" (1956, p. 68).

The role of the caregiving objects in developing the child's feelings about herself has been extensively explored in the psychoanalytic literature. The affective interaction in the mother's mirroring (Winnicott, 1971a) and her affect attunement (Stern, 1985) provide the narcissistic layers for the construction of a girl's body and self-representations. In the give and take of the sensual and verbal interactions between mother and child, there will be a multitude of identifications which will shape the mental representations of her self and her body (Sandler & Rosenblatt, 1962; Joffe & Sandler, 1967).

As noted, internalization over time of the relationship between mother and daughter will influence the young girl's relation to herself, and the way she takes care of her body and takes over the maternal role towards herself and towards others (A. Freud, 1965c; Furman, 1982; Mahler, 1975; P. Tyson, 1986; Winnicott, 1963a).

Case history: Michaela

Michaela, the adolescent I present here, is at this point in her life in the process of "taking ownership" of her body (Laufer, 1968). She uses desperate measures to seek independence through refusal of identification with her mother (Laufer & Laufer, 1984; Ritvo, 1984).

Her adolescent struggle is exponentially intensified due to a history of conflict with her mother. How she feels about herself is the result of hypercritical introjects which counteract her attempts to increase her self-esteem by using external sources. Unresolved "rapprochement" conflicts can be glimpsed in the poor integration of her ambivalence (A. Freud, 1949a, 1965c), which in turn influences the way she relates to others and to herself.

In the past, Michaela's exhibitionism may have served to gain approval and positive responses from her mother and later her father (Edgcumbe & Burgner, 1975). At present, using the same strategy but with a different body she realizes that boys, men, and other girls are reacting to it differently. Even her mother is reacting to Michaela's sexualized displays, which only increases the tension between them.

I will only speak about one side of the story, Michaela's version, which could be partially constructed after many months of therapeutic work. However, one should also consider the mother's contribution to the separation-individuation difficulties (Mahler, 1963, 1971; Mahler & Furer, 1968; Mahler et al., 1975): not only when she was absent and unable to meet Michaela's needs, but also now, in her fifties, when she is dealing with menopause at the very point of her daughter's pubertal flowering, and her own reactivated past conflicts, consciously and unconsciously evoked by her daughter's adolescence (Benedek, 1950; Berkowitz et al., 1974; Brandt & Silverman, 1985; Sprince, 1962).

Often during Michaela's analysis I wondered about the emotional whereabouts of her parents. When a young girl is confronted with intensification of her aggression and her sexuality, the road towards finding an identity for herself will be more painful if she feels alone with no one to guide or meet her half way. With Michaela I often felt that as her therapist I was handed responsibility for her actions, while her parents were too involved in their own difficulties to help, but could not work on themselves despite my suggestions.

Even though Michaela's treatment ended prematurely, I believe there was a shift nonetheless, in that as she was gradually able to see parts of herself within the mirroring process of the analysis, she could contain her desperate search for love and admiration in the transference relationship while it lasted.

Referral

Michaela was referred at age fourteen and a half for treatment by her school principal, Mrs L, because of her difficulties at secondary school. At first glance, Michaela's behaviour did not come across as unusual for her age. She was constantly seeking attention by dressing inappropriately for school, by shouting and running in the corridors, and by exaggerated flirtatious and teasing interactions with peers and some of the male teachers. Her grades reflected long-standing difficulties with conceptualization and focusing on her work. Michaela received remedial help throughout the upper primary years though no definite diagnosis of learning disabilities was ever confirmed. Teachers felt that Michaela needed one-to-one help with her work outside her home environment in order to mitigate the ongoing battling relationship over homework between Michaela and her mother. The twice weekly learning support Michaela received for a period of almost three years did help her to put her ideas on paper, to improve her organizational skills and to increase her understanding of maths concepts. The school's main concern was related to Michaela's emotional well-being. Mrs L, who had known Michaela for many years, was of the opinion that her difficulties reflected the impact her father's absence from home had on her and the longstanding tension between Michaela and her mother. She felt that despite the extraordinary closeness between mother and child, Mrs G still found it difficult to accept her daughter for who she was.

Michaela is an only child. Her father, Mr G, distanced himself from the family as his work required him to travel oversees from the time Michaela was nine years old. Although he continued to support his wife and daughter financially, his periodic absences from the family lasted sometimes up to two or three months. Father's intermittent separations from home were initially seen as a temporary arrangement; however, even by the end of Michaela's treatment the father's living circumstances remained the same.

Michaela's analytic treatment lasted nearly three years. Mr G supported and financed treatment until the last session, but it was Mrs G who drove her daughter to sessions or arranged the transportation for her. The four times a week sessions often decreased in frequency because of Mrs G's strong ambivalence to treatment. Michaela's mother persistently declined the possibility of therapy for herself. Apart from the occasional meetings of the analyst with the parents, the school principal's role as a mother substitute provided Mrs G with some of the containment and support she so desperately needed throughout her daughter's analytic treatment. Ideally, a simultaneous analysis of mother and daughter (see Burlingham, 1955; Hellman, 1960; Levy, 1960; Sprince, 1962) perhaps would have fostered mother's separation from her daughter by addressing Mrs G's own history of loneliness and disappointment. Nevertheless, the imminent threat surrounding Michaela's wish for closeness and passive surrender contributed to the premature termination of her analysis.

Background summary

Mr G often voiced his concern about Michaela's difficulties at school, and with remorse wondered whether her struggle with discipline was related to his absence from home. He was deeply worried about the fact that his wife had become "obsessed" with religion ever since her own father died, when Michaela was six years old.

Mr and Mrs G had known each other since childhood as their parents had mutual acquaintances. They met again in their mid-thirties and after a few months of dating Mrs G fell pregnant with Michaela. The couple decided to marry, as it was "the best thing to do". Michaela was named after her grandfather as Mrs G was convinced during her pregnancy that her baby would be a boy.

According to Mrs G, Michaela had been an easy baby. She was looked after by a series of nannies while her mother continued with her artistic work. She suffered from separation-anxiety for several months upon entering nursery school at age three. Mrs G described Michaela's relationships to her nannies and to other children as "clingy" and demanding. Mrs G often felt exasperated with her daughter's reluctance to follow rules. The latest argument she had with her daughter was over her wearing tights (instead of socks) for school. She regretted the fact that Michaela was not brought up in the Catholic school she herself had attended when she was young. Although the same order of nuns still owned Michaela's school it was now co-ed (mixed gender) and much more liberal. Mrs G and her own ten years younger sister Lala were never particularly close as they are "opposite poles" to each other. She felt that in some way Michaela could have been Lala's daughter, as they both are "forgetful, stubborn, and flaky".

Mr G, a successful executive in his own field, had to focus on his studies from very early on as he was sent abroad after his mother died. He identified with his daughter's "jolly character" although he wished she could be more interested in her academic work at school. He described Michaela as insecure and vulnerable to peer pressure, as she usually has difficulties with standing up for herself vis-à-vis her girl friends.

The ever-present animosity between Michaela's parents was pervasive throughout all our interviews; this could be seen in their non-verbal communications and in their inability to agree on many details of events or the overall description of their daughter. Mrs G's annoyance with her daughter turned out to be more than a phase-related reaction to her daughter's adolescent behaviour; this was corroborated by the school teachers, by Mr G, and by Michaela herself.

The manifest demand for treatment from both parents was to bring Michaela "back on track" to get on with her studies. They were also concerned about her lack of interest in school and her exaggerated interest in boys. In my opinion, both parents had the unconscious realization that the tension between them and their own difficulties had taken a toll on their daughter's emotional development.

Michaela's analysis

The following is a schematic presentation of Michaela's treatment organized sequentially around themes, which concentrically overlap in Michaela's use of her body as a scenario where multiple ramifications of past and present conflicts are represented.

Michaela's experience of her mother

Although Michaela welcomed the fact that in analytic sessions she had a "special place" of her own, it was initially hard for her to feel comfortable in this one-on-one situation, and she felt she could not totally trust me to keep the information she gave me away from her mother.

During the first months of treatment, Michaela tested my loyalty to her by bringing into the sessions detailed altercations with her mother where she wanted me to take sides and validate her sense of constantly being belittled at home.

At school, since her later latency years, Michaela had always been part of a group. Her difficulties with developing mutual and empathic relationships with others contributed to her social conflicts as she could not establish a "best" friend. In order to obtain approval and recognition from her peers, she followed and idealized the group's leader and ignored the girls whom she considered stupid or immature.

Michaela's advanced physical development contrasted with the immature way in which she expressed herself. She was not used to thinking about herself and had difficulty describing herself or others. I often felt that I needed to connect her scattered ideas for her before I could attempt to give any interpretation. As treatment progressed, I wondered whether Michaela's difficulties in thinking about herself had become defensively stunted or were the result of not having had an intimate relationship where her feelings were translated for her (Edgcumbe, 1993; Fonagy & Moran, 1991; Fonagy et al., 1991, 1993). Michaela's shallowness and sometimes concrete grasp of ideas became, with time, sporadically interrupted by revelations that made sense to her. I could see that father's role as her ongoing "homework helper" gave Michaela an opportunity to be close to him, and his support helped her to "make up" her mind, as she often demanded from me. Although there were times when her father's exasperation left her feeling helpless or abandoned, the experience of having someone thinking *with* her may indeed have fostered some aspects of her ego functioning.

Michaela sometimes equated me with her school principal or her aunt Lala in that both were able to acknowledge Michaela's own wishes without being punitive and critical. However, derogatory aspects of herself were often part of her ambivalence in the transference, where she projected her own perception of being unintelligent and not good enough. She feared that during my moments of silence or when I did not respond to her direct questioning as to whether her actions were right or wrong, I was in fact also being critical of her and would be judging her behaviour as immature or simply stupid.

Michaela often complained about her mother's critical attitude towards her and perceived her mother as angry and miserable. She was unable to see in her mother any positive qualities which she might want to admire or emulate. However, she did remember that as a young girl she admired her mother's artistic talents as a performer. Although she experienced her father as more benign, she also regretted the fact that he could be manipulated by her mother, as he almost always ended up doing what Mrs G wanted.

Michaela's attempts to find the limits between herself and her mother

During the first year of treatment, Michaela related an incident where she and her friends were hiding from a nun who wanted to measure the length of their skirts. I then linked the material to her feeling that her mother always wants to have control of the way she uses her body. In this session, Michaela confessed to me that she had gone to a mall with her friends to have a belly button piercing. She was anxious about the fact that the area of the piercing was sore and she feared it might be infected. The symbolic piercing of the umbilicus metaphorically represented Michaela's attempts to cut loose her ties by choosing that part of her body that signified connection to the life-giving mother.

As she revealed her abdomen to me, I could sense her anxiety about having brought on herself an uncontrollable damage, which originated in her attempts to make herself sexually appealing to others. Guilty feelings regarding her exhibitionistic wishes were reflected in her fear that the infection would worsen. By externalizing her own superego anxiety onto her mother, she feared the infection would lead her mother to discover the piercing and that she would react by "grounding" her "indefinitely".

The "belly button incident" became a turning point in the treatment, as we went back to this instance when she invited me to rescue her from something dreadful that she had brought upon herself. Gradually, we could connect Mrs G's preoccupation with her own body with Michaela's attempts to bring her objects closer by endangering or causing damage to herself.

Although Michaela spoke at length about her mother's "migraines", it was only during the second year of treatment that Mrs G, after a series of repeated cancellations of Michaela's sessions, spoke to me about her chronic fatigue and lack of stamina, which had kept her bedridden for days throughout the past years. Her doctor had told her that her migraines and lack of energy had to do with a hormonal imbalance due to the menopause.

Michaela had spoken about her mother's unavailability through material that focused on her mother's "tiredness" and involvement in events organized by the church. Initially, Michaela would express anger towards her mother by accusing her of being "theatrical", exaggerating her inability to function. At the same time, Michaela's preoccupation with her mother's depressive moods were re-enacted in the transference whenever I was emotionally less responsive or recovering from a week's absence due to illness. Michaela's defensive manic accounts of her ordeals were understood as her wish to make me happy and to decrease her anxiety lest something happen to me.

The extent of mother's unavailability throughout Michaela's development was not revealed in the history taken from the parents during the initial interviews before treatment began. It became clear, however, that ongoing marital tensions and father's intermittent physical withdrawal from his wife and daughter had taken a toll on Mrs G's emotional availability throughout Michaela's early years.

When she referred to her father's absences, Michaela herself made the connection between her mother's present complaints about tiredness and her own feeling that mother had always been distant from her. She remembered how her mother had missed a couple of her performances at school because she was always "too busy not feeling well" at home. She was convinced that her mother "pretended" to be ill and exhausted in order to bring her father back earlier from his trips: "She could fool me because I sometimes was worried about her, but not him: he knows her better."

Quite often Michaela felt she needed to compete against mother's narcissistic preoccupation with her own needs as if she was competing against a baby sibling who was being looked after and cared for at the expense of her own emotional and physical needs.

Her identification with her mother's theatricality was not only evident in Michaela's exhibitionism, but also in what seemed to be disconnectedness with what she felt and thought. Speaking about Winnicott's concept of the true self (1960a), Modell (1985) reminds us that the mirroring process depends on the capacity of the mother accurately to perceive the child's affects, and that the exchange of false or compliant affects places both the child's and carer's self out of reach. Following this line of thought, I am reminded of the many times in treatment when Michaela was confused by her mother's refusal to talk to her "for days", as a recurrent way to punish her, and of Michaela's own feeling of "paralysis" as she usually remained silent and unable to respond to her mother's recriminations. She felt she could never confront her, as she dreaded she would cause both irreparable damage to her mother and then also to herself, because of her mother's response. To my mind, the prolonged experience of heightened anxiety over loss of mother's love and Michaela's attempts to placate and appease her mother with compliance and submission, also contributed to the development of a false sense of self.

The second year

During the second year of treatment, Michaela had a reaction to antibiotics prescribed for a throat infection. She was hospitalized for two nights. Upon returning to treatment, Michaela was thrilled that many members of her family, including her father, had visited her during her stay at the hospital. She felt triumphant about the fact that her mother looked scared. She was thrilled that Mrs G must have realized that it was not only she, mother, who could be physically ill.

Michaela's experience of heterosexuality

In the transference, the battling and competitive overtone that permeated Michaela's relationship with her mother took over as she began to be more open about the risky nature of her experiences outside treatment. At one level, there was her wish to show me that she was able to elicit sexual responses from boys and men of different ages, thinking that I, like her mother, would be "jealous" and envious of her body.

On another level, whilst including me in the intimacy of her coupling encounters, Michaela also communicated how she endangered herself by frantically going from partner to partner, responding impulsively to their invitations but unable to remain under control once she was alone with them and, had "gone too far" (as she once described it). I saw Michaela equipped with a fully developed feminine body launching herself into situations without the ability to establish a dialogue and/or read the intentions and motives of the others. Now and again, like the car rides Michaela accepted from youngsters who had drunk too much, she seemed to be propelled by a newly acquired freedom, which she was unable to direct or calibrate.

The excitement about having "scared" her mother resembled the way in which I reacted to Michaela's behaviour outside treatment. I found myself anxiously preoccupied with the way she endangered herself. Awareness of my countertransference led me to understand that Michaela wanted me to control and restrict her while she was battling her way out from an interlocked anal-aggressive relationship with her mother.

Before the analysis started, Michaela had already had her first heterosexual encounter while she was away with a girlfriend and her family during the summer. She had reacted to the boy's incessant insinuations because he had commented on how good she looked in her bikini while they were all together in the swimming pool. Michaela did not think he was particularly attractive, but the fact that he had "noticed" her amongst all the teenagers in the pool had excited her and made her curious. She arranged an "escapade" in his room where they felt each other's bodies and she masturbated him.

Further incidents continued to present a pattern: maybe there was a strong attraction from Michaela's part, but the fact that other girls found a boy attractive led her to take the decision to have more intimate contact with the youngster. By the time Michaela started treatment she had already had a similar experience with an adult, the manager of a restaurant next door to her friend's holiday home.

When Michaela had intercourse for the first time at age fifteen years and nine months, with an eighteen-year-old whom she had not seen for a long time, she found herself in a situation where the excitement of teasing and petting evolved into having intercourse without any precautions. This incident was not isolated; she repeated involvement in unsafe intercourse several times after this, even after she had obtained contraceptives through an older girlfriend.

In the cultural milieu of Michaela's school, friends, and family, her behaviour stood out. All the incidents took place in the context of a holiday or a weekend with a friend. Michaela's parents were not aware of their daughter's behaviour but, as it often happens, Michaela's peers were speaking about it and her wish to be noticed and be popular came true. Unfortunately, she was not the triumphant Oedipal princess of her story; Michaela realized that behind her back she was seen as and called "a slut".

Many authors have conceptualized heterosexual acting out in adolescence as a defence against the regressive pull towards the pre-Oedipal mother (Blos, 1962; Dahl, 1993; Ritvo, 1984; Pines, 1993). In his article on female delinquency, Blos (1957) explained that the resistance against a strong fixation to the mother can be seen in the girl's illusory maintenance of an Oedipal situation.

In Michaela's desperate attempts to resist regression and identification with her mother, she unconsciously modelled the image of herself into the opposite by acting against the perceived expectations of her mother. The level of structuralization of her superego can be inferred by her attempts to escape the severe-nun-religious introjected aspect of the mother by expressing her libidinal wishes in an unregulated manner.

What was particularly striking in all Michaela's sexual encounters was the lack of emotional closeness to her partners. The narcissistic gratification derived from people's reactions to her erotized displays of her body served as a transitory compensation for a deeply rooted feeling of being unlovable and worthless.

Through Michaela's sketchy communications we came to understand that, although she felt reassured by the excited response she elicited through her body, she was anxious about being rejected by her partners for many reasons; for example, when she spoke about her vaginal odour or about how sex sometimes hurt, alluding to fantasies where intercourse can become violent and sadistic. The initial excitement about being seduced disappeared as she ended up "doing to" or "being done to" with another body. Who the person behind the body was did not seem to be as relevant as what he represented.

At some point Michaela metaphorically used the dichotomy "outside" versus "inside" in order to portray the way she felt about herself. With vivid images, aided by few words, she explained that while from the outside she seemed happy and proud of her looks, behind the screen there teemed a messy disgusting part of herself.

As in the past, Michaela continued to rely on turning passive defences into active, in order to find reasons for not developing a relationship with the teenagers whom she initially considered as steady "super boyfriend" candidates. The excitement about the possibility of a relationship contained fantasies about conquering the "handsomest guy" and provoking admiration and envy from others.

As Michaela came back from weekends and holidays with her "exciting/scary" news, I was able very gradually to link her "fear" of my being angry about her not taking care of herself to her own anger about my "dumping" her and being with someone else (see M. E. Laufer, 1996).

Michaela's fantasies about my holidays without her conveyed jealousy and envy of a perfect life with a perfect husband and perfect children (boy and a girl) who fulfilled all my needs. More in-depth description of my idealized family contained all or nothing qualities, where gradations or the "good enough" elements were not considered (Novick & Novick, 1996).

There were times when Michaela suddenly removed her pullover in the session displaying to me her low-cut blouses that revealed her cleavage. Clearly her excitement had to do with the way she thought I saw her when she used displacement to talk about the envy and jealousy of other girls who had "smaller breasts" than her or when she thought about what her girlfriends would say when she had been with someone valued by them.

Michaela's wish to be rescued

Michaela's difficulties with looking after herself and her propensity for seeking high-risk situations revealed paradoxical wishes: on the one hand she wanted to hurt her object by turning the aggression against herself, yet she also wanted to be passively looked after and "mothered" on the other.

A fantasy she brought at different stages of the treatment used a hospital as a background scenario where Michaela would see herself surrounded by friends and family as she recovered from a "minor operation". Alongside Michaela's ideas on how she would manage to get hospitalized (for example, as a result of a car crash, or due to appendicitis or "mild pneumonia"), she described how each one of the characters (among them her mother, her father, and me) would be so overcome by guilt that we would devotionally look after her and pamper her.

The common denominator among multiple scripts of this fantasy was pre-Oedipal longings, with a figure who, at the end, would rescue her from her pain. Yet Michaela constantly defended against such longings in her relationship with her mother. In the last stages of Michaela's treatment the hospital fantasy shifted into her wish to become pregnant and get married in order to be looked after "forever" by her husband. The material that preceded this new solution was the unplanned pregnancy of a teenager acquaintance. Michaela's fascination was definitely not with the baby, but with the fact that the mother became the centre of attention by proxy because the baby was so beautiful and perfectly dressed.

In her studies of women's unconscious uses of the body, Pines (1993) speaks about the effects of the developing body on the adolescent's self-esteem. The response to the girl's physical attraction and acknowledgment of her body as a source of pleasure, may confirm for the adolescent a sense of existence. She refers to a study on adolescent promiscuity (Mehra & Pines, 1972), where the wish for a baby represented a "search for an object which is never found in actual experience and contains the underlying fantasy of being looked after, cuddled and fed" (Pines, 1993, p. 70). Although the unconscious ramifications to this fantasy might have been Michaela's attempt to re-create her mother's unplanned pregnancy and give birth to a new model of herself, her overwhelming need to feel important to others was once again in the centre of our sessions.

Michaela's experience of her father

Work in the transference regarding her wish to be rescued and cared for brought Michaela closer to her disappointment and anger about her father, and a concomitant curiosity about his life, which until now had been denied. Michaela's partial idealization of her father protected her against the pain and the realization that he was not the reliable loving figure to whom she could turn.

Michaela's relationship with her father merits another paper. It is important to say that despite his inconsistency throughout Michaela's life, she perceived he had more real qualities than her mother, with whom she was often immersed in a confusing entanglement of ownerships, not only regarding her body but also her thoughts and wishes.

Michaela's unresolved Oedipal relationship with her father bore the stamp of many other cases mentioned in the psychoanalytic literature (e.g., Burgner, 1985; Burgner & Gavshon, 1981; Neubauer, 1960), in that she often conveyed her feelings of being trapped in a situation from which she needed rescuing and guidance. As a young child Michaela must have received some admiration that confirmed her femininity and her overall feelings of self-worth and self-esteem; but she did not manage to consolidate a good enough loving relationship with her objects, which could accompany her in her attempts to establish intimate relationships with others (Kernberg, 1984). Michaela desperately needed her father, not only in her relationship to him, but also in his relationship with her mother as a couple, to convey and model what a loving and caring relationship was like.

This was particularly illustrated in a dream just before a three-week break (a couple of months before stopping treatment), where she dreamt of some classmates inviting her to the beach. I was in the distance and then disappeared. Michaela's associations regarding beaches and holidays led her to speak about her fear of going into the ocean and how she remembered that it was her father's grasp of her hand that had made her feel secure to face the force of the waves. She felt that her mother was too weak to be able to save her if they were both "swirled" inside a wave. In fact, she would end up saving her mother, who did not have a clue how to resist the current, and would drown. If no lifeguard were there, at least her father could pull them out ... or (she added), maybe not.

Discussion

In the turmoil of adolescence, when the integration and reorganization of past and present self-representations and fantasies are taking place, the adolescent's behaviour reflects different gradations of disturbances which may point to temporary solutions or to long-standing difficulties which are carried over from the past (A. Freud, 1958, 1969; Blos, 1962, 1967; Laufer & Laufer, 1984).

A good enough relationship with the caregivers generates built-in mental representations which accompany the adolescent through a gradual detachment from their infantile internal objects, while at the same time enabling transformation of the updated relationship to and from the external parents.

In cases where the adolescent is caught in the grip of an intense anal-aggressive mode of relationship, conflicts regarding closeness-distance are exacerbated, driving her to use desperate defensive measures, like those Michaela employed, in order to take flight from her objects. As Anna Freud (1958) poignantly pointed out in her description of reversal of affects:

> ... the adolescent imagines himself to be "free" but, unluckily for his peace of mind and sense of conflict, this conviction does not reach further than the conscious surface layer of his mind. For all deeper intents and purposes he remains as securely tied to the parental figures as he has been before; acting out remains within the family; and any alterations achieved by the defense turn out to his disadvantage. There are no positive pleasures to be derived from the reversed relationships, only suffering, felt as well as inflicted. There is no room for independence of action, or of growth; compulsive opposition to the parents proves as crippling in this respect as compulsive obedience to them can prove to be (p. 158).

Michaela's narcissistic vulnerability revealed a faulty internalized self-esteem regulatory system which propelled her search towards validation and recognition from the external world. A response from the other which would help her construct and solidify a coherent and good enough ideal of herself. In this adolescent's quest for "optimal distance", we are reminded of Anna Freud's paradoxical phrase: "Mothers have to be there in order to be left" (Furman, 1982).

References

Benedek, T. (1950). Climacterium: a developmental phase. *Psychoanalytic Quarterly, 19*: 1–2.

Berkowitz, D. A., Shapiro, R. L., Zinner, J. & Shapiro, E. R. (1974). Family contributions to narcissistic disturbances in adolescents. *International Journal of Psychoanalysis, 1*: 353–362.

Blos, P. (1957). Preoedipal factors in the etiology of female delinquency. *Psychoanalytic Study of the Child, 12*: 229–249.

Blos, P. (1962). *On Adolescence*. New York: Free Press.

Blos, P. (1967). The second individuation process of adolescence. *Psychoanalytic Study of the Child, 22*: 162–186.

Blos, P. (1983). The contribution of psychoanalysis to the psychotherapy of adolescents. *Psychoanalytic Study of the Child, 38*: 577–600.

Brandt, D. & Silverman, H. (1985). The impact of maternal personality on individuation during adolescence. *Psychoanalytic Psychology, 2*: 267–273.

Burgner, M. (1985). The Oedipal experience: effects on development of an absent father. *International Journal of Psychoanalysis, 66*: 311–320.

Burgner, M. & Gavshon, A. (1981). Study group on one-parent families. *Bulletin of the Anna Freud Centre, 4*: 292–294.

Burlingham, D. (1955). Simultaneous analysis of mother and child. *Psychoanalytic Study of the Child, 10*: 165–186.

Dahl, E. K. (1989). Daughters and mothers—Oedipal aspects of the witch-mother. *Psychoanalytic Study of the Child, 44*: 267–280.

Dahl, E. K. (1993). The impact of divorce on a preadolescent girl. *Psychoanalytic Study of the Child, 48*: 193–207.

Edgcumbe, R. (1993). Developmental disturbances in adolescence and their implications for transference and technique. *Bulletin of the Anna Freud Centre, 16*: 107–120.

Edgcumbe, R. & Burgner, M. (1975). The phallic narcissistic phase—a differentiation between preoedipal and Oedipal aspects of phallic development. *Psychoanalytic Study of the Child, 30*: 161–180.

Erikson, E. H. (1956). The problem of ego identity. *Journal of the American Psychoanalytic Association, 4*: 56–121.

Fonagy, P. & Moran, G. S. (1991). Understanding psychic change in child psychoanalysis. *International Journal of Psychoanalysis, 72*:15–22.

Fonagy, P., Moran, G. S., Edgcumbe, R., Kennedy, H. & Target, M. (1993). The roles of mental representations and mental processes in therapeutic action. *Psychoanalytic Study of the Child, 48*: 9–48.

Fonagy, P., Steele, M., Moran, G., Steele, H. & Higgitt, A. (1991). Measuring the ghost in the nursery: a summary of the main findings of the Anna Freud Centre—University College London Parent-Child Study. *Bulletin of the Anna Freud Centre, 14*: 115–131.

Freud, A. (1949). Aggression in relation to emotional development; normal and pathological. *Psychoanalytic Study of the Child, 3*: 37–42.

Freud, A. (1958). Adolescence. In: *The Writings of Anna Freud, Vol. V* (pp. 136–166). New York: International Universities Press.

Freud, A. (1965). Normality and pathology in childhood: Assessments of development. In: *The Writings of Anna Freud, Vol. VI*. New York: International Universities Press.

Freud, A. (1968). Acting out. *International Journal of Psychoanalysis, 49*: 165–170.

Freud, A. (1969). Adolescence as a developmental disturbance. In: *The Writings of Anna Freud, Vol. VII* (pp. 39–47). New York: International Universities Press.

Furman, E. (1982). Mothers have to be there to be left. *Psychoanalytic Study of the Child, 37*: 15–28.

The Hampstead Psychoanalytic Index (1981). *Bulletin of the Anna Freud Centre, 4*: 279–287.

Hellman, I. (1960). Simultaneous analysis of mother and child. *Psychoanalytic Study of the Child, 15*: 359–377.

Joffe, W. G. & Sandler, J. (1967). Some conceptual problems involved in the consideration of disorders of narcissism. *Journal of Child Psychotherapy, 2*: 56–66.

Kernberg, O. (1984). *Object Relations Theory and Clinical Psychoanalysis*. New York: Jason Aronson.

Laufer, M. (1968). The body image, the function of masturbation, and adolescence—problems of the ownership of the body. *Psychoanalytic Study of the Child, 23*: 114–137.

Laufer, M. & Laufer, M. E. (1984). *Adolescence and Developmental Breakdown*. New Haven, CT: Yale University Press.

Laufer, M. E. (1982). Female masturbation in adolescence and the development of the relationship to the body. *International Journal of Psychoanalysis, 63*: 295–301.

Laufer, M. E. (1986). The female Oedipus complex and the relationship to the body. *Psychoanalytic Study of the Child, 41*: 259–276.

Laufer, M. E. (1996). The role of passivity in the relationship to the body during adolescence. *Psychoanalytic Study of the Child, 51*: 348–364.

Levy, K. (1960). Simultaneous analysis of a mother and her adolescent daughter—the mother's contribution to the loosening of the infantile object tie. *Psychoanalytic Study of the Child, 15*: 378–391.

Mahler, M. S. (1963). Thoughts about development and individuation. *Psychoanalytic Study of the Child, 18*: 307–324.

Mahler, M. S. (1971). A study of the eparation-individuation process—and its possible application to borderline phenomena in the psychoanalytic situation. *Psychoanalytic Study of the Child, 26*: 403–424.

Mahler, M. S. & Furer, M. (1968). *On Human Symbiosis and the Vicissitudes of Individuation*. New York: International Universities Press.

Mahler, M. S., Furer, M., Pine, F. & Bergman, A. (1975). *The Psychological Birth of the Human Infant*. New York: Basic.

Mehra, B. & Pines, D. (1972). Study of promiscuous girls under the auspices of the Centre for Adolescent Research [unpublished]. Cited in: D. Pines (1993). *A Woman's Unconscious Use of her Body*. New Haven, CT: Yale University Press.

Modell, A. H. (1985). The works of Winnicott and the evolution of his thought. *Journal of American Psychoanalytic Association, 33S*: 113–137.

Neubauer, P. B. (1960). The one-parent child and his Oedipal development. *Psychoanalytic Study of the Child, 15*: 286–309.

Novick, J. & Novick, K. K. (1996). A developmental perspective on omnipotence. *Journal of Clinical Psychoanalysis, 5*: 129–173.

Pines, D. (1993). *A Woman's Unconscious Use of her Body*. New Haven, CT: Yale University Press.

Ritvo, S. (1984). The image and uses of the body in psychic conflict—with special reference to eating disorders in adolescence. *Psychoanalytic Study of the Child, 39*: 449–469.

Sandler, J. (1960). On the concept of superego. *Psychoanalytic Study of the Child, 15*: 128–162.

Sandler, J. & Rosenblatt, B. (1962). The concept of the representational world. *Psychoanalytic Study of the Child, 17*: 128–145.

Sprince, M. P. (1962). The development of a preoedipal partnership between an adolescent girl and her mother. *Psychoanalytic Study of the Child, 17*: 418–450.

Stern, D. N. (1985). *The Interpersonal World of the Infant*. New York: Basic.

Winnicott, D. W. (1960). Ego distortion in terms of true and false self. In: *The Maturational Processes and the Facilitating Environment* (pp. 140–152). London: Hogarth and The Institute of Psychoanalysis.

Winnicott, D. W. (1963). The development of the capacity for concern. In: *The Maturational Processes and the Facilitating Environment* (pp. 77–82). London: Hogarth and The Institute of Psychoanalysis.

Winnicott, D. W. (1971). *Playing and Reality*. London: Tavistock.

CHAPTER TWENTY FOUR

"The terrorist and the boffin"—a two-year intensive psychotherapy with a thirteen-year-old boy

Helen Ritzema

Introduction

William was a thirteen-year-old boy who had not only experienced three years of emotional and very likely sexual abuse, and neglect while living with his birth mother, but he had also, at the age of nine, been rejected by his adopted parents due to his "unmanageable behaviour". I wish to describe William's seemingly interminable conflict between two very different states of mind that we came, over the course of his psychotherapy, to refer to as being a "terrorist" and being a "boffin". For William, occupying a state of mind aligned to a "terrorist" offered a defensive delinquent solution to his profound sense of loss and unmet need, providing the opportunity for him to join with his peers and gain attention, albeit negative, from the adults around him. On the other hand, being aligned to states of mind of a "boffin", making use of his therapy and cognitive capacities to engage with his academic life, meant "working really hard and doing well in class" to achieve the job and independence he wanted in life. The reappearance of William's birth mother during the second year of treatment only served to heighten this conflict further. While psychotherapy is clearly not the treatment of choice for every delinquent, I believe this paper provides evidence in accordance with Horne's (2004) statement that "It remains a vital provision of treatment for those individuals for whom delinquency is a defence or a response to a deficit, and where there is conflict" (p. 344).

Referral

William was referred, for a second time, to the local child and adolescent mental health service (CAMHS) when he was twelve years old. This was just five months after the ending of his previous non-intensive psychotherapy, which ended due to the child psychotherapist leaving the service. A social worker who met with William at that time expressed great concern over his behaviour. William had been verbally abusive towards her and had been observed to "constantly rock back and forth" throughout their meeting. His foster carers, Mr and Mrs A, felt "pushed to the edge" by his relentless question asking, silly behaviour, noise making, and his getting up at night to "raid" the kitchen cupboard. William was said, by Mr and Mrs A, to struggle to make and maintain friendships.

Following this referral, an assessment of William's emotional, psychological, and cognitive needs was carried out by a consultant child and adolescent psychotherapist at the clinic. William was described as a boy who was "still very deeply troubled by his past experiences which he had been unable to comprehend and digest in a way that would guarantee him some developmental and rational freedom. Instead, all his current actions and ways of being and relating were entirely determined and governed by his past experiences." Intensive long-term psychoanalytic psychotherapy was recommended for William, given that he was at the beginning of the adolescent process: a process that would further test his emotional capabilities, especially in relation to his sexuality, peer relationships, and individuation and separation. His previous experience of psychotherapy was reported to have been a positive one and William had explicitly asked to be seen again. I was pleased to be in a position to offer William three times a week psychoanalytic psychotherapy. This started soon after William turned thirteen years.

Family background

The information concerning William's early life with his birth mother was sparse and left much to one's imagination as to the extent of his deprivation (Winnicott, 1956), abuse, and neglect. William had two half sisters: Sarah, four years his elder, and Lucy, three years his junior. All three children had different fathers. William had never met his birth father. When William was two years and two months old he and his sister Sarah were voluntarily given into the care of the local authority and placed with foster carers, Mr and Mrs A. At this time William was described by Mr and Mrs A as "hyperactive, bad-tempered, and incontinent". He was also observed to bang his head on the door and floor. Whilst he was in their care, Mr and Mrs A reported William made "gradual progress: he stopped head-banging, his temper calmed, and he achieved control of his bowels".

When William was seven years old he and his sisters were adopted by Mr and Mrs B. Two years later William's adoption placement broke down irretrievably. Mr and Mrs B claimed they could no longer cope with William's behaviour. While they retained Sarah and Lucy, they returned William to the care of the local authority. William was described by Mr and Mrs B as displaying sexualized behaviour and he was said to be violent towards other children. He had urinated against the wall of the toilet and needed a high level of supervision with self-care. He soiled, lied, and stole food. He was also reported to prefer to sleep fully clothed and he was said to have an inability to fully engage in emotionally meaningful and gratifying exchanges with others. William was once again placed with Mr and Mrs A.

Throughout his education William experienced severe and inhibiting developmental difficulties. He was not able to follow the education curriculum in an age-appropriate way and he found it very difficult to socialize with other children; he was being bullied and he also bullied other children. When he was ten years old William was diagnosed with attention deficit hyperactivity disorder and prescribed methylphenidate, or Ritalin. The following year he was given extra academic support through the "educational statementing" process. In addition at eleven years old William was involved, along with a friend at that time, in a sexually abusive encounter with an elderly man in the neighbourhood.

Beginning treatment

William and I met for his first session having had no prior introductions. He had a black coat on over his blazer and this was zipped all the way up to his chin, giving me the sense he felt he needed to take care of himself against the elements and protect himself while meeting a new person. William had short brown hair, brown eyes, and fair skin with freckles on his cheeks. He was fairly tall and slight. He had a warm, slightly unsure look about him, and his eyes, although slightly narrow, had a sparkle about them:

> After a time of William looking about the room I reflected it may feel difficult meeting someone new. William replied: "Yeah, it's always like that, you say hello and then you don't know what to say". (Session 1)

Having had the experience of working with an adolescent who was almost always non-verbal, I felt a sense of relief in William's response. Gradually, the first session took form as William requested I join him where he was sat in order for us to play hangman. He demonstrated his hyper-vigilance and capacity to read others, as he explained he had managed to guess the word I had chosen, without needing to guess any letters, as "people always looked at what it was they had chosen. So you followed the line of their eyes to see what it was."

Games and action became a major preoccupation of William in the therapy room. Each activity he started alone then became a shared one as he asked me to join him. Cars, tunnels, garages, people, and board games were made from the card and tape provided. In the fourth session I was assigned the role of the "rescue lorry" used to tow his broken car back to the garage to be fixed, providing a sense of William's understanding of our relationship and his wish to be rescued by me. William impressed as being very resourceful as he adapted whatever he had in his box to meet his needs. However, through his resourceful actions he also demonstrated his inability to ask for anything new for his box, giving the sense he felt he had to "make do" with what he had been given for fear of pushing me away through his neediness.

As the first term of treatment progressed, William began to talk about his central preoccupation, over what kind of a boy he was, disguised within displacement through his use of descriptions of his friends. Lanyado and Horne (1999) suggest "Adolescents may talk of 'a friend who …' and may need the vehicle of the friend for several weeks before they can own the anxieties disclosed as their own" (p. 66). In his fourth session, William spoke of a boy at school who had a "girl's name". He commented that perhaps the boy should come here and talk about his problems. This was an indicator of William's wish to speak to me about his concern over his identity as a boy, and his fear over his sexuality and what kind of a male he may be. As William made use of his tales of his friends to bring his worries into the room, there was the overriding sense that negative affects were to be avoided at all costs. Painful incidents were described as "funny" as he demonstrated his use of the defensive "reversal of affects" (A. Freud, 1966). Following such an exchange William would retreat to playing games.

William's use of games in the sessions continued for many months and appeared to provide a defensive retreat from talking and thinking as I felt pulled into playing the games with William. Often I was left with a sense of being prevented from thinking in the room as William's games became more elaborate and I was drawn into the concrete action, rather than being able to maintain a space where I could think about the meaning of the material. Volleyball, basketball, and football became firm favourites. Many of the games played also appeared to have been games William had played with his last therapist, and as such he appeared to be attempting to re-create what he felt he had lost. It took many months, and much self-reflection on my part, for me to resist his transferential pull (Sandler, 1981) into playing the games and acting out rather than talking and thinking.

Holding back, and not joining in games, quickly brought sexual material into the sessions. In session 39 William drew a picture which appeared to graphically demonstrate his fear of what type of a man he would become:

> William drew a very fierce-looking man and added a body which looked like a penis. To this he added arms and legs which were also penis shaped. He added nipples, a belly button, and female genitalia. On drawing William's attention to this he tried to rip the bottom of the sheet off but didn't take it off fully. He then added a boy bending over showing his bottom, as a "moony", next to the man.

This disturbing communication happened at the very end of the session as if William wanted to leave, to "evacuate" (Bion, 1963) the disturbing feelings with me and disown the accompanying affect. William wanted to leave me with his powerfully painful anxieties over what type of a man he would become: a castrated sexual predator, or a sexual object offering his anus to be buggered. Within this profound and torturous confusion William also conveyed his fears over how to find a way to be close to an adult without being abused and betrayed. In relation to Winnicott's theory of the "antisocial tendency" (1965), Gordon (2002) suggests it is in the hopeful moment that the child stirs up the environment to make it alert to danger. It appears William was beginning to trust me to be an adult with whom he could express his inner fears, hopeful that together we could work through them. Several weeks later William returned to this topic as he spoke of the incident of abuse which had occurred two years previously.

Another feature which appeared early on in William's therapy, and became a central theme throughout, was his need to cause irritation in the other. I began to gain a sense that William's need to irritate people was born out of his attempt to rid himself of his unbearable sense of loss and unmet need. His winding up became known as "terrorizing".

The terrorist

William's sessions started early in the morning before the clinic was open and I was the one who let him into the clinic. Shortly before the first break, William began to ring the bell continuously until I got to the door to let him in. On the first occasion he appeared shameful and ducked down as I approached the door. He giggled nervously as he said, "The bell got stuck, or something, it wasn't me." My interpretations of his need for me to come quickly to the door to let him in appeared futile, as this mode of beginning the sessions became fixed and continued for many months. William seemed to feel the need to disturb the other in order to get noticed. This created a feeling of being intruded into and a sense of confusion in the countertransference, as I felt at a loss to know what interpretation to make to stop the incessant ringing, which would continue even after we could see each other through the glass in the door. Wilson (1999) describes the key therapeutic task as being the therapist's resistance to the young person's implicit invitation to repeat the past. William appeared to be expressing the belief that he could only make contact with me if he disturbed me. William conveyed a wish to see how I would react when intruded, penetrated into in a violent way.

William's compulsive need to be noticed, to terrorize, and to set up a reaction in the other was also acted out in the sessions, as anyone who passed the window of the therapy room was called out to. The sexual excitement which seemed to accompany these incidents appeared to demonstrate a developmental path where sexual excitement was used to deal with conflicts of separation and loss (Ruszczynski, 2007). At such times William seemed to be attempting to elicit me as an adult who would stop him as he appeared out of control and unable to stop himself. He was seeking what Winnicott (1956) described as "environmental stability which will stand the strain resulting from his impulsive behaviour". His excitement appeared to be very close to physical aggression, suggestive of violent enactments. Indeed, William would speak of having broken material objects at home, such as his game console, due to being unable to tolerate frustration and feelings of being a failure. For a time William also spoke of "terrorizing" the teachers at school. However, as more aggression and talking came into the therapy room, so it appeared William was managing better at school. He spoke of his parents having been informed that his teachers were pleased by the improvements he was making.

As we moved towards the first long summer break, William's fear of this separation caused him to revert to old modes of relating in the room as he requested we play hangman. Hangman was increasingly used to bring topics of concern into the room as full sentences were introduced by William rather than single words. Moves towards delinquent preoccupations appeared to emerge as the summer break drew ever closer. William brought pictures of marijuana and pornography on his mobile phone, into the room to show me. Within this exchange he asked if I knew of the "Mr Lonely" song; it appeared drugs and sex offered a "delinquent solution" to the loss and lonely feelings that would be felt over the summer break. Hodges, Lanyado, and Andreou suggest, "If a child has had no opportunity during development to internalise parental representations as sources of security, it impairs the growth of his own capacity to contain painful and aggressive thoughts" (1994, p. 290). William was left with scarce resources with which to manage his depressive affects.

The boffin

Following the first summer break, William returned fearing his return to school. He described school as "boring and stupid" as he attempted to mask his worry over being able to manage. Once he was back at school, William seemed to struggle between avoiding being pulled into behaving badly, and trying hard in class. It seemed he was attempting to engage with academia as he spoke of having done his homework. However, on the day William was due to hand a piece of homework in he announced he had lost it:

> William said he didn't want to go to school; I linked this to his missing homework. He said that it didn't bother him as he was used to it, he never did homework. I reflected, "But this time you did." William said, "Yeah, but it's only lunch break in detention. I'm okay with that. I'm used to it. I'm not a boffin". (Session 70)

Fear of becoming a "boffin", someone who worked hard all the time and had no fun, appeared to have caused an internal sabotage to take place resulting in William losing his homework. This self-defeating aspect of William was suggestive of a deep-rooted fear of humiliation and failure. Over the next few sessions William spoke of aspiring to get a good job. He didn't want "to sweep the roads, work in McDonald's, or be a dustbin man". He had in fact managed to find his homework and handed it in, and for this he had been awarded two house points. However, he appeared highly anxious that his hunger to do well may be too much, and he may not be able to manage. He began to express fears of being envied as a "boffin" and being fearful of what his peers would think. His sessions appeared to oscillate between discussions of wanting to do well, and descriptions of his delinquent solution to failure, as he spoke of his friends smoking marijuana and watching pornographic films. William appeared to be describing his conflict of loyalty between his identification with his "terrorist" friends and his identification with me "the boffin".

Within school William appeared to be managing this conflict, albeit precariously; by half-term he spoke of having received thirty-five house points. However, William's tales of his recreational time increasingly involved delinquent acts as he "terrorized" adults, causing them to set limits; he had been banned from McDonald's for "throwing chips and swearing at a security guard with his friend". Friendships appeared to be bound up with delinquent activities, leaving a sense of William continuing to struggle with creating a coherent sense of himself and the type of man he would like to be. He was caught between identifications with his peers which would lead to delinquency, and identification with me which he felt would lead to hard work devoid of peer relationships. William spoke of his conflict between liking being the bad William, who got told off—as he said, the telling off lasted longer than the praise and he didn't like the praise, and being good, which he didn't want to be. However, he reflected he did like it when his foster mum was called and informed he had been good.

Around the time of William's fourteenth birthday he spoke of having been given an award for the most improved pupil. He informed me that "lots of girls" had "shouted for" him and "cheered" as he had gone up to collect his award and this had been "embarrassing". William seemed to be describing a defensive move away from his sexual feelings for the girls in the audience, as he used "embarrassment" to cover over his feelings of excitement. This incident appeared to signify a move towards heterosexual relationships as William began, albeit tentatively at first, to talk about girls he liked.

As we moved towards the end of the first year of treatment and the Christmas break, William brought his mobile phone to the therapy room. William's fear of separation and being left alone with his conflicts and confusions during the break appeared to be expressed through the use of sexual material as he showed me clips and pictures on his phone of men and women having sex. The pictures felt relentless and the session seemed uncontained as William used "sexualization" (Ruszczynski, 2007) to generate excitement in order to move away from the painful feelings caused.

The second year of treatment

Following the break, William continued to bring stories of having spent his time with peers who could offer the delinquent solution to his predicament of being left alone with his anxieties. William's battle between being a terrorist and being a boffin persisted and his fears over what kind of a man he would turn out to be continued to be a preoccupation. Not long after he spoke of his wish to do well, he drew a picture of a man, to which he added arrows and darts through the man's head, knives in the chest, a gun next to the man's head, a noose around his neck, and a bomb above his head. William was conveying his sense that being a terrorist, i.e., terrorizing others (projecting and enacting internal violence onto others), is mixed up with a fear of persecution that is intolerable; and that means he is ultimately terrorizing himself by self-destructiveness.

William began to talk about his obsession with taking things apart; calculators, watches, mobile phones, and MP3 players were all dismantled as William appeared to be compelled to try to see the inner workings of the object: demonstrating his wish to know not only how physical objects work but how minds work; how thoughts and feelings are generated and expressed. The problem, William described, was that he was "never sure how to put them back together again". Together we began to think of his fear of "disintegration" (Winnicott, 1962), as we spoke of his worry that if we looked at his thoughts and feelings then he might be left not being able to put himself back together again. Exploration with William over his multi-determined wish to take objects apart led to interpretations over his fear with regards to his developing body and his penis.

A change in the escort who transported William to his sessions brought about a change in the manner in which he began each session, as he often arrived more than fifteen minutes before his session. He sat in the waiting room "munching out" on food, appearing to need to fill himself up to stave off his empty, lonely feelings while he waited for me. During this time, perhaps as a reaction to the loss of his previous escort, William struggled with letting me know he was unhappy about cancellations, holidays, and having to wait for me to start the session. For many months any attempt on my part to discuss this with William was met with defensive "rationalization" or "reversal of affects" (A. Freud, 1966), as he spoke of filling his time with activities and being happy for the "lie in". Gradually, over time, he would tentatively state he was "not a happy chappy" as I encouraged him to speak of his affects. He appeared to be expressing his conflict over how to be angry at the people you are dependent on. Around this time William stopped ringing the doorbell continuously, following a time when he thought he had broken the bell. This was interpreted as a communication of his belief that everything has a breaking point, which he believed he exceeded due to his greed and sense of unmet needs.

Over time William's aggression and disappointment with me was expressed through his support of a Premier League football club. He would talk at length, at the start of each session, about the games they had won and lost. He decided I supported an opposing team. Through these identifications battles could be fought, in displacement, as he would tell me with great delight: "My team are playing the team that you support and they're going to thrash them" (session 125). This appeared to be an identification with his foster father who also supported his chosen team. Outside the therapy room Mr and Mrs A described William as withdrawing from friendships and choosing to spend all his free time at home. They described him as having "gone mad and over the top" about football. William seemed fearful of the type of friendships he would get involved in and his being drawn into terrorizing. The only friendships he spoke of in his sessions were formed at a weekly youth club run by social services for fostered children. Here, William seemed to feel safe, as he mixed with children who had similar backgrounds to his own. During this period his masculine identification with his foster father increased, as he spoke of using his aftershave and wanting to have Mr A's car when he could drive. He began to form heterosexual relationships, as he spoke of having girlfriends. In the therapy room William relied on the games less and less as he was able to talk directly about his experiences and take in my interpretations.

The arrival of a letter from his birth mother, several months into his second year of treatment, coincided with a move towards delinquent acting out at school, as William increasingly spoke of skipping classes with his "mates". Terrorizing at school continued to offer the function of defending against boredom and depression. Woods (2003) describes how more often than not society overlooks the intrinsic value of the adolescent's protest expressed through their delinquent act. William spoke of his fear of succeeding at school. This fear appeared to centre on his sense that this would be a feminine retreat and he would be at risk of being attacked if he was studious. William began to express a wish to identify with delinquents, his peers, who were seen to create excitement, and annoyance in the adults, therefore they were noticed. People he did not like were described as "gays" and "pussies", as he appeared to try to distance himself from them and identify with a more masculine role model. The delinquent pull again felt very strong as William appeared to be struggling to find a masculine identification in his external world. As I took up William's concerns over what kind of a man he would be he agreed and said, "I think I'm normal though, and I just want to be happy and to be myself."

Reappearance of birth mother

Following the letter from his birth mother William expressed his fear of her finding out where he lived. He stated angrily that if she "missed him" as she had said in her letter then why did she give him up. He described his thoughts that his mum would turn the animals she lived with "mad". His fears soon became a reality as a few weeks before the long summer break, when William was fourteen years old, he came to his session and announced he had seen his "real" mum. The meeting with his mother appeared to have a severely destabilizing effect on William. It left him fearful over what would happen at home, as he spoke of his sense that there was a limit to how much he could antagonize his foster family. As he spoke he started to play with a lighter, moving his finger through the flame:

> I suggested that William felt there was something quite fiery and hot about the situation with his mum. William said, "I like it when you do that, you take something that I say and look at what I am doing and join them together." He said he would like to be able to do that, and he

> thought he would tell his mum (Mrs A, foster mother) to do that as his niece is badly behaved and his mum thinks it's the food that she eats but he thought that there was something else going on. [Session 160]

Even through this very unsettled time, William appeared to be able to maintain the thinking in the room with me. However, his lack of control over when his birth mother would turn up, coupled with the fact that this was happening just prior to the long summer break, when I would be leaving him, left William feeling very unsafe. Once again William seemed unable to tell me directly how angry he felt with me for leaving him over the summer break, as he feared destroying the relationship we had.

Following the summer break, William's birth mother continued to make clandestine meetings with him. Through these meetings he was informed about his birth father, who was said to have held a knife to his birth mother's throat. William spoke of the great difficulty he had in hearing this information. Again he had to consider his heritage and was struggling to know what kind of a man he would be. As this stressful situation continued, school life became increasingly difficult and William was pulled into a delinquent mode of behaving, as he spoke of bunking his lessons, swearing at teachers, being caught smoking, hiding in a caravan, and fighting with others at school. His conflict over being "Einstein" the boffin or "Bin Laden" the terrorist (his terms) continued, and it seemed as though his ability to maintain the advances he had made at school was beginning to be severely compromised. Wilson (1999) suggests the delinquent acts of stealing, deception, and/or physical or verbal violence are intended to attack and confound those perceived to be responsible for the individual's difficulties. It appeared William wished to reverse the experience he had with his birth mother through his risk taking activities; in reality it was the adults around William who were failing to keep him safe.

The network around William became increasingly concerned by his withdrawal from school, and meetings were held to try to contain some of his behaviour. William remained extremely traumatized by the events around him as his birth mother continued to make contact and tried to entice him to live with her. William arrived at his sessions in a state of turmoil, providing me with the sense he truly felt terrorized by his mother. He spoke of his worries that I was the only person who knew all he did and I was also going to be present at one of the meetings. We spoke of his fear that I would also become a frightening, unpredictable female in his life. Parsons and Dermen suggest "The psychotherapist's job is not to justify the unacceptable; it is to discover the meaning of the act from the point of view of the subject (1999, p. 329)". Indeed, interpretations over William's wish to create anxiety and worry in my mind when his mind felt flooded seemed to calm him down.

Social services arranged for a homework tutor for William to help him with his school work. William again spoke of a wish to get good grades so he could go up a set in maths. However, William's internal saboteur seemed to be at work as he failed to hand in his homework. The wish to be seen not working was too powerful and William often expressed his anxiety over growing up and changing. He appeared to fear both doing well at school, which he believed would mean his sessions with me would come to an end, and the humiliation of failure. William continued to bunk from his lessons. As we moved towards the Christmas break, William started to talk explicitly about his concerns over what state I would be in when he returned, as he described me answering the door with dark rings under my eyes from all the marijuana I would have been smoking over the holiday, as he projected on to me his internal image of a maternal object: who is immersed in self-involved, mad, drug-altered states of mind, where there is no space left for true maternal preoccupation. This was coupled with his increased ability to tell me I had "hurt his feelings" and he was going to "sack me".

Following the break, William announced he had made New Year's resolutions to "be good *and* terrorize" and we spoke of his conflict between passivity and aggression. William appeared to fear giving up terrorizing as he felt it to be a loss of his ability to actively protect himself. He said he knew he wouldn't be able to be good all the time so he would be good one day and terrorize the next. William described his fear of going back to school after the break as feeling as though he had "a big lump" in his throat. He then informed me his birth mother had turned up at his school the day before the Christmas holidays. He said she was "really mad". William was fearful he too would become stuck, terrorizing and out of control like his birth mother. As the meetings with his birth mother started again it was not long before William had been excluded from school due to breaking a table and swearing at a teacher. William's mother provided him with cigarettes and allowed him to drive the car when they met; life with her was a life of lawlessness and delinquent solutions. William seemed torn between ego ideals (Freud, 1914): the ideal formed around an image of his birth family, he "the terrorist", and the ideal formed around an image of me, his foster family and teachers, he "the boffin". William began to view me as being joined together with his teachers, as he saw me as someone who wanted him to become a boffin. At such times it felt as though we lost a connection in the therapy room.

Working towards an ending

In this time of turmoil I struggled with letting William know I would be leaving work. I informed him a few weeks after the Christmas break that I would be leaving in May. His reaction only served to confirm his level of commitment to the treatment:

> William said for me to shut up, this wasn't true. He asked why I was leaving, and stated I hadn't been here for long enough; I had only been here for a few years. I took up that he felt it was too soon to end and he was not ready for me to leave. He said it was alright, he knew what car I drove and he would find out where I lived and then he would find me. [Session 205]

His sense of loss prevailed throughout this session. In the sessions that followed, William brought tales of animals being killed, as he expressed his worries over how he was going to survive without me, imploring me to acknowledge he felt his life to be at stake. His calendar was counted with thirty-three sessions until we said goodbye. I spoke of his feeling that this was not enough and I was really letting him down. William increasingly spoke of friends, peers who he was spending time with. Akin to the breaks my leaving appeared to be causing him to turn to his peers for support, as they continued to offer a delinquent solution to his loss. William openly spoke of increasing his terrorizing activity when we stopped seeing each other.

My worry over what state I was leaving William in continued. The advances he had made during his treatment appeared extremely fragile. William expressed his belief that it was due to him having done something "stupid" that our work together was ending. William's sessions continued with his preoccupation on the oscillation between being a "boffin" and "terrorizing". It was evident that the ending was occurring before consolidation had had a chance to take effect. This situation appeared to be exacerbated by adolescence and the regressive pull and progressive push (Laufer & Laufer, 1984). William increasingly told me of events outside the session when he was involved in delinquent activities. He seemed to be joining with peers who were schooling him in their delinquent activities of stealing. William appeared to be pulled into stealing as he felt I was stealing from him—his sessions and his chance for a different type of relationship (A. Freud, 1965). He conveyed his anger with me, as he spoke within the same session of the progress he was making with his homework tutor and he expressed his sense that becoming a boffin had caused him to be dropped by the person with whom he was identifying. Therefore, he wished to hurt me through attacking the thinking. William spoke of having wasted his time at school and also with me as he said he "should have been a boffin this year rather than last year".

Conclusion

Over the two years and five months I saw William he never missed an appointment through either illness or a reluctance to come. He remained highly committed to the relationship he built with me during that time. William spoke with ambivalence about continuing his therapy with another clinician; at times he spoke of wanting to and at other times he was unsure. Unfortunately, there was no provision, at that time, for the treatment to continue and I was only too aware this left William in a precarious state, one where the delinquent solution continued to offer a defence against his feelings of loss of his therapeutic relationship.

Woods (2003) suggests the delinquent adolescent has a desire to have their actions translated by an understanding adult, and their attacks on the environment signify a need for human contact and meaningful interaction. With regards to psychoanalytic work with children and adolescents who demonstrate delinquent, acting out tendencies, William's willingness and wish to engage in the therapeutic process never ceased to amaze me. He truly demonstrated both a wish to be understood and a wish to understand himself; as he stated very early on in the treatment (session 3): "You're clever. I would like to have your brain. I know we could swap." It appeared our work together was to become a process whereby the main aim was, as it is in many other psychoanalytic treatments, to begin to enable William to have his own mind.

References

Bion, W. R. (1963). *Elements of Psychoanalysis*. London: Maresfield Reprints.
Freud, A. (1965). *Normality and Pathology in Childhood: Assessments of Development*. London: Karnac.
Freud, A. (1966). *The Ego and The Mechanisms of Defence* (revised edition). London: Karnac.
Freud, S. (1914). *On Narcissism: an Introduction. S. E., 14*: 67–104. London: Hogarth.
Gordon, P. E. (2002). Naughty girls: commentary on paper by Jackie L. Cohen. *Psychoanalytic Dialogues, 12*(4): 627–641.

Hodges, J., Lanyado, M. & Andreou, C. (1994). Sexuality and violence: preliminary clinical hypothesis from psychotherapeutic assessments in a research programme on young sexual offenders. *The Journal of Child Psychotherapy, 20*(3): 283–307.

Horne, A. (2004). "Gonnae no' dae that!" The internal and external worlds of the delinquent adolescent. *Journal of Child Psychotherapy, 30*(3): 330–346.

Lanyado, M. & Horne, A. (1999). The therapeutic relationship and process. In: M. Lanyado & A. Horne (Eds.), *The Handbook of Child and Adolescent Psychotherapy: Psychoanalytic Approaches.* London: Routledge.

Laufer, M. & Laufer, M. E. (1984). *Adolescence and Developmental Breakdown: a Psychoanalytic View.* London: Karnac.

Parsons, M. & Dermen, S. (1999). The violent child and adolescent. In: M. Lanyado & A. Horne (Eds.), *The Handbook of Child and Adolescent Psychotherapy: Psychoanalytic Approaches.* London: Routledge.

Ruszczynski, S. (2007). The problem of certain psychic realities: aggression and violence as perverse solutions. In: D. Morgan & S. Ruszczynski (Eds.), *The Portman Papers: Lectures on Violence, Perversion and Delinquency.* London: Karnac.

Sandler, J. (1981). Character traits and object relationships. *Psychoanalytic Quarterly, 50*: 694–708.

Wilson, P. (1999). Delinquency. In: M. Lanyado & A Horne (Eds.), *The Handbook of Child and Adolescent Psychotherapy: Psychoanalytic Approaches.* London: Routledge.

Winnicott, D. W. (1956). The antisocial tendency. In: D. W. Winnicott (Ed.), *Through Paediatrics to Psycho-Analysis* (pp. 306–315). London: Karnac, 1958.

Winnicott, D. W. (1962). Ego integration in child development. In: D. W. Winnicott (Ed.), *The Maturational Processes and the Facilitating Environment* (pp. 56–63). London: Karnac, 1965.

Winnicott, D. W. (1965). *The Maturational Processes and the Facilitating Environment.* London: Karnac.

Woods, J. (2003). *Boys Who Have Abused: Psychoanalytic Psychotherapy with Victim/Perpetrators of Sexual Abuse.* London: Jessica Kingsley.

CHAPTER TWENTY FIVE

"Speaking with silence and tears"—psychotherapy with an adolescent girl

Norka T. Malberg

Introduction

In her 1958 essay on adolescence, Anna Freud describes the analytic treatment of this age group as "a hazardous venture from beginning to end, a venture in which the analyst has to meet resistance of unusual strength and variety". Indeed, it is a time in development in which the influence of early experiences on the present state of affairs is significantly relevant. Not only are they vital in understanding what is being manifested in the therapeutic relationship, but also in trying to sort out what is needed of the therapist as a new and different developmental object. There are many ways of thinking about psychotherapeutic work with adolescents. The focus of this clinical paper will be on understanding affective states within the therapeutic relationship and on the importance of countertransference to guide the process of understanding what is being communicated.

Krystal (1985) proposed two developmental lines of affect. The first one—"affect differentiation", is the development of an array of distinctive emotions which form the diffuse early affective states of pleasure and unpleasure. The second—"desomatization and verbalization of affect", means the evolution of affect states from their earliest form as exclusively somatic into emotional experiences that can be verbally articulated. Socarides and Stolorow (1988) expand Krystal's developmental model of affects by further exploring how this developmental progression takes place within a relational medium, an intersubjective context. From this perspective, it is the caregiver's attuned responsiveness appropriately conveyed through *words* that facilitates the gradual integration of the child's bodily emotional experience with symbolic thought, leading to the crystallization of distinctive emotions that can be named as feelings. In the absence of such verbally expressed attunement, or in the face of grossly misattuned responses, derailments of this developmental process can occur, whereby emotional experience remains largely expressed bodily. When there is an expectation that symbolically integrated feelings will be met with rejection and scorn by the other, the person may revert to exclusively somatic forms of emotional experience. The case explored in this paper is an example of such a process in which Sophie, a highly anxious fifteen-year-old young woman chose to express her feelings through the use of silences and tears. She did so while struggling with fears of rejection and uneconomical defensive attempts to contain her aggression at the expense of her capacity to sleep, and her overall sense of safety in relationships.

In the following pages, I intend to relate the process through which my patient Sophie and I struggled to find words for her emotions in twice weekly psychotherapy for a period of two years. Our work together was, as Anna Freud described, "a hazardous venture", in which silences and tears came to have many meanings. At times, they became a way of seeking union as well as an expression of infantile longings. At other times, tears signified feelings of rage, anxiety, and disappointment over the archaic object's lack of attunement and empathy. But above all, they served as an invitation to the therapist to pay close attention to the patient's *unspoken* affective states and the strength of her unmet early needs. These needs manifested themselves in a tendency to both withhold and seek reaffirmation of an internal representation of the maternal object as ineffective and misattuned. I wish to illustrate how my countertransference played a pivotal role in understanding Sophie's use of somatic forms of expression of emotion, and of her masochistic stance in relationships.

Referral and family background

Seeking answers to tears: Sophie's referral

Initially, Sophie referred herself to her school's counselling service. However, after a few sessions, the school counsellor became concerned regarding Sophie's capacity to contain her anxiety after sessions and decided to make an external referral for after-school counselling. It was at this time that the Anna Freud Centre was contacted and a diagnostic process took place followed by a recommendation of twice weekly psychotherapy.

According to the school counsellor, at the time of referral Sophie (who had just turned fifteen) described herself as being depressed and suffering from frequent anxiety attacks. During her first meeting with the counsellor, Sophie expressed feelings of helplessness regarding her incapacity to withstand the stress of school work. She spoke of not being able to stop thinking about her work and of experiencing constant stomach aches, sweaty palms, and headaches which she associated with what she called "panic attacks". She often became, in her own words, "very worried and annoyed" at her incapacity to stop her thoughts and feared being seen by others as stupid and whining. Furthermore, she spoke of her difficulties falling asleep, as she was haunted by fears of not waking up on time or forgetting important school tasks. She spoke of putting herself to sleep by listening to audio books, as she found the narrator's voice soothing and the storyline captivating and hypnotic. Sophie reported waking up at night and going to her parents' bed, fearing a male burglar could come into her room and rape her. In response, her mother would often come to her bed and wait until she fell asleep.

Sophie was regarded by her teachers as a serious and responsible girl who was somewhat anxious but not enough to affect her school performance. Sophie reported having a group of girl friends with whom she spent a lot of her time. She enjoyed swimming and playing the saxophone. In fact, her schedule was so full of special tutoring sessions and extra-curricular activities that it made one wonder when she ever had time to eat or sleep.

The school counsellor described Sophie as complex and difficult to reach. Sophie was constantly in tears during sessions and barely managed to think about her worries. Concerned, the school counsellor contacted Sophie's parents to discuss the situation and recommend the possibility of long-term psychotherapy. The parentss seemed confused and bewildered when confronted with the counsellor's description of Sophie as a highly anxious and depressed adolescent girl who felt very lonely and misunderstood. However, they expressed their desire to help their daughter and their willingness to support psychotherapy. Two weeks later, in accordance with Anna Freud Centre custom, I met Mr and Mrs F in order to gather a social history, and introduced them to a senior colleague who would be working with them in order to support my therapeutic work with Sophie.

A different picture of Sophie emerged during the process of listening to her parents, who spoke of long-term difficulties falling asleep, as well as her tendency from a very young age to become very distressed when separating from her mother. Mrs F remembered Sophie chewing her jumper and the buttons on it, and getting very upset with her daughter over this. I wondered about Sophie's struggle with regulating anxiety from an early age, and about her mother's lack of sensitivity, responding with disappointment and anger when confronted with her three-year-old daughter's expression of nervousness over being at school for the first time. It also emerged that Sophie's parents had been contacted by her teacher at a younger age, due to her concerns over Sophie's class journal having a lot of self-hating messages. At the time, mother felt Sophie's low self-esteem was the result of bullying for being overweight. Mrs F spoke of her worries over Sophie's loneliness during that period, and how difficult it had been for her to have a working mother, being an only child, and having experienced multiple carers throughout the years. Quite recently, Sophie and her mother had decided that they were not going to employ more au pairs as Sophie had become too old for this. Mrs F had cut down her hours at work in order to spend more time with her daughter and seemed genuinely concerned.

On the other hand, Mr F felt that Sophie's difficulties were typical of an adolescent, and openly expressed his concerns over Sophie becoming dependent on psychotherapy. He spoke of his wife attending psychotherapy for the last seven years as a result of her fears over becoming depressed like her father. Mrs F, on the other hand, seemed conflicted between her guilt as a working mother and her own needs for recognition and safety. She spoke of the frail state of their marriage and of having spent many years attending marital therapy. She described feeling ignored and not understood by her husband who she felt was a distant and self-absorbed man. Mrs F spoke of Mr F's tendency to become demeaning towards both her and Sophie when things were not going well in his own life. He would stay silent and withdrawn which often felt like a torture to her.

Considering the parents' difficulties, was Sophie allowed to have her own thoughts, her own difficulties? Was her self-referral considered an unconscious betrayal by these parents? In general, it seemed that Sophie's initial comment to me during our first meeting, that "Nobody can understand how difficult it is to live with these problems," was somewhat confirmed by her parents' ambivalent reaction to her self-referral at school, and to her interest in seeking twice weekly psychotherapy at the Anna Freud Centre.

Sophie's place in the family: the only child

Mrs F came from an intact, working class family; she was the middle of three daughters, and the first woman in her family to go to university. Sophie believed that, as a result, her mother looked down on her sisters. Mrs F had a difficult and somewhat distant relationship with her own father, who was a very depressed man for most of his life and had a severe breakdown resulting in hospitalization during his late adulthood. Mrs F's sisters also suffered from depression and had been on medication most of their adult lives, hence her own fears of becoming depressed like them.

Sophie was born when her mother was in her late thirties. Mrs F described herself as a career woman. The couple had not wanted children, but as Mrs F got older she decided she wanted a baby. One can only speculate as to what it meant for this woman whose narcissism relied so heavily on her career accomplishments to come into motherhood at this late stage in her life. What did this baby mean for her? And what motivated her change of heart? These questions came to mind while experiencing the strength of Sophie's unmet infantile needs in the transference later on in the treatment.

Sophie's mother returned to work when she was six months old, but continued to breastfeed until Sophie was thirteen months old. As a result of mother's early return to work, Sophie was cared for by nannies from a very young age. Many of them became Sophie's surrogate siblings, particularly later on during the latency years. Sophie kept in touch with a particular nanny (Maria) with whom she felt she had established a long-term close attachment.

Mr F was very quiet and distant during his meetings with the parent worker, and as a result very little was known about his childhood and his family of origin, other than the fact that he too was an only child. Sophie seemed to remember better days when her paternal grandmother was well (she died shortly after we began our work together), but no mention was ever made of paternal grandfather. Mr F had never really changed his mind about not wanting children and even after Sophie's birth he did not desire to be a father. However, he reported that as Sophie grew up and became more of a "little person", he felt more comfortable with his role as her father.

During the diagnostic discussion at the Anna Freud Centre, interesting questions were raised regarding the source and meaning of Sophie's anxiety and symptomatology—namely her silence and tears during sessions. These questions guided my own thinking regarding Sophie's difficulties with aggression and her tendency to assume a masochistic stance in relationships. Also, the question was posed about the role this child played for her parents, who seemed so over-involved in their professional lives and difficult relationship with each other. Did they have the capacity and willingness to enter into an intersubjective dialogue with their child?

Treatment

Baby tears and whispers: finding Sophie's voice

I met Sophie on a bright spring day, a tall fifteen-year-old girl, with brown curls adorning her head, dressed casually in bright pastel colours. She was escorted to her session by her mother, a rather thin and attractive middle aged woman who greeted me with a big smile.

Mrs F explained that Sophie would be coming on her own after this first meeting but that she would be picking her up. Meanwhile, Sophie smiled shyly, managing to produce enough eye contact to avoid being rude, but staying safely away from my gaze. Her feline blue eyes and attractive face were given a rather babyish look by two flushed cheeks. However, once away from her mother, Sophie transformed into a young adolescent, crossing her arms while glancing at me with an avoidant gaze and quite frequently looking out of the window. She seemed unreachable for most of our first session.

After a long awkward silence, Sophie began to speak with difficulty of what she called her "daytime and night-time worries", becoming tearful and looking away quite often. There were long and uncomfortable silences in-between as Sophie looked truly frightened and upset. Feeling overwhelmed by the flow of tears and silence, I found myself asking her in a rather concrete fashion to tell me more about her worries. In retrospect, I wondered about my uncharacteristic lack of warmth and sensitivity towards this girl who seemed to be in so much pain. What was being enacted at this moment in the early stages of our relationship? Was Sophie conveying to me the experience of a mother unable to understand her emotional needs? Sophie felt herself in safe and familiar relational territory, while I continued to struggle to understand my perceived lack of empathy towards such an open display of distress. The following excerpt from my process notes of our first session illustrates this state of affairs:

> I wondered about school. S said that she was pretty good as a student, but that she always worried about failing. Tears began to fall as she spoke of being quite messy with her school work when she was younger, but becoming better at it as she got older. Sophie said she considered herself really organized, a perfectionist. I wondered what motivated this change. S said that it was partly her mum, who was always paying attention to her when she worked. "I guess that is one of the curses of being an only child, you get attention even when you don't really fancy it." A long silence followed, tears continued to fall. I was struck however by the lack of empathy I felt for Sophie's tears. The stream of tears just fell down her face as S looked to the floor. "I guess it feels a little lonely at times," I said. "Maybe," Sophie replied, shrugging her shoulders. There was a long silence. I wondered aloud what she thought was upsetting her right now? With great difficulty, she spoke of how she felt it was never good enough for her mother. She gave the example of her writing and how her mum felt that S did not put enough effort into it and did not express herself well enough. I wondered how she responded to this criticism. S replied that after a while she just stops listening, it is useless. Tears overwhelmed S's face and a long, uneasy silence followed.

After this session, I tried to understand my countertransference, namely my detachment and feelings of helplessness. I wondered about the affective meaning of Sophie's copious tears, and as I thought of my own feelings I wondered if the tears represented her feelings of anger and grievance, and her way of exerting control over the object. Sophie's complaints about her mother's judgmental and persecutory stance, the mother "looking over her shoulder demanding perfection in her writing", made me wonder about Sophie's tears as a symbolic way of making a mess. Sophie held on to the unconscious belief that her words were not good enough for me and that I would think of her as a silly, whining girl. So perhaps, like a stubborn toddler, in that first session, Sophie was exerting her right to stay away, to say no to my advances and to make a mess of the therapy and anything I could offer. This message was certainly experienced in the countertransference, as indeed I felt like a mother who tries hard but fails to understand what her baby needs, being left with a crying and angry infant.

This early period of the therapy was filled with silences and tears. I found myself paying close attention to the links between Sophie's material and the sudden change in her affective state. She often seemed to move from verbal expression (regardless of her shy demeanour) to becoming completely withdrawn, silent, and tearful. I often found myself lost and frustrated, without my own words to help her to think. Sophie would often speak in quite a condescending tone about her parents' arguments. She often spoke of them as two stubborn teenagers always trying to get their own way, and how happy she felt going away from them during holidays and leaving them to deal with their "mess". However, alongside these feelings of adolescent triumph, there were Sophie's feelings of fear of loss, more archaic and infantile in nature. It was during these times that Sophie's tears would flow, manifesting what I thought was her frustration and embarrassment over being needy and dependent. Sophie's silences on the other hand, I came to understand as a way of expressing her longing and fantasy for union in the transference, where words are unnecessary.

It seemed to me that Sophie's struggle with finding the words to express her feelings and her fears of exclusion and rejection impinged on her adolescent feelings of self-worth and separateness. She regressed to an earlier way of functioning in the transference, a time before language. Her thumb sucking during sessions when discussing painful topics such as her difficulties with menstruation seemed an indication of how helpless she felt in terms of her ability to cope with the strength of her instinctual urges. Overall, she seemed to use early, somatic ways of self-soothing and discharge such as tears, biting, and thumb sucking. In the same manner, she assumed a passive and masochistic attitude in her relationships and often placed herself in a position of helpless victim only to be left feeling let down and frustrated. The following excerpt from my process notes illustrates these patterns:

> ... Sophie said that when she had gone camping with her friends last weekend, she had fallen and was rather scared. She told me she stayed on the ground, in the rain, waiting for about two hours until her friends came looking for her. As she was saying this she became tearful and silent, looking away as in a trance. After a few minutes, I wondered aloud what the silence was saying. Sophie looked away and shrugged her shoulders. I waited. "I think that I was embarrassed," she whispered. She spoke of having a black bruise on her leg as a result and was quite embarrassed to show her mother. She looked down and tears came down her face. "It is difficult for you to ask for help sometimes," I said. She looked at me with what I thought was a resentful look but did not reply. There was another long silence. "But sometimes, like when you asked for counselling at school, you are able to ask for help," I added. After a long silence, Sophie replied while looking out of the window: "I just could not take the sadness alone any more!" We stayed in silence while a tearful Sophie looked down and tried to contain her tears and clear her eyes, putting on a brave face. S looked down and shrugged her shoulders again: "I am just fed up with being the responsible one, the one that other parents want their children to be like. I don't even like being like this. I hate who I am! I just don't know,

> I don't know! I am just so tired of feeling sad, I am just so tired …" Sophie fell into a long silence until the end of the session.

Sophie's words in this session seemed to indicate feelings of confusion between her early unmet narcissistic needs for asserting separateness while still seeking approval from the object (like a toddler), and her feelings of helplessness when confronted with the demands of her external adolescent world. As in her relationship with me, she resorted to passive-aggressive ways of recruiting the object which often resulted in others feeling confused and frustrated. In this situation, she had sat on the ground and waited silently for two hours waiting to be noticed by someone, confirming once more her feelings of not being seen or heard by the other.

Bion's (1999) belief that "There can be neither learning from experience nor mental development unless there has been a maternal container at the outset" came to mind at this time during my thinking after sessions. Sophie seemed to find in the therapeutic environment a place where "one does not have to take the sadness alone any more", where distress could be contained.

In general, Sophie's material could be understood as a sense of herself as slave to her parents' wishes; she indicated her perception of their narcissistic needs as her responsibility. This was exemplified by Sophie's constant fear of failure, and anxiety, for example over her writing, that mother never seemed satisfied with her efforts, accusing her of not working hard enough and wasting her talent. I began to explore the feelings of my being alone in the room during my clinical supervisions. I acknowledged the level of hostility I often felt in Sophie's presence when she assumed her passive and masochistic attitude. For instance, I became aware of the fact that the box of tissues had run out, and for weeks I had forgotten to get more, so Sophie was left without anything to dry her tears. Using these feelings and my unusual lack of sympathy, to aid my understanding of the meaning of Sophie's tears and silences, proved instrumental, as I began to find the words to speak about them during sessions without feeling like an impinging and persecutory object. As a result, I found myself thinking of her tears in my presence as her chance to seek and find a "shoulder to cry on", not only as an angry expression. Consequently, the possibility of me as a different developmental object, a non-judgmental person who could help offset the impact of her harsh and restrictive superego on her maturation, became more tangible in my mind.

I continued to invite Sophie to think with me about her silences and tears, and survived my own feelings of inadequacy and boredom in the room. In response, Sophie began to allow herself to explore our relationship in the transference in what felt like a more real exchange. The following excerpt from a session during the summer illustrates this emerging capacity:

> Sophie said she felt sorry … "Why?" I wondered. She said she knew how boring it was to talk to her with all her whining. She could never understand how people like me did this job. "Sorry!" she repeated. I commented on how Sophie had started the session today apologizing for falling down the stairs on the way up, which could have happened to anybody, and now she was apologizing about expressing her true thoughts and feelings in her therapy. She smiled: "That is me! Always worried!" "Worried?" I wondered. She shrugged her shoulders, looking tearful, … that maybe you are going to get sick of me and not want to see me …" She became silent and I replied by thinking of the break and how difficult it was for her to believe

that I would remember her after all that time. She smiled shyly and looked away. "Maybe ..." she replied, "maybe." Tears kept falling down her face and she fell silent for a long time ....

Overall, during this first period of the therapy, Sophie's silences and tears often felt like an act of defiance, as if she was breaking the rules of "talking therapy" by being extremely withdrawn and silent. Sophie's punitive superego seemed satisfied as the silence stimulated the punishment of abandonment, of being left out of my mind. However, as I began to disconfirm Sophie's expectations of being rejected and regained my capacity to think and feel when confronted with her silences and tears, I was more able to provide Sophie with the possibility of finding a space to make meaning, to find her own psychological voice, to find the words.

First moves: beginning to learn to be alone without feeling orphaned

I found Sophie's use of audio tapes to fall asleep or calm herself when upset a very useful way to explore her fear of loss and feelings of exclusion in displacement. As a result, we spent a lot of time discussing Huckleberry Finn and Sophie's impressions of the book and her favourite chapters. Sophie spoke of the scene when Huckleberry Finn fakes his own death and spies on everybody. I thought Sophie was telling me about her wish to be able to see what everybody did when she was not around, including me perhaps? She smiled shyly and agreed reluctantly. She spoke of wondering what her friends talk and think about her when she is not there, and managed to express her belief that they probably do the same things they do when she is there, just watch movies and talk about people at school. I wondered about her parents. As she was leaving them for two months this summer did she have any thoughts about what they did when she was away? Her answer was simple and to the point: "They work a lot and try to stay out of each other's hair, and then find many projects they can both work on." When I reflected on the lack of thinking, feeling, and intimacy in both these fantasies, Sophie responded with tears and a resentful statement: "It is not like I think I am so important they are all going to be missing me!" However, when I tried to explore repeatedly Sophie's identification with Huckleberry Finn as a child who discovers he has been abandoned by his father, she became silent and looked out of the window.

On one occasion, and after a long silence, I reflected out loud about Sophie's wish to fly out of the window and be safe, away from the mean therapist who wanted her to think and feel and get to know her embarrassing side.

She agreed and in a genuinely sad tone spoke of her wish that she could stay little, and expressed her sadness over having to grow up and deal with difficult relationships and feelings. I considered this a turning point in our work together as well as an indication of the emergence of a genuine therapeutic alliance. I replied by reflecting on how our relationship often felt very confusing, and spoke of Sophie's worry that I might decide to go away if she were to tell me how she really feels about some of my annoying comments. Perhaps, I suggested, she was worried about becoming an "orphan patient". She nodded and smiled shyly: "That sounds a little strange but rather close to the truth," she concluded before falling into a long silence.

In the following sessions, Sophie spoke of her feelings of exclusion in relation to her friends and of her constant fear of being left all alone. She told me how her friend Jessie had invited everybody to her party at the skating rink, and although she knew it was during Sophie's therapy time, she went ahead with it. I wondered: "Why do you think Jessie did that?" Sophie replied: "Because she is mean like that sometimes and I hate her for that; she is always only thinking about herself." Aware of Sophie's feelings of confusion and fear in the transference about what kind of object I would become if she allowed herself to come closer and acknowledge the existence of an attachment to me, I was very careful in my approach to this material during this session. I focused on her feelings of being disappointed and wondering if, like her friend Jessie, I would disappoint her—or remember her, like Maria had always done. Lost in her parents' narcissism, I thought Sophie tried to find a space where she felt herself truly capable of standing on her own. She needed this feeling in order to move on developmentally and accomplish tasks that her adolescent environment demanded of her, such as dealing with peer conflict, sexually active boys, and the increasing demands of school. All these pressures continuously put the strength of her own narcissistic supplies to the test and made Sophie feel in her own words "exhausted all the time, tired ...".

Upon her return from the summer break, there was a significant change in Sophie. Although she frequently became silent, the nature of the silences felt different and the tears began to disappear. It felt more intense, but it felt real, like we were actually together in the room all the time.

Middle phase

Unspoken and unthinkable truths: beginning to make sense of relationships

During this second phase of our work, after the summer, Sophie began to explore her feelings of longing, anger, and disappointment in the context of her parents' own narcissistic needs and their inability to get along as a couple. She expressed her confusion over being caught in the middle of this needy and demanding parental pair, and about her worries about not giving them what they need. The following excerpt reflects her struggle to separate her own needs from those of her parents, and her grief over mother's perceived incapacity to empathize and understand her difficulties:

> Sophie said that last Saturday she was going with her parents to visit some friends. But while the three of them were on their way, Mum started to feel sick and Sophie began feeling sick too, and they decided to go home. When they got home Dad said he was going to go out with his "mates" (pals). Sophie told him that he should not go out and was quite annoyed with him. Dad ignored her and left. Sophie was left on her own with a sick mother, and after a while went to her room and listened to her Harry Potter tapes. I said, "feeling like an orphan ..." She nodded and stayed silent for a long time, then told me that most weekends they are all together but that her parents are always fighting and this drives her crazy. She said her mother is quite unassertive with Dad and at work, and when she gets home she gets angry with Sophie for no reason. Sophie said that Dad moans to her about her Mum, but then if Sophie says something to him about Mum he tells her not to disrespect her. "It is very annoying!" she said, becoming silent for a long time, looking lost in her thoughts. "I'm going to stay with my grandmother this weekend, I really like it, there is a real family feeling there." She smiled and looked away. Sophie said that her mother had a tough time growing up, being the middle

> child and feeling ignored and abandoned by her father. I said it must be difficult feeling like that, and Sophie added: "I don't understand how she can ignore me and make fun of me if she knows exactly how it feels. …" She began to cry and fell silent for the rest of the session. I offered a tissue.

As exemplified by the previous vignette, Sophie struggled with her parents' rejection of her infantile needs for protection and safety, feelings with which they themselves seemed to struggle. For instance, father tended to quit his job every time his sense of omnipotence was challenged and mother seemed constantly to assume a rather masochistic stance at work in order to gain the support and protection of others. Thinking about these issues had a significant impact on Sophie's capacity to listen and accept my interpretations of how her tears and her silences represented her ambivalence and aggression towards these parents. Furthermore, by acknowledging their narcissistic way of functioning, a recognition of her "otherness" began to emerge. Sophie began to be aware for instance of her identification with father's silent and withdrawn defensive stance as well as his lack of frustration tolerance. She spoke of how he had never been able to study with her, becoming sarcastic and cruel in his comments towards her when she asked him to explain a concept again. She began to link this experience to her own behaviour with peers, and spoke of exploring new ways of coping with her feelings of anger and frustration in the context of her relationships, such as verbalizing her discontent instead of assuming a passive and masochistic stance. At the same time, she began to go out with friends after her sessions instead of being picked up by Mum.

Thankfully, Sophie's attempts for individuation were being received with support by her mother, partly as a result of her commitment to "parent work" sessions. However, father's attempts to "stop time" and regain the blissful relationship he maintained (in his mind) with Sophie over her latency years was in full force and became the central theme of Sophie's work for months to come. Mr F refused to attend parent work sessions, always finding excuses, whereas Mum attended sessions and tried to understand her reactions to Sophie's attempts for independence and autonomy.

The theme of Sophie's relationship with her father, in particular her difficulties moving on by identifying and internalizing new ways of functioning without feeling guilty, became central. After nearly a year of treatment, Sophie announced she was going away with her father for a weekend, leaving mother behind at home. She thought of having time to go to the museum and to a famous shopping centre where her father, less "stingy" with money than her mother, would buy her some nice clothes. Sophie seemed to enjoy her sense of Oedipal triumph in light of her fantasy of her mother being bored all weekend. However, upon her return, she described enjoying the museum, but the mall was closed, the food was not good, and when she arrived she found her mother rested and happy. "From now on", she declared, "she deals with him! She is married to him, not me!".

Although at first glance the disillusion of her Oedipal fantasies seemed to be the pivotal issue, Sophie's tendency to "rubbish" whatever attention and honest understanding the other offered was, I thought, more central to her conflicts. I connected my early countertransference feelings in response to Sophie's description of her father as someone who can never get it right, and although there was the reality of father's narcissistic way of functioning, the fact remained that no matter what people tried, in the end Sophie made sure they disappointed her. This was the case with her friends, with teachers, and with her parents. Perhaps, the only way in which she could keep the relationship with me safe was not to give too much. The only viable solution seemed to be staying silent and using our relationship as a safe place in which to discharge through her tears deep feelings of grievance and rage towards the maternal object.

However, as our therapeutic alliance became stronger, so did her capacity to speak openly about these feelings, as exemplified by the next excerpt:

> Sophie said she was angry, mainly over an argument with her mother because she had promised her a new coat and now said that she should buy it with her own money. Her mother always did this, she said—she promised and never delivered. She described her mother as "cheap" and said she felt that she always put money into the wrong things, like the stupid carpet Mum and Dad had spent a whole Saturday buying together. Sophie showed me her shoes and how they were broken and hurting her feet. She said she did not work, so she had no money to buy shoes. "These are basic needs!" she said enraged. I reflected on her feelings of being mistreated, and of her needs not being understood, like here when I go on holiday or make an annoying comment. She looked at me with a rather adolescent: "You are annoying me" look and added: "My Mum has always been really selfish. …" She continued to complain. I wondered if we could think together about Sophie's tendency to often feel mistreated and let down by people, and wondered what that was really about. At first Sophie looked away and stayed silent. However, I could see in her eyes the rage and the wish to scream and tell me to shut up. When I reflected out loud about this, she smiled, but did not reply. There was a long silence followed by a short comment: "Yes, maybe sometimes I do that, I don't know why." Tears fell down her face.

Putting words to her masochistic tendencies and to her feelings of envy and reproach towards her mother was an arduous task for Sophie and myself. Sophie regressed during this period and became very tearful again. However, she was able to accept my interpretations about the anger behind the tears. In the countertransference, I still often felt cruel and punishing, but came to understand that responding differently to Sophie's expression of these feelings was pivotal in my role as someone who was giving her the chance to revisit what felt like pre-Oedipal unsatisfactory experiences, and providing her with the hope that she could find the "I" in herself. As a result of a stronger therapeutic alliance and sense of safety within the therapeutic relationship, Sophie began to speak more openly about her fears over sexuality and what I thought was her confusion between maternal and sexual love.

The third phase of treatment

Feline love: aggression and sexuality

Anna Freud (1948a) reminds us that "The fusion of sexual instincts with aggression makes it possible for the child to assert his rights to the possession of his love objects, to compete with his rivals, to satisfy his curiosities, to display his body or his abilities." When early object relations do not provide the basis for further structural development to allow this process of fusion to occur, it impacts significantly on the otherwise budding emergence of a sense of agency, which promotes such developmental progression.

During what I consider the third and final period of our treatment the themes of growing up, aggression, and sexuality became central in Sophie's material. Following the spring break, Sophie did not return to her appointments for two weeks. I had sent her a letter to which she did not reply. Perhaps, I thought, as the therapeutic alliance had become stronger and she found herself missing therapy and her therapist, Sophie had to defend herself against her dependency needs. After three weeks I phoned Sophie who greeted me and said she had received my letter, but she had been "really busy" with work and did not feel like coming to see me. In other words, she was showing me she could drop me whenever she wanted. I spoke of the importance of continuing our meetings regularly and let her know that I would be waiting for her here next time. She said she knew I would be there when she decided to come back, and on second thoughts she should have let me know. She arrived on time for our following appointment and greeted me with warmth and spoke in a relaxed way on our way to the consulting room. However, once she entered the room, she was silent for a few minutes, but not absent as had been the norm until now following breaks.

During this returning session and after a few minutes of silence, I picked up her fear that I would say goodbye soon, and her choosing to run away before that happened. She ignored my comment but spoke of her new kitten, a "little baby boy". She spoke of him being very friendly and needy of her and gave examples of her capacity to satisfy his needs. However, she said, cats are very independent animals and one must let them find their way too. I tried to link her own need to be allowed to find her way and she smiled, but did not reply. Instead, she spoke of her father's annoyance over the cat's mischief and said that it reminded her of Sophie when she was little, always finding trouble before trouble found her. She said her Dad had taken some home movies of him and Sophie when she was a toddler and she thought it was funny how her father spoke to her as if she was ten and not two. Sophie became very sad, tears coming down her face; however, she managed to continue thinking and said she could not imagine her parents as children. I spoke of how difficult it is to let go of the little kitten inside her when she feels maybe she was not satisfied enough. She smiled and said if she ever had children she would always be there for them. I thought of Sophie's precocious ego development and how previously at times it had felt not genuine as a way of protecting against feelings of neediness and security—her "kittenish" feelings. However, I also began to think about it as a defensive move in the context of her parents' narcissistic functioning. I thought that Sophie's tears represented her need for a transitional space in the therapeutic context, what Winnicott (1971) calls a "potential space".

Thinking of herself as a potential mother who could sooth her baby was a hopeful sign in my mind, as this indicated her capacity to think of herself as a different type of woman than her mother, but yet identify with the positive aspects of womanhood. However, her identification with the aggressive rather than the benign and loving side of cats indicated the fragility of her progress.

Sophie's fears over the exploration of her sexual body, and her unconscious belief that only by murdering her mother would she be able to freely explore her sexual longings and possess what was rightfully hers, ran deep and fuelled her fantasies and her writing. My interest in her writing freed her to explore her capacity as a poet and short story writer. She started a club at school and often brought examples of her writing to sessions. On one occasion, she wrote a story based on a picture of a tiger sitting next to a boat in a dock. The story was filled with Sophie's primitive fears and fantasies of being devoured by the object, and her intact Oedipal omnipotence which fuelled her feelings of being cheated of what was rightfully hers. In the story, the tiger stood for the punisher, all powerful and unforgiving, Sophie's punitive and cannibalistic superego. However, he was portrayed as waiting for his love, and feeling lonely and sad trapped in his rage and need to devour. In my countertransference, I felt somewhat bothered and tired while Sophie read her story and showed me the picture in question. I realized I was defensively reacting to the level of aggression contained in the story and decided to speak openly about what I thought were Sophie's fears over sexuality and aggression. Sophie responded by crying and becoming visibly shaken: she spoke of her fear of socializing and recurrent anxiety over being raped when inebriated, as illustrated by the following excerpt:

> I really would like to go to parties, but I can't. I'm so afraid of what can happen. It is so dangerous my friends get really drunk, and it is so stupid. I once got very drunk but I become very sad and I cried a lot, and got very scared." When I invited Sophie to tell me what dangers she meant, she became very tearful and felt silent for a while. The room felt like the early days. Sophie had become cut off. After a few minutes I pointed this out to her. She cried inconsolably: these were not empty tears, there was a sense of real fear. Sophie spoke of her fear of being raped at a party, said she just freezes when she enters a full room of young people. She said: "All the bad things that can happen go through my mind all at once" …

As this vignette shows, Sophie worried constantly about losing control and struggled to understand her primitive fears. However, her capacity to use her writing to communicate and work in displacement served as very useful means of discussing what she felt was not allowed to be spoken about, namely her fantasies regarding sexual intercourse as highly aggressive and dangerous. These beliefs were exemplified by her story about two cats, a girl and a boy. The girl cat was always scratching and hurting the boy until one day he got tired of the abuse and ran away with the girl's food, leaving her lonely and hungry. This story, in my mind, demonstrated Sophie's confusion between early needs of hunger and safety (usually satisfied by the maternal object) and more physical and active needs of a sexual nature, which she perceived as extremely dangerous. Sophie's progressive moves to explore and understand her confusion brought tears and silence back to the room; however, there was a sense that some thinking about these matters was taking place, and exerting changes in the external world.

Finding a space to be separate and create: the emergence of a potential space

After the Easter Break, Sophie began to come only once a week, regardless of her knowing that I was there, waiting for her, twice weekly. She would often call or show up late, and I would try to speak of her desire to let me know that she could come and go as she pleased, and that

I would still be there. In return, she would assertively remind me of her busy life and all the new things happening socially now that she was in her final year of school (studying for A levels). I found myself enjoying Sophie's adolescent acting out, reinforcing my sense that she was moving forward in her capacity to feel safe in the context of separation.

However, Sophie's fears over being rejected, and her defensive arrogance and tendency to make the object into a rejecting one, came to the fore as she began to express interest in Robert, a boy at school. She manifested extremely ambivalent behaviour and feelings towards this boy, but managed to attract him and went out for the first time on a couple of dates. She had a lot in common with this boy, specially his interest in her writing. As she continued to bring her short stories and poems to our sessions, she spoke of her experience of this boy as understanding her thinking and her feelings. She attended her first party with Robert and managed to stay there without running away as she often did by calling her mother. She felt proud, yet still quite apprehensive.

Along with Sophie's wish for independence and what I thought was a fragile wish to explore her sexuality, her wish to end the therapeutic relationship emerged. At first, I struggled to understand her motivation for terminating treatment—wondering whether perhaps my own excitement over hearing Sophie speak her mind after so many months of silent communication was blocking my capacity to appreciate her wish for letting me go and her need for me to let her go.

A couple of months before the summer break, Sophie spoke of being in the middle of a difficult decision: she wrote this great short story and wanted it published, but knew it would hurt her mother's feelings. Sophie said that it was based on her thoughts about mother's experience of being a working mother. Robert had read it and seemed touched by it. She told me that lately she felt this urge to talk about how she has felt in the past and that she feels it has to do with coming here. There was a silence. Sophie became tearful. When I wondered what was so scary or worrying about what she had expressed in this piece of writing, she replied she thought it was very sarcastic. I suggested that Sophie was talking about her sadness, but also her anger. Sophie said she thought it was about her anger with her Mum over leaving her alone when she was little: "She chose herself over me, she always does. I am just a burden". She cried inconsolably. Sophie spoke about her Mum and how it is impossible to tell her how lonely she feels because she will end up making it about herself. She said: "Now, this *is* going to be about her and she is going to know how I feel, and she is going to pay!" She became visibly angry and added: "I usually punish her with silence. I ignore her, she hates that, but she makes me feel sorry for her. But now, I am really paying attention, and let's see what she does."

I thought of this session as the final turning point in our work, as Sophie's material shifted and she allowed herself to bring into the therapy room all her feelings of rage, envy, and disappointment. Also, it confirmed my understanding of her silence as a powerful way to punish her mother, to let her know how she felt. Weeks later, Sophie arrived triumphantly announcing that over the weekend she had "pulled" a boy for the first time. She spoke openly about enjoying the experience but feeling somewhat shocked the next morning about her courage to try it out with a boy she did not know well. In the countertransference, I felt myself seduced by the excitement of the adolescent story. However, as Sophie expressed her satisfaction at Robert finding out and realizing that he had missed out on the opportunity of being "pulled" by her, my interest shifted. I thought of the aggression contained in this statement and wondered after the session about Sophie's attack on this boy who had been a real source of support for her. Who was she really attacking? I felt concerned about the fragility of Sophie's progress and thought about the imminent end of our therapy. I found myself trying to think of ways in which I could convince Sophie to stay. During this period, I often felt very maternal in the transference, feeling concerned about Sophie's risky behaviour and the fragility of her sense of safety.

During our last session together, Sophie spoke of her university application and her parents' disapproval of her choice. However, she expressed her wish to become a writer and to continue to express herself this way. She told me that she would miss therapy, which for her had meant a place where she could think and not worry about me thinking she was "silly or just a baby about things". Most of all, she added, she liked it that I did not mind her quiet side. She said she had come to appreciate that side and that she thought it was that side that came out in her writing. Perhaps, I thought to myself, her writing has now come to represent a way of containing her tears and finding the words. However, I still felt that by choosing creative writing as her degree course she was indicating having found another way of defying her mother. I was left with the feeling that she might return to therapy later on in life as the strength of her unmet early needs and her strong ambivalence towards the parental couple remained underground but close to the surface. In general, some restoration of the developmental path had taken place as indicated by Sophie's emerging interest in film and poetry as well as her frequent outings with friends to places she had considered very dangerous before. She also reported being able to fall asleep easily, especially after having transformed her childhood room into a tribute to adolescent rebellion: purple and pink with pictures of such legendary rebellious figures as James Dean and Marilyn Monroe.

Some final thoughts

Winnicott (1958) wrote about the function of the mother as "guardian of the instinct-barrier". Through her devotion the mother can anticipate and divert almost all stimulation reaching her baby, or ration it so that it is enough, but not too much. In this way she sets up what Winnicott has called "a good enough holding environment". Like Anna Freud, he felt that a mother who provides this acts as an "auxiliary ego", protecting the baby from both under- and over-stimulation, and from premature development of its own resources. Consistent failure to guard the instinct-barrier happens when, for reasons either of her situation or of her personality, the mother's cathexis of things other than her baby predominates and, as we say, she "has something else on her mind".

As illustrated by Sophie's case, often my role in the transference was that of the mother who provides a good enough holding environment where this young woman could feel safe to explore new ways of regulating difficult affects, many of which were associated with early, preverbal experiences of not feeling kept in mind.

The experience of a different kind of holding developmental object and environment provided Sophie with the experience of a relationship where her thoughts and feelings could be spoken and thought about without being overshadowed by the other's own needs. What I considered technically challenging in this case was Sophie's tendency to turn interpretations into judgments, making me into a persecutory and dangerous object. In other words, words could easily hurt and destroy the relationship, resulting in what Sophie herself depicted as "walking on broken glass all the time". This was an experience which she described constantly in relation to her parents, and that I myself came to experience frequently in my relationship with her.

I came to understand Sophie's need to let me go by terminating therapy as her way of safely expressing her wish to grow up and leave behind her infantile needs of dependency and fear of being alone. Sophie left therapy feeling stronger, optimistic, and empowered to embrace the challenge of growing up. Her writing seemed to have provided her with the opportunity to integrate herself and create something that belonged to her. In fact, following the end of her formal education, she continued to explore her outstanding literary abilities and decided to pursue an academic path in the field of literature.

In her 1969 paper on "Adolescence as a Developmental Disturbance", Anna Freud explores the concept of transitory developmental disturbance which she links to the process of development in the context of new emerging demands that bring imbalance to the internal functioning of the child. In adolescence, the reorientation to object attachments and social relations is a primary source of anxiety for the young person. In Sophie's case, the degree of unmet pre-Oedipal needs impinged significantly upon her capacity to manage powerful emerging adolescent instinctual drives. She reverted to early ways of self-soothing and communication which proved ineffective when faced with the external demands of her adolescent world. I understood my role as a "new developmental object" with whom she could explore different ways of interaction, and safely mourn losses and what she felt she had never had. Together, we survived a period of developmental disturbance. But a question remains as to how much our relational journey together prepared her for the future developmental challenges of adult life.

References

Arlow, J. A. (1961). Silence and the theory of technique. *Journal of the American Psychoanalytic Association*, 9: 44–55.

Bleandonu, G. (1999). *Wilfred Bion: His life and Works*. London: Free Association.

Freud, A. (1948). Notes on aggression. In: *The Writings of Anna Freud: Indications for Child Analysis and Other Papers, Vol. IV* (pp. 60–73). New York: International Universities Press.

Freud, A. (1969). Adolescence as a developmental disturbance. In: *The Writings of Anna Freud. Vol. VII* (pp. 39–47). New York: International Universities Press.

Hurry, A. (1998). *Psychoanalysis and Developmental Therapy*. London: Karnac.

Krystal, H. (1985). Genetic view of affects. In: *Integration and Self-healing: Affect, Trauma, Alexithymia* (pp. 38–62). Hillside, NJ: Analytic Press.

Mahler, M. (1963). Thoughts about development and individuation. *Psychoanalytic Study of the Child, 18*: 307–324.

Socarides, D. D. & Stolorow, R. D. (1988). Affects and self-object. *Annual of Psychoanalysis, 12/13*: 105–119.

Winnicott, D. W. (1958). The capacity to be alone. In: *Psychoanalytic Explorations: Winnicott*. Cambridge, MA: Harvard University Press, 1989.

Winnicott, D. W. (1971). *Playing and Reality*. London: Tavistock.

Outreach

CHAPTER TWENTY SIX

"Adolescence as a Second Chance"—AFC training for practitioners working with pregnant teenagers and young parents and their children

Joan Raphael-Leff

> *"… more than any other time of life, adolescence with its typical conflicts provides the analyst with instructive pictures of the interplay and sequence of internal danger, anxiety, defence activity, transitory or permanent symptom formation, and mental breakdown".*
>
> —(Anna Freud, Adolescence, 1958, p. 258)

Introduction

Adolescence is indeed a time of "internal danger", and of external enactments. As such, teenage mothers and their infants are at risk. The United States and Britain currently have the highest rate of teen births in the Western world, with most girls now keeping their babies. Today's focus on infant mental health issues has heightened governmental awareness of the necessity to support young people who deal simultaneously with the double demands of adolescence and parenthood—striving for their own individuation while meeting demands, and providing emotional sustenance for a dependent baby or individuating toddler.

In 2007, the Anna Freud Centre received government funding to design, implement, and evaluate a psychodynamically informed training course to enhance emotional understanding among practitioners working with this complex client group.

In keeping with the Anna Freud tradition, the original course, "Teenagers Becoming Parents", was devised through a "think tank" approach of brainstorming, weaving together new and old paradigms into a comprehensive model of teenage pregnancy and parenting. This process involved many self-selected participants, some of whom later became presenters or ran reflective work groups. In that sense, the course is true to the essence of the Anna Freudian vision of disseminating psychoanalytic understanding to professionals in other fields.

In 2008 two pilot courses were delivered to eighty-five participants. The teaching faculty included clinicians, practitioners, and academics, lecturers from the Anna Freud Centre, and from the Portman Clinic, the Tavistock Clinic & Centre, and a variety of NHS and voluntary sector organizations. They included Drs Carol Broughton, Anita Chakraborty, Sue Gerhardt, Zack Eleftheriadou, Viviane Green, Leezah Hertzman, Earl Hopper, Helen Johnson (Ritzema), Valli Kohon, Egle Laufer, Norka Malberg, Maggie Mills, Dana Shai, Natalia Stafler, Ju Tomas-Merrills, Isca Salzberger-Wittenberg, Jenny Stoker, Susan Straub, Margot Waddell, John Woods, and Marie Zaphiriou Woods.

Course evaluation consisted of detailed feedback of all components in each study day; mid- and end of course appraisals from participants on a variety of measures in both the spring-summer and autumn-winter 2008 trainings, and follow-up of the first cohort nine months later. In line with these, as project leader, I condensed the original eight full study days delivered over sixteen weeks by some twenty teachers—into a more manageable five half study days, run by a single leader, which was piloted and evaluated. This shorter version, "Adolescence as a Second Chance", is now in the process of roll-out, by means of training leaders at the Anna Freud Centre and elsewhere, to disseminate the five modules of the course (see below) to a variety of practitioners working in their own locality. Training also occurs abroad, in both low and high income societies. Group instruction and dissemination of complex psychoanalytic ideas to "front line" workers is elucidated through observation, self-reflection, and interactive learning, in keeping with the Anna Freudian tradition of training in the War Nurseries (see Chapters One, Two, Three, and Four).

"Adolescence as a Second Chance"

This AFC training course focuses on enhancing infant mental health. It aims to increase practitioners' understanding of the typical emotional states, psychodynamic processes, and developmental issues of teen parents and their offspring—how a newborn baby comes to develop an awareness of self; how the growing child consolidates his or her understanding of the world of emotions; and how in adolescence, s/he must rework many of the issues of toddlerhood before becoming an adult. With the objective of helping professionals break the trans-generational "cycle of disadvantage", the central focus of this course is on the internal world's external consequences when a teenager, in the throes of adolescent turmoil, simultaneously takes on the tough demands of parenting.

Practitioners

One aspect of working with teenage clients is their keen ability to pit one professional against another, exacerbating a tendency for splitting within multi-agency teams of practitioners who have different ways of understanding emotional issues. By bringing together a variety of practitioners at many levels the AFC course offers an opportunity to network, understand individual, group, and institutional dynamics, and benefit from an integrative multidisciplinary view of this complex clientele.

Course participants vary from people with minimal training but wide experience (e.g., hostel staff or youth workers, who may not have completed secondary education), to professionals with specialized qualifications, master degrees, or even doctorates. Disciplines range from parent-project coordinators, "early years" professionals, specialist midwives, health visitors and nurses, child protection or family support workers, workers with young fathers, group leaders, personal advisors or counsellors to child and adolescent mental health practitioners, including social workers, clinical psychologists, child psychotherapists, and others. Participants in UK courses come from all over the British Isles, and from as far afield as Australia, Holland, and Germany, but courses are also run in a variety of countries as dissimilar as Italy, Madeira, Morocco, Poland, and South Africa.

This variety of backgrounds means that the training must meet a broad spectrum of requirements, without anyone feeling patronized, bored, or out of their depth. And provisions must be made for practitioners to benefit from their colleagues' varied experience. To accommodate these multiple needs the course is highly interactive, and structured progressively in both form and content: the nature of learning material and group exercises increases in complexity and depth from the beginning of each session to its end, and from the beginning of the course to *its* end, to allow each participant to find their own "comfort zone" and "voice". Above all the course provides containment—a space to contemplate anxiety provoking issues, and to imbibe some psychoanalytic ways to continue thinking about these when engaged at "the coal face".

Each study day is comprised of two interrelated sessions (an "Interactive Workshop" and a "Skill-building Seminar"), with the large group often breaking into smaller units of varying sizes for exercises and role plays; and an intimate "Reflective Work Group" of seven to nine members who meet regularly each study day with an experienced leader to discuss their own cases, becoming more aware of some of the unconscious configurations, defensive mechanisms, and underlying fantasies that make up the human psyche.

In the intervals between the fortnightly study days, participants engage in "Self Study", the units of which include preparatory reading, internet lecture videos and self-reflective exercises. In addition, all course participants are asked to keep a private journal to chart their own emotional journey on the course, including countertransferential responses to their challenging teen clients, whose intense feelings often provoke strong reactions, involving irritation, concern, anxiety, and sometimes, secret admiration and envy. Again, this is in keeping with the Anna Freudian model of self-observation and self-reflection.

Course modules

1. **Interrelationships**
   Interactive Workshop: Teen clients—expectations and meaning making
   Skill-building Seminar: Co-constructed interactions and mentalization
2. **Adolescents**
   Interactive Workshop: Maturational tasks of early and late adolescence
   Skill-building Seminar: Psychological processes of pregnancy and teen mothering
3. **Babies in Teen Families**
   Interactive Workshop: Attunement, attachment and affect regulation
   Skill-building Seminar: Babies—and reflective function in teen parents
4. **Toddlers and Teen Mothers and Fathers**
   Interactive Workshop: Extending boundaries: separation-individuation and imaginative play

Skill-building Seminar: Contemporary parenthood and emotional disturbance in teen parents

5. **Families, Groups and Organizations**

Interactive Workshop: Family dynamics and psychosocial narratives

Skill-building Seminar: Teams, groups and institutional defences

Take-home messages:

a. Teenage parents are teenagers.

b. "... we do not deal with the happenings in the external world as such, but with their repercussions in the mind" (Anna Freud, 1960, p. 54).

c. Precisely because both adolescence and parenthood are transitional states reactivating unresolved emotional issues, they provide a "second chance" to work through conflicts belonging to the past, while processing current demands.

These hopeful messages are embedded in the full title of the Anna Freud Centre's course—"Adolescence as a Second Chance: working with the emotional needs of teen parents and their children". Practitioners also learn to work with cultural diversity, to identify disturbances during pregnancy and postnatally and to refer clients for appropriate therapeutic help, including perinatal counselling, group, individual, couple, or parent–infant psychotherapy.

In sum, teen pregnancy is a societal issue that brings with it higher levels of maltreatment, childhood pathology, parental disturbance, and a series of adverse issues that weigh heavily on society and resources. Service projects of any nature must involve an understanding of the emotional issues involved. An integrative training which includes these as well as an exploration of the participating practitioners' own feelings not only is truly Anna Freudian, but most importantly, contributes to more empathic forms of early intervention.

Disseminating psychoanalytic thinking to non-analytic practitioners aims to enhance their own practice according to the demands of their own disciplines, rather than turning them into mini-therapists. The following exposition will touch upon some of the course content as taught, such as maturational tasks and the challenges this clientele poses to practitioners; anxieties that adolescence evokes in the teens themselves, and in their carers; conscious and unconscious motivations for conception in adolescence, and concepts such as defence mechanisms, "generative identity", primal scene, and "contagious arousal".

Adolescence

Heralded by the appearance of secondary sexual characteristics and the onset of menstruation/nocturnal emissions, the main features of adolescence may be defined as potency and power—the potential realizability of desires and aggressive impulses—exciting, but for teenagers who are unsure of their internal restraints, frighteningly real. Childhood preoccupations resurface, as the troubled teenager seeks new resolutions to the eternal universal problems of "birth, copulation and death" (to use T. S. Eliot's felicitous phrase).

Maturational processes

Disillusioning doubts, the capacity to procreate, and untested physical strength mean that the teenager's destructive rage or defensive sexuality can now have real consequences. Young people are prone to experimentation, and most societies provide auxiliary social controls and acceptable outlets. Thus, worldwide, adolescence is shaped by cultural patterns and specific social constraints. Yet, despite these differences, having worked professionally with primary health carers on six continents, I find that developmental goals are remarkably similar cross-culturally (albeit varying in definition, content, and centrality) (Raphael-Leff, 2005):

- *Emotional maturation*: Self-reflection vs. acting-out. (Developing realistic self-esteem. Ownership of previously dangerous and overwhelming feelings and/or developing socially acceptable expression of hostility in symbolic ways.)
- *Intellectual tasks*: Self-discipline and motivation. (Search for meaning. Consolidating adult knowledge and work patterns.)
- *Social tasks*: Control over antisocial impulses. (Appropriate disengagement from carers and development of more complex relationships.)
- *Sexual representation*: Gender and generative identity. (Incorporation of bodily changes. Achieving sexual intimacy and procreative responsibility.)

However, in contemporary Western societies, media glorification and commodification of youth and sex eroticizes experience. Leisure activities, clothes, toys, games and movies aimed for pre-teen "Tweenies" promote premature sexual engagement without the supportive mechanism of more traditional societies. Surveys on underage sex find that three quarters of eleven to fourteen year olds in the UK wish they had more guidance and find it difficult to talk to parents about sex. Today's precocity short-circuits the slow process of accommodation to altered relationships, and gradual mourning of the loss of childhood and of the pre-teen body prescribed by Anna Freud.

In contemporary adolescence, girls may conflate sexual arousal with anxiety, while boys might respond to anxiety with sexual and/or aggressive behaviour. Research studies find that troubled adolescent girls tend towards *internalizing behaviours* (withdrawal, depression, anxiety, eating disorders, and somatic problems), and boys towards *externalizing behaviours* (antisocial behaviour and aggression), probably linked to ubiquitously female primary caregivers, and their varied effect on girl and boy babies respectively. As we know, the archaic mother's misperceptions, disapproval, demands, over-involvement, bodily shame, or rejection during the child's early use of her mind, are absorbed and retained as procedural rather than semantic memories, expressed somatically (and retriggered when she has a baby herself).

Generative identity

The thrust towards psychic maturation and growth is especially impeded when adverse experience during toddlerhood has prevented establishing a solid sense of self, gender, and generative identities. What I term "generative identity" proposes that beyond one's "core" embodied sense of femaleness or maleness, and in addition to mental representations of femininity/masculinity, and articulation of erotic desire, there is a further gender component—a psychic construction of oneself as *a potential [pro]-creator*.

In toddlerhood, and again in adolescence, consolidation of generative identity entails recognition of sexed restrictions and of distinct reproductive capacities:

> *Sex* ("I am either female or male, not the other sex, neither, or both")
> *Generation* (Adults make babies; children cannot)
> *Genesis* ("I am not self-made. Two people made me")
> *Generativity* (Females gestate, give birth, and lactate; males impregnate).

These limitations also raise "genitive" anxieties about finitude (death and the irreversibility of time) and arbitrariness—the chance meeting of parents, and gametes, alike. Paradoxically, acceptance of sexed restrictions enables fluidity of gender. The more varied the range of identifications with non-reproductive aspects of carers, siblings, and others, the richer the self-concept of gender (Raphael-Leff, 2007, 2010b). Conversely, when, rather than generalized creativity, generative identity remains restricted to procreativity (as in many traditional societies), and/or linked to Oedipal desires for a *real* baby, precipitous reproduction may ensue.

Indeed, empirical studies show that in Britain, care leavers are disproportionally represented among teen mothers. In the USA girls whose fathers left the family early in their lives have a five-fold rate of early sexual activity and teenage conceptions (Ellis et al., 2003). Where paternal presence has been peripheral or absent, young girls often treat their male peers with considerable contempt, turning to older men, who, themselves suffering from lack of self-esteem and inadequate role models, privilege sexual conquest above intimate relationships (Waddell, 2009).

The primal scene revisited

For the child, initiation of selfhood resides in acknowledging difference and separateness. The primal scene is not merely sexual—but reproductive. Recognition of the parental capacity to make babies initiates recognition of generative restrictions (above). The Oedipal moment consolidates "triangular space" (Britton, 1989). This encounter with the caring parents' erotic preoccupation may seem "enigmatic" in that it sensually arouses the child's awareness of secret sexual knowledge beyond his/her understanding (Laplanche, 1995). But, in my clinical experience, exclusion from the parental couple's union has another, equally dramatic effect—recognition of one's (temporary) obliteration from the coupling parents' minds. This emotional absence may be experienced as a human "void" generating dread, and initiating those "genitive anxieties" about unconnectedness, the arbitrariness of genesis, the ungraspability of life's finitude, and the irreversibility of time (Raphael-Leff, 2010a). Depending on the degree of attunement of early carers and/or experiences of failed dependency, the subjective meaning of this "abyss" ranges from tolerable dread, to traumatic "black hole" terrors of catastrophic loss, or even annihilation. These anxieties are revisited when puberty lifts the enigmatic veil. (Indeed, when extreme psychic defences of dissociation and encapsulation have been employed against anxiety of annihilation, in pubertal fantasies the bleeding of menstruation may unconsciously signify dissolution of the encapsulated trauma (see Hopper, 1991)).

In adolescence, the Oedipal triangle is triumphantly rotated when, rather than excluded, the fecund teen becomes an *active* sexual participant. The solidity of the teenager's generative identity and security of attachment will determine whether she or he succumbs to sexual excitement as addictive. In vulnerable adolescents, reawakened genitive anxieties may lead to escapist solutions—substance abuse, pregnancy/impregnation, "invincible" risk-taking (or even suicide as an act of "mastery" over death)—all misguided ways of asserting physical "self-sufficiency" in the face of the relational abyss (Raphael-Leff, 2008).

Teenage alcohol addiction, anorexia, compulsive binging or bulimia, as well as self-cutting or burning, suicidal and aggressive tendencies are now so commonplace that many adolescents are unlikely to recognize these problems as bodily expressions of depression, persecutory disorders, anxiety states, and/or PTSD following childhood deprivation or abuse. The AFC course trains practitioners to better understand such defences, and to encourage their clients to seek psychotherapeutic help for incapacitating problems.

Defences in adolescence

While re-appraising his/her personal identity, the teenager fluctuates between child-like and adult feelings. Previous defences prove inadequate against the threat of intrusion of repressed Oedipal feelings (and genitive anxiety).

Anna Freud regarded this emotional upheaval of adolescence as part of the maturational process—and, indeed, its absence as a possible indication for treatment (1958). Already in 1905 Sigmund Freud had noted the losses attendant on "transformations of puberty" as qualitative changes in internal pressures, and that their intensification requires an adolescent to renounce the incestuous objects of childhood. His daughter ascribed a "state of mourning" to this emotional struggle of detaching libido from the parents and cathecting new objects (possibly involving teenage "crushes"). She added that mental suffering and an urgent wish to be helped are insufficient motivations for therapeutic success since, as in bereavement and unhappy love, the immediate lost object must be given up before analytic treatment could become effective.

At a symposium held in 1957 in Worcester, Massachusetts (home of Clark University where her father gave his 1908 lecture), Anna Freud described four types of defences characteristic of adolescence (used together or singly):

- *Removal* (withdrawal of libido from the parents).
- *Reversal of affect* (intense love for the parents is felt as hatred).
- *Withdrawal of libido to the self*—ideas of grandeur and extreme narcissism, or hypochondriacal symptoms (and see somatic manifestations above).
- *Regression* to the undifferentiated phase of ego development, resulting in a dissolution of boundaries between self and object, leading to disturbances in identity and a fear of surrender (see Geleerd, 1964).

Today we may add the further defence of *escapism*—defensive sidestepping of maturational tasks. To truly establish "adult" status, the youth's physiologically mature body representation must come to include physically mature, sexually "alive" genitals (Laufer, 1996). However, cumulative research into psychosomatics shows that bodily sensations and action may be substituted, to keep painful emotional states split off and denied awareness.

Findings suggest that in both sexes implicit "fault lines" occur when early collaborative dialogues with carers have failed to provide attuned mirroring and satisfactory emotional understanding of internal contradictions. Unconscious enactments ensue in adolescence when procedural representations have remained segregated, fragmented, and unprocessed, with few chances to update or integrate these as new developmental capacities become available (see Lyons Ruth, 1999). A teenager may avoid depression by concretely expressing her conflictual feelings of love and hatred towards herself and/or others through compulsive sexual acts—which unconsciously serve as a means of self-punishment, while satisfying unfulfilled early longings for the (pre-Oedipal) mother (Balint, 1973; Pines, 1988). Eating disorders often reflect difficulties in differentiating from the same-sex mother. Cutting can be a disguised attack on the maternal body, or the pubertal body that still "belongs" to mother. And similarly, premature pregnancy is an unconscious communication to the mother, and/or a means of refusing adolescence. Inadequate consideration by professionals of the contrast between women's "whole body" and men's phallocentric sexuality led to the failure to recognize a wide range of symptoms of physical self-harm (e.g., self-mutilation and starvation) and of mothers' attacks on their babies as extensions of their own self-hatred, and/or as manifestations of intergenerational propagation of pathological or perverse mothering (Welldon, 1988).

Teenage Pregnancy

Motivations for conception in adolescence

In an age of educational parity and readily available safe contraception, conception may offer a life choice made under pervasive romanticization of motherhood to gain prestige and consolidate selfhood, especially when faced with educational failure, constrained ambition, or limited occupational opportunities. In industrialized societies around half of all pregnancies to under-eighteen year olds are concentrated among the most deprived population, with increased financial worries, poor housing, and isolation from peers. A quarter of such adolescent mothers will have a second child within two years of the first!

Unconscious motivations for teenage conception vary from blissful ignorance, through omnipotent risk-taking, a desire to be loved unconditionally, or to become "fully adult", to emulate or surpass parents, or as a magical means of rewriting history ... Conception also may be used to ratify doubted fertility (Pines, 1988) or to defensively avoid the emotional reality of adolescence. Pregnancy can alleviate a pubertal girl's anxiety about losing her mother's care. Refinding maternal support during pregnancy and mothering offers reassurance that she has not killed or damaged her mother by usurping her (Laufer, 1996). Likewise, a teenage boy's desire to prove his virile masculinity through impregnation reflects complex identifications and motivations.

While in some families in industrialized countries, teenage motherhood is ego-syntonic and recurs normatively over several generations, where this is not the case, even "planned" pregnancy tends to be associated with pathogenic factors. Multiple studies indicate a threefold incidence of childhood sexual abuse, domestic violence, conduct disorder, and paternal absence in the family of origin of adolescent mothers (Adams & D'Souza, 2009). Ditto young fathers, especially those who have grown up in the "care" system.

Double crisis—adolescence and gestation

Specialist midwives and nurses may expect pregnant teenagers to behave like other expectant mothers. However, a pregnant adolescent crosses the boundary between being a child herself, and birthing a child. The young girl is subject to all the usual upheavals that pregnancy evokes in older women—anxieties about altered sensation and shape, unfamiliar body-image, fantasies of corporeal exploitation, and the universal mysteries of formation, transformation, and preservation found through observation, and qualitative and quantitative research (Raphael-Leff, 1993). However, these are juxtaposed on the pubertal body's rapid changes. And the pregnant body's bulging belly, blue-veined breasts, nausea, uncontrollable foetal movements, tiredness, and swollen ankles is extraordinarily confusing and antithetical to an ultra-slim teen-ideal.

Anxieties

It is important for antenatal practitioners to recognize that like other adolescents, a pregnant teenager is still trying to come to terms with pubertal body ownership, and reactivated issues of sex, gender, and sexuality. But her swelling shape discloses her sexual activity to all and sundry, and gaining possession of her own body is complicated when it has two occupants. Control over psychic and corporeal space is jeopardized. Doubts about her capacity to cope with labour pains and a vaginal birth are accompanied by fantasies of tearing, bursting, being emptied, internally damaged, and damaging. Invasion of privacy by the baby kicking inside her most intimate cavity feels especially fraught for girls who have suffered sexual abuse or violation (Raphael-Leff, 2005).

Persecutory anxieties that the baby knows her inside out and will reveal her hidden feelings after the birth, exacerbates a desire for, yet dread of, separation. Furthermore, these anxieties echo her difficulties in achieving separation from her own mother now that she feels vulnerable and tethered to the fragile yet powerful baby inside her. At the very point of trying to define a separate identity and hoping to become individuate, the pregnant teenager finds herself intensely dependent on others and faced with a future dependent baby. If for both sexes pubertal anxiety relates to the fear of the newly sexual body providing the power to usurp the archaic parent—pregnancy offers the teenager triumphal supremacy, to replace and internally destroy her mother by *becoming* her, competing with her, and showing her what she did not provide. A pregnant daughter's conscious anxiety now inverts: fear of damage by her mother's anger and rejection as a deserved punishment for what she has done.

Practitioners

Those working with young mothers often treat them with a "you brought this upon yourself" attitude. A pregnant teenager may feel condemned not only by her mother but also by society, which sees her as an irresponsible child who should be punished for her delinquent act of not making sure that her baby will have what it needs—a "happy mother and father", and a home of their own for the baby (Laufer, 1996). The AFC training helps practitioners to see how their own punitive responses may feed into such (unconscious) fantasies.

As noted, the pregnant body may be used to express internal struggles. Risk to the foetus is increased by common adolescent lifestyles of bad eating habits, smoking, alcohol, and substance misuse. Giving birth before the age of fifteen confers a five-fold risk of maternal death in childbirth, yet despite a higher incidence of pregnancy loss, birth damage, prematurity, low birth-weight, and a twofold increased rate of infant mortality, teens are less likely to attend antenatal clinics on a regular basis.

Additionally, many teenage girls are rejected by their families and/or partners when they become pregnant, which provokes an emotional crisis for the already overburdened young woman. In low-income societies, HIV testing occurs during pregnancy. In some townships two thirds of pregnant women may receive a HIV+ diagnosis, followed by abandonment by partners and/or family. Timing is particularly poignant given the young woman's sense of betrayal (by her partner's toxic infidelity as well as his desertion), shame where AIDS is stigmatized; her anxiety, and complex feelings of guilt towards the baby, as well as fears relating to her own mortality. The AFC course trains practitioners to see the dual and triple burdens of adolescence, pregnancy, and motherhood, with a focus on feelings—their own as well as their clients', and repercussions of these on body and mind.

Teen Parenting

Young mothers

Practitioners tend to forget that very young mothers may often be unable to recognize distress signs or symptoms of illness, and lack practical skills to access health services on behalf of their children, or indeed themselves. An increasing prevalence of undiagnosed sexually transmitted infections (STIs) can affect the newborn, as do easily missed fatal conditions such as meningitis. Maternal eating disorders are associated with feeding difficulties and most Western young mothers decline to breastfeed, feeling unable to be both a maternal and a sexual woman. This ambivalent split also feeds intimate partner violence which increases during childbearing.

Thus parental immaturity poses a developmental threat, putting the vulnerable infant at risk of erratic, neglectful, or damaging care. Yet despite being in the medical high-risk category worldwide, children of teenage mothers receive only half the level of medical care and treatment compared to those of older mothers (UNICEF, 2010).

In the UK and elsewhere, the AFC course helps midwives, primary health attendants, and other relevant practitioners to engage pregnant adolescents and teen parents on their own emotional level, encouraging them to be reflective, and providing emotional guidance to safeguard the baby's psychic and physical well-being as well as their own.

Young fathers

Research finds that fewer than half of all young fathers have ever lived with their child. Non-resident biological fathers are at risk of losing contact, as 20%–40% see their children less than once per week, 20–39% not in a year. In the UK and USA such under-involved teen fathers are found to have been brought up in stressful environments with insensitive, harsh, or unpredictable carers in poor neighbourhoods in large, low socio-economic status families with lone mothers who have low educational aspirations.

Compared to resident fathers they have insecure attachments, low threshold for anxiety and anger; high alcohol and marijuana dependency. Often disabled by mental health or drug problems, they engage more in illegal or abusive behaviour, and have more criminal convictions (Jaffee et al., 2001).

Lone mothers without partners are generally poorer, isolated and more likely to suffer from depression, stress, and other emotional, psychological, and health problems. Children living without their fathers are therefore more likely to live in poverty and deprivation. They have more trouble at school and socially; have more health problems, and are at greater risk of suffering physical, emotional, or sexual abuse. They are more likely to run away from home, and as teenagers are more likely to smoke, drink alcohol, take drugs, play truant, be excluded or leave school at sixteen. Therefore, they have lower qualifications, low income, or are unemployed or live on income support. They are more likely to experience homelessness, to be caught offending, and go to jail. Finally, they tend to enter and dissolve partnerships earlier, have children in adolescence and become absent fathers themselves (O'Neill, 2002)—thereby perpetuating the cycle in their own offspring.

Contagious arousal

As noted by Therese Benedek over fifty years ago, parents tend to retrace their own developmental steps with their child, whose difficulties will therefore relate specifically to the carer's weakest areas of unresolved developmental conflicts (1959). Studies show that babies of depressed mothers develop a hyper-sensitive stress response, with a threefold risk of emotional disorders in childhood and depression in adulthood. Children of angry parents have difficulties soothing themselves or others, poor anger control, and deficient understanding of emotional states. Violent or abusive parents play out their sadism with the child, who projects it onto toys and others, who then become hostile persecutors rather than comforters.

During parenthood, unprocessed infantile issues (of companionship, security, separation, boundaries, and control, as well as Oedipal and other conflicts) are enacted externally and imposed upon the baby as "ghosts in the nursery" (Fraiberg et al., 1980). A teenage mother may identify interchangeably with an idealized version of mothering, and with her baby who is felt to enjoy devoted care. The latter can provide a vicarious source of infantile fulfilment, but also often arouses envy for what the young mother feels she herself never had (Raphael-Leff, 2005; Waddell, 2009). These anxieties and deficiencies of the carer are absorbed and introjected by the infant. Research shows that effects of parental disturbance persist into late childhood, as less responsive, misattuned, rejecting, hostile, inconsistent, or ineffectual parenting leads to emotional, cognitive, and psychosocial developmental deficits in the child, including a propensity to depression (Murray, 2011).

However, clinical experience of working with new parents reveals a dynamic two way process—of influence on the baby, but also the profound emotional impact of the baby on the primary caregiver. I have termed this "contagious arousal", suggesting it happens through emotionally arousing interchange—exposure to, and trying to fathom the baby's "primitive" pre-verbal communications. But moreover, close contact with primal substances (amniotic fluid, vernix, colostrum, breast milk, lochia, puerperal secretions, baby urine, posset, faeces etc.) can retrigger the carer's own sub-symbolic infantile experience (Raphael-Leff, 2002). In young caregivers, this heightened arousal is aggravated by ongoing adolescent turmoil. Identificatory fusion/confusion with the romanticized or denigrated infant, coupled with imagined representations of her own baby-self in the eyes of her archaic mother at a time of powerful teenage conflicts with her present-day mother, provokes a spectrum of grievances, depressive affects, persecutory experiences, and extreme anxiety, with protective obsessional rituals, defensive disassociation, or withdrawal from the powerful infant, who represents idealized or split-off repudiated aspects of the infantile self. When the baby is deemed malevolent (among extreme "regulator" and "conflicted" parental orientations as opposed to "facilitator" or "reciprocator" ones), the perceived threat is minimized by the carer defensively maintaining an emotional distance from the infant, through routines, regulation, and detachment.

Young mothers with low self-esteem, who doubt their ability to mother, often hand the baby over to another carer, usually their own mother (Raphael-Leff, 2005). Distorted primary relationships often manifest in infant disorders of sleep, failure to thrive, persistent crying, and sleep—both expressing and further contributing to family disturbance (Hopkins, 2001).

In sum, pregnancy and parenting require tolerance and deferment which contrast with the adolescent's needs for immediate gratification and tension-release. Looking after a baby is always extremely demanding, and lone parenting is doubly so. When youth is added to the mix, it is hardly surprising that epidemiological studies find a threefold rate of postnatal depression in young mothers who lack a confidante and guidance. A survey of teenage mothers found most complained of anxiety, self-harm, eating disorders, and risk-taking behaviours (Sure Start Plus evaluation, Institute of Child Health, 2006).

Excluded from school, and lacking childcare provisions, young mothers feel isolated and shut out from the ordinary carefree activities of their peer group. Colleges with crèches are rare in the UK and USA. Seven out of ten adolescent mothers drop out of their schools, and fathers, too, tend to curtail their education. Multiple studies show that children of teenage mothers consistently score lower at school than children of older mothers. Even though a high proportion of the babies born to teenage mothers in the UK are conceived within an ongoing relationship and most of these young couples register the birth together, young fathers are less likely to live with or even to maintain regular contact with the child; and as noted, father absence is associated with poor outcome. This perpetuates a cycle of low income, few resources, and emotional deprivation. Once again, the preventive support of trained practitioners can help young fathers take an active role and ameliorate distress.

Brain development

Today's neurobiological research confirms psychoanalytic tenets of the centrality of interactive engagement in organizing patterns of connectivity of the neonate's "personality". However, it also reveals that the brain architecture is actually moulded by interaction. Circuits themselves are affected, as neural networks (proliferating at the truly extraordinary rate of 1.8 million new synapses per second until two years after birth) are activated, reinforced, or pruned within primary object relationships. During this critical period of prolonged dependence, the infant's neuroplastic malleability calls for both protective care and lively emotional responsiveness from others in order to promote healthy flexible connections. Conversely, emotionally damaging effects of parental depression, abuse, and neglect are found, amazingly, to be associated with permanent maladaptive "wiring" of neural response patterns (see Karmiloff-Smith, 1995; Balbernie, 2001; Trevarthen & Aitken, 2001). (At the AFC, the PIP therapeutic model provides a means of early intervention to alleviate such problems. See Chapter Ten.)

However, like the growing brains of infants, adolescence too involves neuronal "sculpting" and "pruning" into a more streamlined and efficient form, on a "use it or lose it" basis. The medial prefrontal cortex, the region important for planning and executive functioning is still developing through the teenage years. This brain reorganization increases the tendency of young adolescents to react in an emotional and impulsive way, relying on their more primitive "gut" reactions, instead of using the higher frontal lobes, thus reducing their capacity for mentalization, empathy, self-control, and prediction of the feelings of others. We are familiar with these as manifestations of impetuousnous, emotional hypersensitivity, problems concentrating, containing excitement, confusion, resentment, etc. In teen parents these affect the infant in their care.

Some research indicates that teenage mothers are less sensitive and attuned to their babies, and more "switched off" physiologically by comparison to adult mothers, who show increased heart rate and cortisol in response to baby's cries. Similarly, when filmed, they spend less time interacting with their child, and more looking away. These differences are ascribed to the neural immaturity of the teenage mothers' brains (Giardino et al., 2008). In addition, many of those who go on to become teenage parents have insecure emotional development in the first place. All the deficits of insecure attachment—poor self-soothing, anticipation of rejection, problems in managing conflicts co-operatively—are brought to their relationship with the infant. Nonetheless, although teenagers who have not been well cared for themselves are at risk of passing on their difficulties to their babies, the hopeful aspect is the very fluidity of their maturation.

The most important message of the course is that the adolescent's relationship with the baby offers a "second chance" to re-experience infantile emotions. Precisely because new pathways are being formed in the teenage parent's own brain relatively rapidly at this time of turbulence and malleability, s/he may be able to create a new "template" (what Bowlby, 1969, called an "internal working model") of a soothing caring relationship. With enough positive support for their own needs, teens can re-think their basic assumptions about the world being critical, hostile, or disinterested (Gerhardt, 2004)—which, with help, s/he can then offer the baby. Indeed, parenthood offers a "second chance" to rework unresolved conflicts. It constitutes an incentive to provide better nurture than they received, and an impetus to improve their own lives.

Mentalization

Mentalization means keeping the other's mind in mind. Mature caregiving implies using one's mind to mentally elaborate one's own experience, and that of the infant, so as to better understand the baby's feelings and help him or her to process the world. Parental reflective function rests on a capacity to think about the baby's desires, intentions, and vulnerability—and to cope with this without becoming overwhelmed by the baby's feelings or one's own unintegrated anxiety or hostility (Fonagy et al., 2002). This in turn enables a carer to soothe the baby and regulate his or her fear and distress without frightening or disrupting the infant further. Conversely, when a mother or father is stressed, they move into "survival mode" (Allen, 2006), and anxiety inhibits their capacity to mentalize. Reflective functioning pivots on the mother or father's ability to take a different perspective, to think of the child's needs as *separate* from her/his own (Slade, 2005). This capacity is affected by the development phase (of carer and child), current stressors, and negative experiences in the past. In adolescents, prevailing states of mind tend towards action rather than reflection and, under duress, provoke egocentric and thoughtless reactions, which exacerbate parenting difficulties.

This is where the AFC training course comes in—providing practitioners with understanding of reflective function and skills to increase mentalization in young parents. Furthermore, the course is designed to activate reflectiveness in practitioners themselves. Through interactive workshops and skill-building seminars it raises awareness of multiple perspectives and emotional complexities, encouraging the course participants to wonder what their own young clients might be feeling and what their own effect on these feelings might be. In addition to more theoretical input, each study day consists of a series of group exercises and games, including DVD material to enhance observation, role play to increase empathy, listening and communication skills to hone mirroring, contingent responsiveness, and the capacity to think about feelings. The self-study element helps participants to recognize and use their own affective reactions (countertransference), and to step back from these to think about the subjective intentions of both clients (baby and carer/s), especially during moments of stress or periods of conflict. By sponsoring curiosity in practitioners, the training also explores ways of engaging teen mothers and fathers by arousing *their* curiosity about feelings, their own and the child's. By having their own feelings validated, practitioners can better give the young parents in their care the language tools to think about their own minds, thereby encouraging them to think about the mind of the infant. In sum, the course hones the practitioners' reflective thinking, caring, and mirroring processes which are implemented in their workplaces, and gradually internalized by the young parents who are better able to keep their own child's mind in mind.

Teen parents and toddlers

Finally, in addition to adolescence and babyhood, the Anna Freud Centre course for practitioners also focuses on toddlerhood. This area is particularly difficult for teen parents since the toddler's struggles for autonomy so closely mirror their own (as the clinical chapters of this book attest). Issues include attachment, separation-individuation, omnipotence, and challenges to the illusion of magical control, necessitating recognition of the other as a distinct person with a mind of her own. Similarly, there exist issues of sexuality and eroticism; sexual difference and gender inequalities; and concerns about control, separateness, independence, and competence. The eighteen-month-old toddler is often volatile, struggling with powerful contradictory impulses from within, and difficult realities without, and raging as the adults around him increasingly impose social constraints and set safety limits (Lieberman, 1997; Stoker, 2005). In time, growing tolerance of frustration contributes to the child's ability to maintain self-esteem, to be alone, and eventually to manage longer separations and separateness (Winnicott, 1958).

However, the contrariness, opposition, and tantrums of the "terrible twos" often echo and clash with similar issues of the "terrible teens". The child's resistance to help and emotional provocation intensifies the young parent's own anger, which may touch on her/his own unresolved early issues to do with anality, sexuality, and aggression. Full responsibility for the intimate care and safe protection of the little child's body offers opportunities for unconscious enactments. The toddler's demand for independent bodily ownership may aggravate the young parent's possessiveness rather than a desire to hand over. But failure to do so results in bitter battles for control over essential bodily management of functions such as feeding, sleep, and toileting, and defiance may spread to other areas such as clothes, hygiene, or play.

Misattunements and misunderstandings are frequent and inevitable, indeed necessary, if the toddler is to learn to tolerate anxiety and frustration, and to transform aggression to socially accepted assertiveness. At the same time, reparation of disruptions in attachment is essential for communication to be resumed, to reassure the toddler that s/he is not omnipotently destructive, and that mother or the relationship with her is not permanently damaged (Anna Freud, 1965; Mahler, 1985; Zaphiriou Woods & Pretorius, 2010). While all parents struggle to manage their own feelings in order to stand firm in the face of their toddler's ambivalent behaviour, adolescent turbulence is likely to affect a teen parent's readiness to *repair* the relationship following inevitable disputes.

At the very point when she is expected to be flexible, sensitively responsive, and emotionally available in the face of the toddler's ever-changing developmental needs, a lone young mother may feel overwhelmed. In the absence of a helpful partner or confidante, with whom to "debrief", she lacks a "third" position to help her shift from experiencing the child as an extension of herself, to perceiving him/her as a unique individual, with separate needs, and different from herself.

This period is difficult for any parent, but adolescent parents, who are simultaneously dealing with the reactivation and reworking of many of these same issues, may find that their unresolved history, unformed personality, and difficult external circumstances make them more vulnerable to contagious arousal of the turbulent feelings and fantasies their toddler evokes in them.

In the AFC course, practitioners learn to make young parents aware of underlying processes, assuring them that given a good start, in the third year difficulties will ease with the child's increased command of communicative language and growing ability to play symbolically. Furthermore, they can convey the importance of imaginative play as a "precursor for adult work" (A. Freud, 1981), helping young parents to provide a healthy foundation for innovatory creativity.

Again, the experience of successfully parenting a toddler offers a teen parent a "second chance" to evolve an increasingly complex, solid, and discrete sense of her/him self alongside the toddler doing so. Simultaneously, the child's identification with a receptive carer enhances awareness of feelings as significant.

Conclusion

Elsewhere, I suggested that smaller nuclear families in stratified societies in transition (such as our own), with dispersed extended families and fragmented communities, offer fewer opportunities to work through infantile issues before the birth of one's own child (Raphael-Leff, 2005). In addition to immaturity, young parents are affected by multiple stressors, including the lack of a supportive social network and estrangement from families, placing their infants at risk of a variety of disruptions. These are exacerbated by sparse previous contact with babies; lack of preparation for the emotional impact of a baby, and poor practical support and developmental guidance. Teens with low self-esteem are unready to take on the full heavy responsibility that parenthood entails. Many lack the psychological resources to care for a needy infant, often feeling needy themselves, persecuted and resentful of extra demands. However, even stable and supported adolescents are at risk as parents. In addition to ordinary parenting stresses and sleep-disrupted nights, young mothers and fathers are also faced with their own emotional turmoil and adolescent restructuring of identity.

Aided by a *Theoretical Handbook and Training Manual* (Raphael-Leff, 2011) the Anna Freud Centre course now trains leaders to deliver the course "Adolescence as a Second Chance" to the wide variety of practitioners who work with pregnant teenagers, very young parents, and/or their children in the UK and abroad. It facilitates preventive work by enhancing understanding of the maturational tasks and emotional needs of babies, toddlers, and adolescents, and the psychodynamics of inter-agency collaboration. Thus trained to provide emotional support antenatally and developmental guidance after the birth, practitioners can prevent and alleviate distress, help mitigate negative representations and projections and, most importantly, provide a *model* that fosters in young parents a capacity for self-reflection and empathy with the baby as a small person with human feelings like their own, and a growing mind that cries out to be kept in mind.

References

Adams, A. & D'Souza, R. (2009). Teenage contraception. *General Practice Update*, *2*(6): 36–39.

Allen, J. G. (2006). Mentalizing in practice. In: J. G. Allen & P. Fonagy (Eds.), *Handbook of Mentalization-Based Treatment* (pp. 3–6). London: John Wiley.

Balbernie, R. (2001). Circuits and circumstances: the neurobiological consequences of early relationship experiences and how they shape later behaviour. *Journal of Child Psychotherapy*, *27*: 237–255.

Balint, E. (1973). A contribution to the question "What does a woman want?" *International Journal of Psychoanalysis*, *54*: 195–201.

Benedek, T. (1959). Parenthood as a developmental phase. *Journal of the American Psychoanalytic Association*, *7*: 389–417.

Bowlby, J. (1969). *Attachment and Loss, Vol. 1. Attachment*. London: Hogarth.

Britton, R. (1989). The missing link: parental sexuality in the Oedipus complex. In: J. Steiner (Ed.), *The Oedipus Complex Today: Clinical Implications* (pp. 83–102). London: Karnac.

Ellis, B. J., Bates, J. E., Dodge, K. A., Fergusson, D. M. & Horwood, L. J. (2011). Does father absence place daughters at special risk for early sexual activity and teenage pregnancy? *Child Development* *74*: 801–821.

Fonagy, P., Gergely, G., Jurist, E. L. & Target, M. (2002). *Affect Regulation, Mentalization, and the Development of the Self.* London: Karnac.

Fraiberg, S., Adelson, E. & Shapiro, V. (1975). Ghosts in the nursery: a psycho-analytic approach to the problems of impaired mother-infant relationships. In: J. Raphael-Leff (Ed.), *Parent–Infant Psychodynamics—Wild Things, Mirrors and Ghosts* (pp. 87–117). London: Anna Freud Centre, 2009.

Freud A. (1958). Adolescence. *Psychoanalytic Study of the Child, 13*: 255–278.

Freud, A. (1960). Discussion of grief and mourning in infancy by John Bowlby. *Psychoanalytic Study of the Child, 15.*

Freud, A. (1965). *Normality and Pathology in Childhood.* London: Penguin University Books.

Freud, S. (1905). Three essays on the theory of sexuality. *S. E., 7*:125–244. London: Hogarth.

Geleerd, E. R. (1964). Child analysis—research, treatment, and prophylaxis. *Journal of the American Psychoanalytic Association, 12*: 242–258.

Gerhardt, S. (2004). *Why Love Matters: How Affection Shapes a Baby's Brain,* New York: Psychology Press.

Giardino, J., Gonzalez, A., Steiner, M. & Fleming, A. S. (2008). Effects of motherhood on physiological and subjective responses to infant cries in teenage mothers: A comparison with non-mothers and adult mothers. *Hormones and Behaviour, 53*: 49–158.

Hopper, E. (1991). Encapsulation as a defence against the fear of annihilation. *International Journal of Psychoanalysis, 72*: 607–624.

Jaffee, S. R., Caspi, A., Moffitt, T. E., Taylor, A. & Dickson, N. (2001). Predicting early fatherhood and whether young fathers live with their children: prospective findings and policy reconsiderations. *Journal of Child Psychology and Psychiatry, 42*: 803–815.

Karmiloff-Smith, A. (1995). Annotation: the extraordinary cognitive journey from foetus through infancy. *Journal of Child Psychology and Psychiatry, 36*: 1293–1313.

Laplanche, J. (1995). Seduction, persecution, revelation. *International Journal of Psychoanalysis, 76*: 663–682.

Laufer, M. E. (1996). The role of passivity in the relationship to the body during adolescence. *Psychoanalytic Study of the Child, 51*: 348–364.

Lieberman, A. F. (1993). *The Emotional Life of the Toddler.* New York: Free Press.

Mahler, M. S., Pine, F. & Bergman, A. (1975). *The Psychological Birth of the Human Infant.* New York: Basic.

Murray, L. (1997). Postpartum depression and child development. *Psychological Medicine, 27*: 253–260.

Pines, D. (1988). Adolescent pregnancy and motherhood: a psychoanalytical perspective. *Psychoanalytic Inquiry, 8*: 234–251.

Raphael-Leff, J. (1991). *Psychological Processes of Childbearing.* London: Anna Freud Centre, 2005.

Raphael-Leff, J. (1993). *Pregnancy—The Inside Story.* London: Karnac.

Raphael-Leff, J. (1997). *Female Experience: Four Generations of British. Women Psychoanalysts on Work with Women.* London: Anna Freud Centre, 2008.

Raphael-Leff, J. (Ed.) (2000). *Spilt Milk—Perinatal Loss and Breakdown.* London: Routledge and the Institute of Psychoanalysis.

Raphael-Leff, J. (Ed.) (2003). *Parent–Infant Psychodynamics—Wild Things, Mirrors and Ghosts.* New York: Wiley.

Raphael-Leff, J. (2010a). Contemporary views on femininity, gender and generative identity. In: L. Glosser-Fiorini & G. Abelin-Sas (Eds.), *Freud's "Femininity. New Introductory Lessons on Psychoanalysis"—Divergences and Convergences with Freud's Works According to Contemporary Psychoanalysis.* London: Karnac.

Raphael-Leff, J (2010b). "The Dreamer by Daylight"—imaginative play, creativity and generative identity. *Psychoanalytic Study of the Child*, *64*: 14–53.

Raphael-Leff, J. (2011). *Working with Teenage Parents—Theoretical Handbook and Training Manual.* London: Anna Freud Centre.

Slade, A. (2005). Parental reflective functioning: an introduction. *Human Development*, *7*: 269–281.

Stoker, J. (2005). *You and Your Toddler.* London: Karnac.

Trevarthen, C. & Aitken, K. J. (2001). Infant intersubjectivity: research, theory and clinical applications. *Journal of Child Psychology and Psychiatry*, *42*: 3–48.

Waddell, M. (2009). Why teenagers have babies. *Infant Observation*, *12*(3): 271–281.

Welldon, E. (1988). *Mother, Madonna, Whore: the Idealisation and Denigration of Motherhood.* London: Free Association.

Zaphiriou Woods, M. & Pretorius, I. M. (Eds.) (2010). *Parents and Toddlers in Groups: a Psychoanalytic Developmental Approach.* London: Routledge.

PART III

SPECIALIZED WORK IN THE ANNA FREUDIAN TRADITION: PAST, CURRENT, AND FUTURE

CHAPTER TWENTY SEVEN

"In the best interest of the child"—the pioneering work of Anna Freud in the field of children and the law, and the court assessment project at the Anna Freud Centre

Minna Daum and Linda Mayes

Among the questions that perplex and burden clinicians is how to interrupt a cycle of chronic stress and adversity so that children are not destined to repeat their parents' tragedies. Anna Freud's developmental theory grew out of her work with children and families beset with the most horrible of adversities and chronic stress. Children orphaned or separated from their parents during the Blitz came into her care and gave her first-hand experience with the often devastating impact of abrupt parental loss, while her experience with highly traumatized families who came to the Hampstead Clinic informed her understanding of the often stubbornly persistent trauma-related behaviours in both adults and children and their expression in children's emerging character structure and personality. As evidenced by her creative collaborations with Albert Solnit and Joseph Goldstein at Yale, she became deeply concerned about child protection in the face of unstable, chaotic families and unpredictable or abusive parental care (e.g., Goldstein, et al., 1984, 1986).

Since Anna Freud, considerable work has focused on understanding how adversity and trauma impacts children's development. Findings from a growing body of research suggest that chronically stressful experiences early in life may have long-term consequences for a child's cognitive, social, and emotional health and long-term consequences for both physical and mental health (Gunnar & Vazquez, 2006). So-called "toxic stress" (Loman & Gunnar, 2010) may lead to a detrimental impact on developing brain architecture and on the physiological regulatory systems that help children respond to and learn from challenge and adversity. What makes a situation detrimental or toxic relates to whether the stressful experience is controllable, how often and how long the stress response system has been activated, and whether or not the child has a dependable, stable set of relationships that are able to provide support, protection, and buffer the impact of the experience.

Indeed, as Anna Freud well recognized through her efforts to provide safe homes and reliable compassionate adults for the children in her care, the stability of a child's caregiving relationships is key to buffering and/or minimizing the deleterious effects of chronic trauma. Findings from many studies now indicate that early caregiving conditions establish "set points" for stress system activation and also for the ability of the system—and the body—to return to baseline after a child is no longer in that stressful situation. In the earliest interactions with parents and other caring adults, there is an essential reciprocity of exchanges—what some have called "serve and return" (Shonkoff & Phillips, 2000), in which infants and young children naturally make bids for interactions through their babbling, facial expressions, and gestures. If all goes well, adults respond often with the same kind of vocalizations, gestures, or expressions—sometimes even more marked for emphasis. The consistency, reliability, and affective tone of these types of early exchanges are fundamental to creating relationships in which children's social communication abilities are nurtured and their exploration and learning about the world around them, as well as their own emotional language, is supported (summarized in Shonkoff & Phillips, 2000). Perhaps most salient in the effects of early relationships appears to be the long-term impact on stress reactivity and allostatic capacities in the face of challenge. Failure of the adult caring environment to "serve and return" and buffer stress creates a chronically adverse environment for children and is related to greater permeability and reactivity to stress in later childhood and adolescence (Loman & Gunnar, 2010; Nachmias et al., 1996). In contrast, secure, consistent caregiving is related to more flexible allostatic or stress response capacities that in turn facilitate children's adaptive ability to deal with inevitable stress and challenge.

What is also now clear is that early and persistently unbuffered exposure to chronic stress impacts the child's ability to care for others once he or she is a parent, and studies are now beginning to disentangle the mechanisms accounting for that well-recognized clinical observation that we parent as we were parented, or the intergenerational transmission not just of the effects of adversity but specifically of parenting behaviours. Of course, this observation is one that Anna Freud was preoccupied with and, with her developmental perspective, was always behind her efforts to protect children from the uncontrolled chaos of war or disrupted, unpredictable family life. Even without the support of the emerging basic science of parenting, she understood the pervasive impact on children of chronic, unbuffered stress and this concern was at the core of her efforts to define the child's best interests.

Here we describe a case, not dissimilar to that clinical material that Anna Freud was familiar with, seen in the Anna Freud Centre's court assessment service, the contemporary instantiation of Anna Freud's prevailing concern regarding the impact of chronic adversity. This multidisciplinary team specializes in the assessment of children whose parents have severe personality difficulties. The team works with so-called "multi-problem" families, typically involving drug and alcohol abuse, domestic violence, and emotional abuse and neglect of children who are on the edge of care as a consequence. Its task, funded by the family courts, is to conduct detailed assessments of parental history, parent-child relationships, and (crucially) the child's experience of his/her caregiving environment; to articulate this experience in the court arena; and to give clear opinions on the risk to the child of remaining with his/her carers. The challenge is to describe the impact of emotional abuse and neglect on a child's development, in the context of an adversarial environment (the court) unused to the language of emotions.

A case history

Lee was ten years old when he was referred to the service. His mother Mary had suffered severe abuse and neglect at the hands of both her parents. The only surviving child of triplets, she had been told by her father that she had kicked her two brothers to death in the womb. Mary's account of her childhood was related without emotional expression or a sense of narrative; rather, it was presented as a series of traumatic events, unexplained and disconnected. Mary had become pregnant at fifteen and had two children by her boyfriend Brian. The relationship deteriorated into violence once her first baby was born, and both children were subsequently taken into long-term foster care in early adolescence as a result of neglect. Both had continually run away from their foster placements to return home. Her eldest son Matthew, now eighteen, was already a father; her second son Thomas, seventeen, was back at home with his mother and involved in drug dealing. Mary's third son George, by a different father, had been removed for adoption at the age of five; when asked, Mary said she had no idea why this had happened: "I asked for some help and they took him away."

Lee was born just before his brother George was removed. His father, a young man idealized by Mary as her "perfect man", had nonetheless never lived with the family, had only seen Lee a few times as a baby, and had died of a heart attack when Lee was two. Mary described being depressed and traumatized by George's removal during Lee's babyhood, and was abusing alcohol at this time; she described turning Lee's pushchair to the wall so that she didn't have to look at him, and leaving him to cry for long periods.

Lee had been excluded from two primary schools for attacking both teachers and pupils; subsequently diagnosed with attention deficit hyperactivity disorder, he was about to begin a trial of medication. His mother, absolved by this diagnosis from any responsibility for his uncontrolled behaviour, diagnosed her other sons retrospectively with the condition. At the age of ten, Lee presented as a slight, pale child. He was attending a special school for children with emotional and behavioural difficulties, and could neither read nor write. His behaviour showed a stark mixture of adolescent swagger (abusive to adults and dismissive of help when he clearly needed it), and toddler-like appeal for care and protection (wanting to hold the (male) child psychotherapist's hand to go down the stairs). His constant movement and difficulty in concentrating in sessions seemed directly related to his (understandable) anxiety in the context of his relationship with a mother who felt utterly unsafe herself and who consequently failed to function as a safe attachment figure. With his mother, Lee alternated between "controlling-punitive" attachment behaviours (Wartner et al., 1994), and anxious, clinging embraces. He continued to sleep in his mother's bed.

The team's report explained Lee's behaviour in the context of his highly insecure and disorganized attachment to his mother, and recommended long-term placement in a therapeutic residential setting. Given the nature of his attachment to his mother, it was not thought likely that he would be able to settle with an alternative family. The court accepted the team's recommendations, and three weeks into his placement Lee's behaviour had calmed dramatically; he no longer swore at teachers, had started to learn, and was sleeping at night. His trial of medication was halted. He sees his mother for weekly contact.

The team's approach to Lee's dilemmas illustrates how clinicians continue to work in the tradition of Anna Freud by holding the child's best interests in mind while at the same time recognizing the complexity of a child's emerging internal representations of his caring world and his own capacities to manage the chaos and stress in his day to day life. The team's work also illustrates the challenges as well as the opportunities afforded by efforts to translate the emerging basic science of attachment and parental care into effective and sensitive interventions for troubled children at greatest risk for having their present difficulties continue to burden them into their adulthood. We can only imagine that Anna Freud would be gratified by the continuity of the court service with her early work, and intrigued by the possibilities of how basic science and clinical efforts inform each other in these most challenging and tragic circumstances.

References

Goldstein, J., Freud, A., Solnit, A. & Burlingham, D. (1984). *Beyond the Best Interests of the Child.* New York: Free Press.

Goldstein, J., Freud, A., Solnit, A. & Goldstein, S. (1986). *In the Best Interests of the Child.* New York: Free Press.

Gunnar, M. & Vazquez, D. M. (2006). Stress neurobiology and developmental psychopathology. In: D. Cicchetti & D. Cohen (Eds.), *Developmental Psychopathology, Vol. 2: Developmental Neuroscience* (2nd edition). New York: Wiley.

Loman, M. & Gunnar, M. R. (2010). Early experience and the development of stress reactivity and regulation in children. *Neuroscience and Biobehavioral Reviews, 34*(6): 867–876.

Nachmias, M., Gunnar, M. R., Mangelsdorf, S., Parritz, R. & Buss, K. A. (1996). Behavioral inhibition and stress reactivity: Moderating role of attachment security. *Child Development, 67*(2): 508–522.

Shonkoff, J. P. & Phillips, D. (Eds.) (2000). *From neurons to neighborhoods: The science of early childhood development.* Committee on Integrating the Science of Early Childhood Development. Washington, DC: National Academy Press.

Wartner, U. G., Grossmann, K., Fremmer-Bombik, E. & Suess, G. (1994). Attachment patterns at age six in south Germany: Predictability from infancy and implications for preschool behavior. *Child Development, 65*: 1014–1027.

CHAPTER TWENTY EIGHT

Anna Freud and her contribution to the field of paediatric psychology

Norka T. Malberg

There will, I hope, be a time in the future when all medicine will have a double orientation—namely, an orientation directed simultaneously towards the body and the mind. This will then presuppose that all people who practise medicine will also receive a double training: that they will learn approximately the same amount about the body and the mind.

—(A. Freud, 1961)

Anna Freud believed that psychoanalytic theory could exert a great deal of influence to change the way other applied fields understood the emotional life of children. She developed innovative ways of working in fruitful partnerships with the disciplines of paediatrics, education, and jurisprudence. Her contribution to the field of paediatric psychology is an example of such a process of cross-fertilization. She advocated a flexible and innovative practice which considered the emotional and developmental needs of the child in the context of his/her external reality. Anna Freud's unique ability to draw a picture of such interaction by combining both drive and object relations perspectives is what offered the clinician a valuable and unique way of understanding the emotional needs of the sick child. Her clinical insights still inspire child psychotherapists working in this field, many of whom have continued to expand on her pioneering efforts.

In the following pages I reflect on such developments and illustrate how Anna Freud's work and that of her colleagues informs contemporary interventions in the field of paediatrics. The first case presented illustrates the value of intensive (four times per week) individual psychotherapy for a young patient diagnosed with diabetes at the age of ten. It highlights the importance of working not only with the child but also with the main social systems supporting him. The second example illustrates how a developmental psychoanalytic perspective can inform the design and implementation of a group intervention which seeks to impact both chronically ill young people attending an outpatient renal unit, and the social support systems around them. Both of these clinical examples took place under the aegis of the Anna Freud Centre and exemplify the value of interventions rooted in a strong clinical tradition.

Anna Freud's contribution to our understanding of the sick child

In her 1952 paper "The Role of Bodily Illness", Anna Freud speaks of the ill child's reaction to being cared for by parents and medical personnel. She explains how the loss of gradually attained mastery of bodily functions and self care means "an equivalent loss in ego control, a pull back towards the earlier and more passive levels of infantile development". She proceeds to distinguish between the different reactions children have to the experience: "Some children who have built up strong defences against passive leanings oppose this enforced regression to the utmost, thereby becoming difficult, intractable patients; others lapse back without much opposition into the state of helpless infancy from which they had so recently emerged" (p. 4).

Through the use of clinical examples and detailed theoretical development, Anna Freud explored the emotional reactions often displayed by physically ill young patients in hospital and other settings such as home and school. Her clinical examples highlighted the uniqueness of the experience for each child as influenced by diverse environmental and developmental variables. Understanding the interaction of the child's internal and external worlds in the context of a traumatic experience such as somatic illness or injury has the potential to provide a powerful way of communicating the emotional needs of the child to parents and medical personnel from a unique perspective. This goal presents an ongoing challenge for the child psychotherapist who needs to develop skills not only to work effectively with the child but also with his parents and other caregivers such as nurses and doctors. It is vital in facilitating new environmental responses to the young person's progressive developmental attempts, such as an emerging capacity to verbalize difficult feelings.

Anna Freud's main clinical method was that of meticulous observation, be it in the nursery classroom, the consulting room, or the hospital unit. Through the analysis of detailed process notes, the impact of internal and external influences on the child's functioning is explored and further analysed through the use of methodologies such as the "Diagnostic Profile" and the "Developmental Lines". For example, when presented with a child suffering from chronic illness, although the nature of the illness and its impact on current functioning is examined, it is done in the context of the larger developmental and psychological picture of that child. As a result, the prehistory of each child's emotional development is explored as well.

A wonderful example of such process was given by Thesi Bergman in collaboration with Anna Freud in 1965 in their book *Children and the Hospital*. This book offers the reader an illustration of clinical observation in action—where children's reactions to illness and hospitalization are explored within the hospital context by drawing a picture of the relationships between the children and the medical staff, and the role of parents in the process. Parallel to those descriptions, the authors provide an understanding of how the experience of illness or injury in such a relational context impacts directly on children's defensive responses and personality development. The book concludes with the introduction of what Bergmann and Freud called "Mental First Aid"—a technique which they delineate as flexible and applicable to a diverse range of difficulties when working with children in the hospital setting. As ever, they emphasized the importance of involving parents as well as the nursing and medical staff—in other words, a systemic approach.

This tradition of clinical observation and research was taken further during the 1980s at the Anna Freud Centre by George Moran and Peter Fonagy (Fonagy et al., 1987), who in collaboration with colleagues from the Middlesex Hospital in London carried out a study to measure the effectiveness of individual child psychotherapy with diabetic children. They focused on the analysis of personality structure, prominent conflicts, the age of onset, and degree of diabetic control. They used biological measures to evaluate the impact of individual psychotherapy on adherence to diabetic control regime. Their study confirmed the potential interference of diabetes with the child's impulse control, thinking, perception, and representation of affect. Furthermore, it highlighted how the type and balance of defences, superego structuralization and object relationships are all vulnerable to distortion from the psychological problems associated with the medical treatment of the illness, thus confirming many of Anna Freud's clinical observations and providing strong evidence of the value of the psychoanalytic method in working with this population. In 1984, George Moran published a detailed account of some of the cases included in the larger study (seventy-one diabetic children, aged six to sixteen). In it, he expanded on some of Anna Freud's observations within her study group at the Hampstead Clinic, which focused on the impact of the experience of diabetes on the various aspects of a child's personality. He points out the advantages and disadvantages of offering intensive psychotherapy to the diabetic child, and highlights the value of intensive work with suitable cases in this population as a source of understanding that can be applied to non-intensive therapy and crisis management with other diabetic children. The following section illustrates how such findings informed my work with a young diabetic patient at the Anna Freud Centre.

Clinical applications: working with a diabetic latency boy

Seth was referred to the Anna Freud Centre by a nurse at the hospital where he had been recently diagnosed with diabetes at the age of ten. Discovering he was sick had been highly traumatic as Seth had nearly fallen into a hypoglycaemic coma. He was referred as he had become very depressed following his diagnosis. He refused to inject himself, was clingy with his mother, but rather aggressive towards his father. He was the eldest of two; his younger brother was healthy and excelled in athletics.

We began four times a week analysis following a diagnostic period. Seth presented a rather mixed clinical picture as indicated by his diagnostic profile. He displayed rather uneconomical defences and a great deal of anxiety and insecurity in his relationship with his primary objects. Several external events seemed to have had an impact on Seth's capacity to achieve an age-appropriate sense of agency and self-regard. His mother had suffered a chronic illness during his early childhood which had impinged on the satisfaction of his pre-Oedipal needs. In addition, his father who suffered from depression was extremely envious of the close relationship Seth and his mother enjoyed as he himself had endured the loss of his own mother at an early age. Seth was described by his parents as a challenging child from a young age—often defiant and frequently succumbing to tantrums. These pre-morbid personality traits, present prior to the onset of illness, were now exacerbated by it. Both parents struggled to manage his behaviour but had not sought help as they felt he would "grow out of it". In a sense, ironically, Seth's diabetes had become his saving grace as he was able to access the experience of a new developmental object with whom he could revisit and mourn all that had been missed, and now, all that he felt was being lost—namely his potential to become a strong and healthy man.

Seth was a bright and insightful boy who seemed burdened by the strength of his anger and sadness, which he exhibited openly and rather impulsively without much regard for others. The following excerpt from our first session illustrates the quality of our initial interactions and how openly he was able to explore some of his feelings around issues of loss and self-regard:

> Seth entered the room, looked out at his old playground, and spoke of his sadness and longing about having left his old school. By coincidence, Seth had attended the school located behind the Clinic for five years. I commented on my impression that Seth had difficulty letting go of places and people he had lost. He agreed. He also spoke of his feelings of being left out from his peer group at school and of being different—a weirdo, who still likes to play with Lego and Matchbox cars—not grown up yet. As the session progressed, his anxiety increased. Seth seemed extremely careful with all the toys in the box and very aware of my presence. While exploring the soldiers and the animals, he spoke of liking to pull things apart. I linked this to his wish to pull apart thoughts and feelings that are bringing him down and making him feel like a "weirdo", and he spoke of his feelings of embarrassment about not being as strong and having less energy than the other boys because of his diabetes. He then drew in a small notebook a picture of a small tree and told me he had made one like that for his grandma, who had died recently, and that she had framed it and put it in the living room. I spoke of his feelings of sadness for having lost his grandma, who had made him feel special. Seth replied by speaking of his feelings of being different, not special, and of his special interest in classical music, reading and drawing. He told me his tree was finished and I assured him it would be safe inside his therapy box. He expressed his fear of the dark outside, but told me his mother would meet him halfway to his house (he would have to walk ten minutes in the dark by himself).

I worked with Seth for three years in a four times a week analysis. Our journey together was truly developmental in nature: first by exploring his need to regress to an earlier time where he could be, in the transference, part of a working dyad away from the eminent sense of loss and separateness that he experienced in reality. As Seth entered puberty, the strength of his anger was fuelled by unresolved Oedipal issues, and at times became unbearable. Parallel to this, as his peer group became increasingly focused on their adolescent physical achievements, he struggled more with his view of himself as damaged and weak. However, he discovered in his capacity to draw and act in school theatre plays new ways to express and like himself. As a result, Seth began to make developmental progress, as evidenced by an improvement in his diabetic regime adherence as well as his capacity to verbalize difficult affects, particularly his feelings regarding his "traitor body" without succumbing to a high state of anxiety. The reparative developmental experience within a safe and predictable relationship enabled Seth to leave treatment with a capacity to reflect on his feelings, having mourned the loss of his healthy body.

Due to Seth's poor compliance with the medical regime, working with his parents and the nurses involved in his treatment was pivotal in order to develop a strong support system around him. But it was also at times frustrating as I was not part of the hospital's multidisciplinary team. For example, on one occasion a new case manager was assigned to Seth who insisted that he needed to attend counselling sessions with someone in the hospital. This created a great deal of confusion for Seth and his parents. However, it once more confirmed my conviction about the importance of educating other professionals on the specific needs of this population who often experience frequent changes in medical personnel. The experience proved traumatic for my patient, but it also reinforced his belief that I would fight to preserve our therapeutic relationship, and in the end it provided an opportunity to further explore his feelings of being unlovable and damaged.

My description of this case is at best superficial; however, I chose to summarize it here to illustrate the value of intensive psychoanalytic work when working with a child who, having been exposed to early relational trauma, had poor existing ego capacities at the time of onset of the diabetes, indicating that falling into a depressive state may be the only way he could survive psychologically.

* * *

My work with Seth motivated me to explore further the development of applications of psychoanalytic thinking and technique to the emotional needs of chronically ill children and adolescents. As a result, in 2004, having worked with groups of adolescents in local schools as part of my clinical obligations at the Anna Freud Centre, I began to explore the possibility of developing group interventions in hospital with a focus on the issue of adherence in chronically ill adolescents. This had been a topic that had framed many of my interactions with Seth during his third year of treatment, as he entered puberty and struggled further with issues of diet and insulin intake. For instance, I felt that encouraging Seth's participation in a hospital support group had been instrumental in helping him feel supported and understood by peers. In addition, I helped Seth analyse a chart of blood glucose levels as he was very active in establishing links between what he felt were "triggers" that made him more fatigued. I strongly felt that an emerging sense of agency and a wish to relate in new ways had resulted from these activities, and we managed to identify the symbolic meaning of his difficulty with injections. As a result, in 2004, during my last year of training at the Anna Freud Centre, I began to explore the possibility of developing a group for chronically ill adolescents.

Group intervention with chronically ill adolescents in a hospital setting

Motivated by my clinical experiences working individually with Seth and other chronically ill adolescents, I approached Dr Jill Hodges, a graduate of the Anna Freud Centre, with the idea of developing a research project at Great Ormond Street Hospital, where she had worked as child psychotherapist and researcher for many years. With her support and that of professors Peter Fonagy and Linda Mayes, I began to develop what came to be known as the "Renal Project".

I chose the haemodialysis unit because of the high rate of non-adherence to medical regime and because the complex setting made individual intervention often challenging and ineffective. This project has been discussed in detail elsewhere (Malberg et al., 2009), so a brief description will suffice here to illustrate the value of incorporating both classical and contemporary ideas within a single intervention model.

The construct of mentalization proposed by Peter Fonagy and colleagues at the Anna Freud Centre (2002) facilitated the development of a common language among the different systems involved in the intervention (patients, parents, medical and nursing personnel). We understood and shared with others the concept of mentalization as the capacity to have others' mind in mind (their intentions, beliefs), and with it the ability that we all inherently have to be able to "put ourselves in other shoes". This empathic capacity tends to be inhibited by the experience of relational trauma such as the one experienced when confronted with a chronically ill young person. The theory of mentalization-based interventions is built on the solid foundation of attachment research, and hence lends itself to be presented to medical staff. We explicitly used the word "mentalization" in all our presentations, and invited medical staff, parents, and young people to think about the way they dealt with others when stressed and feeling helpless, and then linked it to the young person's experience in the hospital.

Having an accessible concept such as mentalization allowed us to achieve to a certain extent Anna Freud's goal of inviting medical professionals to become more aware of the relationship between emotions and behaviours, and to reflect on the impact the quality of their interactions with patients can truly have, in making a difference in the context of a loaded subject such as non-adherence to medical regime. By becoming more aware of their tendency to become "non-mentalizing" when confronted with fears of loss of a patient, we were inviting the medical personnel to put themselves in their patients' shoes and try to understand their experience from a psychological perspective. So, in many ways the concept of mentalization aided the promotion of a "Mental First Aid" at a systemic level.

The intervention built on previous work at the Anna Freud Centre, with its focus on the understanding of young people's defensive strategies and the impact of illness in the context of overall ego development. Work with parents and nursing staff was pivotal in order to reinforce young people's developmental progressive moves, and to explore ways of relating away from the reality of illness while trying to ascertain the meaning of young people's non-adherent behaviour.

Brief description of the Renal Project

The Renal Project had a duration of three years. The first year consisted of setting up and developing the intervention; the second entailed the main intervention, and the third could be described as the follow-up and generalization phase (teaching others how to do it).

a. Preparatory phase

The first step consisted of an eight month observation period during which I kept process notes of my experience of the unit itself, of intake and follow up meetings between doctors and families, as well as observations of staff meetings. This process allowed me to familiarize myself with the different systems within the hospital. I became aware of the importance of siblings and visiting peers during my observation, and later tried to bring topics to group discussions which also included this often neglected supportive social network. Furthermore, I was able to observe families during the different stages of the illness, during onset, crisis periods as well as pre- and post-transplantation. This experience provided me with a window into the experience of young renal patients and their caregivers.

The renal unit at Great Ormond Street Hospital (an NHS specialist hospital for sick children) serves a highly culturally diverse population. This presents a challenge in itself for the medical staff and the psychosocial renal team who are responsible for family assessment, follow-up, and liaison with families and medical personnel. In my capacity as researcher I became part of the psychosocial renal team headed by a family therapist and composed of a social worker, a clinical psychologist, and a psychiatric nurse. I relied on their support and guidance during my work in the haemodialysis unit.

b. Intervention

Following the period of observation, an assessment was conducted to establish a baseline of biological measures of adherence. Several instruments were administered prior to commencing and following the end of the twelve week group, to assess changes in the participants' capacity to mentalize. Defensive strategies used by participants were measured on a pilot computerized instrument consisting of fictional vignettes depicting conflictual interpersonal exchanges. Three of the stories depict situations related to the illness and three present everyday situations that most teenagers would confront. The findings of this study supported existing research in the field of paediatric psychology—namely a high incidence of anxiety-related symptomatology found in this population. Several participants showed significant improvement in their adherence to medical regimes as well as an improvement in their capacity to mentalize when presented with stressful "everyday" vignettes. This last finding is significant, indicating the importance of focusing on developmentally appropriate interventions while keeping in mind the isolating impact that chronic illness has on a young person.

Often, these young people are seemingly very efficient in dealing with situations related to their illness; however, high non-adherence rates tell another story—one of attempts at gaining a feeling of mastery over one's life when faced with a helpless situation. In many ways, the renal discussion group was a relational laboratory where young people in the unit could relate through engaging in playful discussion regarding age-appropriate concerns away from their illness.

The renal group lasted twelve weeks and took place on Saturday morning, a time when the unit tends to be quiet as no teachers or other supportive staff are present. All sessions began with the same "icebreaker" which invited participants to share one good thing and one bad thing that had happened during their week. Following this exercise, a topic would be introduced, often accompanied by a playful activity to illustrate the subject discussed. The group had a "here and now" focus which meant that we often stopped to reflect on the impact on someone's comment on another member, or we might reflect on one member being uncharacteristically silent. In other words, the group had as its main goal practising thinking about feelings, and continuing to think while we are having difficult feelings.

Issues around the experience of illness were brought up explicitly. For instance, we had sessions in which we discussed the links between non-adherent behaviour and strong feelings. The concept of the unconscious and its impact on behaviour was brought up in a playful way by asking participants to draw a dream. We discussed how sometimes we behave in certain ways in order to avoid difficult feelings. Young people called these feelings "bad stuff in the back of your head" and proceeded to give examples of ways in which they think this happens to them. In general, the renal group was a place to play with feelings, to relate in new ways, and, at times, to think about the unthinkable. My role as group facilitator and clinical researcher required support from colleagues and supervision. By creating a horizontal relationship with the young participants of the group, characteristic of the mentalization-based intervention, I too reflected on my own thoughts and feelings. This posed a technical challenge and demanded constant exploration of my countertransference. However, I found that group members valued this approach, as they often expressed their annoyance at being spoken to as if they were not there or simply being seen as their illness, and not as thinking and feeling young people.

Parallel to the main discussion group with the young people, frequent exchanges took place with nurses and parents about concerns around the management and the understanding of certain behaviours exhibited by the young people of the renal unit. These discussions, casual in nature, turned out to be extremely valuable in terms of support for the project, but most importantly, in exploring new ways to understanding the individual *meaning* of the experience of illness for the patients, their families, and their nursing staff.

The following example illustrates the importance of understanding not only the inner world of the patient but also its interaction with both the family and the hospital systems:

> Jane was a fifteen-year-old young woman who was diagnosed with end stage renal disease six months prior to being transferred to our unit. The psychosocial renal team had concerns regarding her state of utter helplessness. She refused to assist in preparations for her renal sessions (handling her needle and fistula), and became despondent and rude whenever she perceived the nurse's competence to be less than adequate. She was silent and visibly depressed and refused any attempt at interaction from the other young people in the unit. Most concerning was her poor adherence to medical regime. Efforts to engage Jane in individual work led to some progress in the form of interaction with peers in the unit. However, the real turning point came as Jane engaged in our weekly group discussion during haemodialysis sessions. Even though she was sceptical at first, the group gave her the opportunity to reassert herself as someone reflective and competent, and she quickly became confident and outspoken.
>
> The nursing staff started to witness from afar "the other Jane", and during discussions with me they managed to reflect about the impact of Jane's helpless behaviour on them. One nurse spoke of her understanding of Jane's behaviour as rubbishing anything she could offer and just lying there, waiting to die. The feelings this elicited were too much for the nurse to bear, and in response she had become quite rigid and authoritative when interacting with Jane. Finally, Jane's family's lack of involvement during her sessions and in general with her illness implied that she was to bear the burden of an ill body on her own. A systemic shift took

place in the response Jane got from medical staff, especially the nurses. In response, Jane was able to engage during both individual and group sessions and to achieve some restoration of her previous developmental accomplishments. Most importantly, Jane's adherence improved significantly, as did her condition, enabling her to return to some of the after-school activities she previously enjoyed. Understanding her non-adherent and helpless behaviour as a way of retaining some sense of agency when faced with a situation unthinkable for an adolescent was vital for the system to lend itself as ego-auxiliary and to promote economical defensive strategies.

Concluding remarks

Anna Freud understood the value of interdisciplinary dialogue and the importance of educating and translating our understanding of children's emotional life to workers in other fields. I believe that her main contribution to the field of paediatrics was her tenacity in envisioning specific changes that needed to occur in order to promote mental health in children experiencing somatic illness. She chose to do this by incorporating her psychoanalytic understanding, as well as by borrowing from the findings of contemporaries such as John Bowlby, to promote changes in parental visitations in hospital, preparation for operations, and developmentally appropriate explanations regarding illness.

The task of integrating established knowledge and new ways of serving the needs of an evolving external world is a challenging one, and one that many of us child psychotherapists working in outreach settings often attempt. Anna Freud's legacy does not only rest on her capacity to achieve such a complex task with eloquence and deceptive intellectual clarity, but also on her relentless commitment to the tradition of psychoanalytic research and practice leading to the evolution of new ways to improve the emotional lives of children at risk.

The two brief examples of clinical practice provided here aim to illustrate the value of having a strong framework from which to depart, and the importance of integrating old and new theoretical paradigms. My rigorous training at the Anna Freud Centre and later on, experience as a staff member, taught me the value of having a strong theoretical base. But I also learnt from my supervisors the value of approaching any case or new project with humility, curiosity, and the wish to learn from the child, his/her family, and the context in which the work takes place. I believe this attitude is particularly needed within the context of a hospital setting or when working in collaboration with other agencies to serve the emotional needs of the chronically ill child.

References

Bergmann, T. & Freud, A. (1965). *Children in the Hospital.* New York: International Universities Press.

Fonagy, P., Gergely, G., Jurist, E. & Target, M. (2002). *Affect Regulation, Mentalization and the Development of the Self.* New York: Other Press.

Fonagy, P., Moran, G. S., Lindsay, M. K. M., Kurtz, A. B. & Brown, R. (1987). Psychological adjustment and diabetic control. *Archives of Disease in Childhood*, *62*: 1009–1013.

Freud, A. (1952). The role of bodily illness in the mental life of children. In: *The Writings of Anna Freud, Vol. IV* (pp. 260–279). New York: International Universities Press.

Freud, A. (1969). Adolescence as a developmental disturbance. In: *The Writings of Anna Freud, Vol. VII* (pp. 39–47). New York: International Universities Press.

Malberg, N. T., Fonagy, P. & Mayes, L. (2009). Contemporary psychoanalysis in a pediatric hemodialysis unit: Development of a mentalization-based group intervention for adolescent patients with end stage renal disease. In: J. A. Winer, J. W. Anderson & B. Gerber (Eds.), *The Annual of Psychoanalysis* (pp. 101–114). New York: Mental Health Resources.

Moran, G. S. (1984). Psychoanalytic treatment of diabetic children. *Psychoanalytic Study of the Child, 39*: 407–447.

CHAPTER TWENTY NINE

"From dependency to emotional self-reliance"—the Anna Freud Centre parent–toddler group model

Marie Zaphiriou Woods

Sam (aged one year nine months) is standing at the doll's house, pushing Lego bricks through its window and door. The toddler group leader asks playfully if he is the postman delivering letters … or parcels. Sam mutters "Gone," but then opens up the house and retrieves the brick. "Got it," says the toddler group leader. He posts it again. "Where has it gone?" she asks. He slams the door: "Closed," he says, then opens it. The game gains in momentum and intensity as he repeatedly shoves bricks through the window or door. He sings "Post it, post it," and then "All gone." Breathing heavily and swaying with excitement, he then "finds" the brick. The toddler group leader comments on things appearing and disappearing, coming and going. When she has to attend to another child, Sam's mother who has been quietly watching the play draws up her chair. She has a little boy figure knock on the doll's house door and, with single words supplied by Sam, they play out a "bath", "shower", and bedtime with "milk". Suddenly, mother pauses and asks him if he has done a poo. "No," he says loudly. She leans forward and smells his nappy. "You have done a poo." He goes to run away, and begins to shout and kick as she picks him up and carries him to the lobby. She puts him down to get a clean nappy. A little girl approaches. Quick as a flash he hits her. She howls and her mother rushes to comfort her. The toddler group leader speaks quietly to Sam while his mother holds his hand.

This scene, occurring during the course of a toddler group session, illustrates some typical features of toddlerhood: the growing pleasure in shared communication through language and play; the anxiety about separation, from the parents and from body products; the drive for autonomy and mastery (of openings and closings, appearances and disappearances); the rage about feeling helpless, intruded on, not in control; the impulsivity with regard to aggression in particular. Toddlers' intense and oft-times contradictory passions may arouse similar feelings in their adult caregivers. These may become overwhelming if they touch on unresolved issues from the adults' childhood or adolescence, or if ongoing circumstances are difficult (physical or mental health issues, financial or housing problems, isolated or dislocated lives). The Anna Freud parent–toddler groups, which meet weekly for one and a half hours, aim to provide support for toddlers and their parents during this tumultuous period during which central emotional issues to do with intimacy, autonomy, aggression, separateness, and sexuality are negotiated (Zaphiriou Woods & Pretorius, 2010).

Background

The parent–toddler service has expanded and evolved since *Joyce Robertson* first started a group for mothers and toddlers at the Hampstead Clinic in the 1950s. The first group was an informal offshoot from the Well-Baby Clinic, to help mothers understand and respond to their infants' changing physical and emotional needs once they grew into active toddlers. Since the 1970s, there have always been weekly toddler groups at the AFC, providing a service to local families, and training opportunities for students of child psychotherapy who observed in the groups, and attended seminars run by the group leaders. Some of them went on to run groups themselves.

In the late 1990s, the toddler group service grew to include four generic groups at the Centre, to accommodate required observation by UCL students doing an MSc in Psychoanalytic Developmental Psychology at the AFC. These were followed by two more groups: an outreach group on a local council estate (2003–2008) and a specialist group for visually impaired toddlers and their parents (2005–2007). The groups were usually led by an AFC trained child psychotherapist, assisted by a graduate of our MSc (or equivalent).

Currently, there are two parent–toddler groups based at the Anna Freud Centre and an expanded outreach service in the local community, which changes according to local needs and availability of funding. At the time of writing, funded by the Surestart children's centres, staff from the AFC run weekly groups in a large hostel for homeless families and a nearby children's centre. Holding the AFC model in mind, they adapt it to the exigencies of the settings and populations with which they work. They attend the weekly team meeting at the Centre in order to refresh their thinking and share clinical and management issues.

A former member of the team has also taken the AFC model to a deprived part of south London where she has established a toddler group which now specializes in referrals of parents with significant mental health problems. Referrals come mainly from the NHS Child and Adolescent Mental Health Services, when there are already explicit concerns about the parent-child relationship. All these groups offer psychoanalytically informed support to the parents and toddlers attending them, complemented by individual work if and when necessary.

The parent–toddler group model developed at the Anna Freud Centre and to be outlined in this chapter has inspired the institution and development of toddler groups, not just in south London, but also in Russia, Peru, and Greece. For a fuller account of these varied groups and indeed of the historical background and theoretical underpinnings of the AFC parent–toddler groups, the reader is advised to refer to *Parents and Toddlers in Groups: a Psychoanalytic Developmental Approach* (Zaphiriou Woods & Pretorius, 2010).

In reaching out to children and parents suffering from deprivation, trauma, and loss, the toddler groups continue a tradition begun by Anna Freud, when she started the Jackson Nursery in Vienna in 1937–1938 and the War Nurseries in and around London in 1940–1945. By offering a service and opportunities for training and research, they embody the vision that first led her to establish the Hampstead Clinic in 1952.

The groups: aims and structure

The groups provide a space where, to paraphrase Winnicott (1966), steady experiences in relationships enable toddlers to enjoy the enrichment that comes from discovery of their internal and external worlds, and to progress along the line from dependency to emotional self-reliance (A. Freud, 1965). The consistency of the setting enables much learning and development to take place spontaneously as group members interact, talking, playing, building new relationships, and discovering alternative ways of seeing and doing things. All the rooms in which the groups meet are spacious, and well stocked with attractive, age-appropriate toys and activities. The staff are warmly welcoming. They move freely among the parents and the toddlers, observing and reflecting inwardly, and intervening when necessary. They aim to maintain an "internal analytic setting" (Parsons, 2007) to make sense of the unconscious communications and intense transference and countertransference feelings that inevitably arise. However, group members are not seen as patients and interpretations are rarely made.

The over-arching aim of the groups is to promote the toddlers' development. This includes enhancing attunement and attachment between the parents and toddlers, with a view to strengthening their relationship, and facilitating separation and individuation, so that toddlers can manage the next step towards growing independence, which is a half or whole day at nursery/school. Understanding the developmental needs of toddlers and parents, and the powerful feelings engendered by the toddlers' attempts to assert and define their emerging selves, are essential aspects of the work, informing all interventions.

The groups at the AFC are kept small with a consistent membership of up to eight mother-child couples. The local outreach toddler groups have a more fluctuating membership and permeable boundaries. Each group has a leader and an assistant (more if the group is large), who are responsible for the day to day running of their groups. By being seen to think and work together for the good of the group, the staff provide a model of co-operative partnership that the parents and toddlers may internalize. Inevitably, however, they also attract powerful (grand)parental transferences, which may be intensely ambivalent and hard to manage. They meet together after each group to share their observations and experiences, and may bring them to the weekly team meeting at the AFC. This meeting provides a reflective space where intense transference and countertransference feelings can be processed, sensitive responsiveness enhanced, and the likelihood of acting out reduced.

Sometimes difficulties arise which cannot be contained within the groups. Then parents may be offered individual sessions with the psychoanalytic consultant. For instance, Sam's parents came to see me about his hitting of other children. They quickly revealed deprived abusive childhoods and an ongoing sense of being rejected by society which they re-created in the toddler group. Understanding these dynamics enabled the staff to generate greater warmth and acceptance within the group.

The group setting: fostering attachment and managing separation

The groups meet in the same place and at the same time each week, and prepare carefully for anticipated changes (holiday breaks, changes to the room, arrivals and departures). In this way, they provide a model for the sort of secure base that parents need to provide for their own toddlers. Parents are encouraged to attend regularly, and continuity and cohesion are fostered by remembering what is going on in the lives of group members and making links between sessions ("Oh, you liked that toy last time") and between group members ("Jane was looking for you last week"). Developmental milestones and birthdays are noticed and celebrated.

Fostering the parents' sense of attachment and belonging to the group, of "being in it together" (James, 2005), establishes a camaraderie that enables them to talk more openly about their toddlers' difficult behaviours (negativism, clinging, hitting, snatching, tantrums, etc), their own ambivalence, and the associated shame and guilt. They can draw comfort from observing or hearing that other toddlers and parents feel and behave similarly. The staff convey interest, respect and empathy. They take care not to judge the parents, and not to present themselves as better parents. They may even draw attention to their own fallibility and regressive tendencies.

They also actively encourage parents to learn from one another, reframing problems in shared terms so that they know they are "not the only one" (James, 2005, p. 135). They may bring together two parents struggling with similar concerns or take advantage of snack time to introduce a discussion about important developmental issues (such as toddler aggression, toilet training, or going to nursery).

The growing attachment to the group means that separations from the group are intensely experienced and become a means of exploring this core toddler, and human, issue. The staff prepare carefully for tidying up time, verbalizing the toddlers' feelings about stopping, and reassuring them that they and the toys will be there the following week. The ways in which the staff manage the toddlers' reactions to the beginnings and endings of the group can be a useful model for parents as they strive to understand and deal with their toddlers' (as well as their own) intense reactions to difficult transitions. Sam's outbursts of aggression often occurred during tidy up time. Once his mother recognized they were a reaction to having to stop, she began to prepare him well beforehand.

Individual interventions

These may range from direct intervention with an individual toddler to listening to a parent with a view to enhancing her emotional awareness and availability to her toddler.

Facilitating creative play and playfulness

The toddler group staff encourage parents to share their toddler's play, and communicate with him or her on a symbolic representational level. The toddler may then use this new medium to express excited risky feelings and fantasies in an enjoyable and safe way, and to master age-appropriate anxieties to do with aggression and loss, separation and merging (see vignette above). The child may also play out frightening external events, such as falling out of their buggy, or daddy going to hospital.

Sometimes parental difficulties intrude; *their* anxieties about excitement and mess, separation and loss, their projected aggression, and their need to inhibit and control may prevent them playing with their children. The staff may then join in or even initiate play with the toddler, supplying ideas and materials, and playfully amplifying their actions and affective communications. They also help the toddlers to construct pretend narratives.

In so doing, they model pleasurable, playful ways of being together for both the toddlers and their parents. They may actively *draw in* a parent who is inhibited or depressed, or *draw out* a toddler from an over-enmeshed relationship. Such interventions both strengthen the attachment relationship and promote separation and individuation, as toddler and parent discover, through playing together or apart, that they have different minds (Fonagy & Target, 2007).

The toddler group staff may also facilitate play *between* the toddlers, e.g., by encouraging them to "cook" side by side in the toy kitchen, or to play hide and seek with one another. Through parallel play, the toddlers are helped to discover each other as playmates and companions, and this helps to prepare the way for peer relationships in nursery and beyond.

Verbalizing the toddlers' feelings and wishes

The toddler group staff often verbalize what they perceive as the toddler's feelings and wishes, supplying words to identify and legitimize the child's experience. Finding himself accurately reflected in another's mind helps the toddler to feel less overwhelmed, out of control, and alone. He begins to learn to delay action, to communicate his experience, and to distinguish between fantasy and reality (Katan, 1961; Furman, 1978; Weise, 1995).

The staff may speak directly *to* the child about what he is feeling or *for* or *about* the child's emotional state to the parent. This may be the most effective way of raising parents' awareness of their toddler's state and enlisting a contingent response from them. Such interventions aim to promote effective communication by the toddlers and sensitive responsiveness from the parents. Helping parents to tune in or "feel with" (Furman, 1992) their toddler strengthens attachments. Since the mirroring is not exact and is "marked", that is, slightly exaggerated and at the same time tinged with a contrasting affect, differentiation is also furthered, both for the toddler, and for the parent who is helped to recognize that her toddler's experience is different from hers (Fonagy & Target, 2007).

Managing aggression and setting limits

The toddler group staff sometimes need to act in an immediate way, to protect toddlers from hurting themselves or one another, and to reassure all members of the group that aggression can be safely contained. They may also intervene to prevent fights over toys and to promote turn-taking and sharing. They may verbalize the toddlers' frustration at having to wait, and their pride and pleasure when they manage to be patient or kind. Over time, these interventions can help to build a toddler's capacity for affect regulation, impulse control, and socialization, and to lay the foundations of a benign superego.

When aggressive incidents occur, as in the vignette above, the staff encourage thinking about what has happened: "Susy was just looking for her mummy; she is sad now." "You really did not want to stop playing with Mummy." "Were you cross at having your nappy changed?" This can help modulate aggressive drive and fantasy (Herzog, 1982).

Supporting toddlers' moves towards independence and autonomy

The toddlers' progression along the developmental line towards body independence (A. Freud, 1965) is noticed and celebrated in the groups, as, for instance, they join the other children at the snack table, eat and drink independently, take off and put on their coats, and begin to use the potty or toilet. These progressive moves contribute to the toddlers' increasing sense of competence and mastery and prepare the way for their independent functioning at nursery.

Most parents feel pride as their toddlers begin to take ownership of their bodies, their functioning, and care. However, some parents need support to enable them to "stand by to admire" (Furman, 1992, p. 119), and to gradually let go, especially when their toddler's progressive moves stir up their own unresolved feelings about separation and loss (Furman, 1994). They may lack confidence in their parenting, and ask for detailed advice at each new stage. The staff try to join with them in finding solutions, perhaps supplying some ideas and guidance, but mainly helping them to pick up on their toddler's cues and work out what is best for them. In encouraging the parents' self-reliance, they perhaps enable them to do the same for their toddlers.

Feeding back observations and understanding behaviours

Parents are encouraged to observe their toddlers' behaviours and to think about what might be going on in their minds in order to enhance their emotional awareness of their toddler, and to enable them to understand and respond to the child in his or her own right. The immediacy of the observations may enable them to see characteristics or developments in their toddler that they may have overlooked, because of their own preoccupations and conflicts.

The staff also try to help parents take into account their toddler's age-appropriate emotional, cognitive, and physical capacities so that they can better tolerate both their dependency and attachment needs, and their urge to separate and individuate. This may mean modifying unrealistic expectations and normalizing behaviours which parents find bewildering or unacceptable. To quote Hoffman, many parents "believe that good parenting involves the elimination of aggression, conflict or ambivalent feelings" (2003, p. 1220). Putting challenging behaviours in a developmental context or linking them to external events may reduce parental anxiety, freeing them to be more in touch with their toddler's feelings and fears.

By modelling reflectiveness, and enjoining parents to think about the meaning of their toddlers' behaviour, the staff hope to minimize the blaming and rejecting that arise when toddlers behave in ways that appear incomprehensible. This may enable them to see their child as "developing and separate" as well as "dependent and connected" (Green, 2000, p. 28). Reflective function is enhanced and with it the likelihood of a secure attachment (Fonagy, Steele & Steele, 1991; Slade, Grienenberger, Bernbach, Levy & Locker, 2005).

Recognizing and containing the parents' experience

The toddler group staff offer a supportive relationship to each parent, holding in mind their individual needs, and offering them one-to-one time in each session to communicate their current state of mind. The members of staff listen attentively and sympathetically, so that the parent feels heard, understood, and accepted. This process may help parents to process potentially overwhelming feelings and experiences without having to cut themselves off from their toddlers or externalize and project onto them, condemning, rejecting, and trying to control them. The "good grandmother transference" (Stern, 1995) which develops may enable them to become more accepting of their own and therefore their toddlers' dependency needs, and means that they are less likely to feel envious of the good care their toddlers are receiving. The attention paid to their own feelings may also help them to differentiate better between their own and their toddler's needs and feelings, and to listen more attentively to the child.

Conclusion

It took many months of regular attendance before Sam's mother trusted the leader sufficiently to confide her terror and condemnation of all aggression. Beginning to understand this enabled her to recognize and anticipate Sam's angry outbursts, and to use her own angry response to set appropriate limits. They both developed friendships in the group.

Writing about similar parent-child groups, Hoffman (2004) highlights the role played by both the transferential bond to the staff and the bonds mothers make with one another in enabling new mothers to address their anxieties. It seems to me that parents and toddlers select what they need for their development from the various "therapeutic possibilities" (A. Freud, 1965) provided by the "supportive matrix" (Stern, 1995, p. 177) of the parent–toddler groups. This is perhaps analogous to the process that Anna Freud described (1965) of child patients taking what they need from the more classical child analytic setting.

References

Fonagy, P., Steele, H. & Steele, M. (1991). Maternal representations of attachment during pregnancy predict the organization of infant-mother attachment at one year of age. *Child Development, 62*: 891–905.

Fonagy, P. & Target, M. (2007). Playing with reality: IV. A theory of external reality rooted in intersubjectivity. *International Journal of Psychoanalysis, 88*(4): 917–937.

Freud, A. (1965). *Normality and Pathology in Childhood: Assessments of Development.* Madison, CT: International Universities Press.

Furman, R. (1978). Some developmental aspects of the verbalization of affects. *Psychoanalytic Study of the Child, 33*: 187–211.

Furman, E. (1992). *Toddlers and Their Mothers.* New York: International Universities Press.

Furman, E. (1994). Early aspects of mothering: What makes it so hard to be there to be left. *Journal of Child Psychotherapy*, *20*: 149–164.

Green, V. (2000). Therapeutic space for re-creating the child in the mind of the parents. In: J. Tsiantis (Ed.), *Work with Parents: Psychoanalytic Psychotherapy with Children and Adolescents* (pp. 25–45). London: Karnac.

Herzog, J. M. (1982). On father hunger: The father's role in the modulation of aggressive drive and fantasy. In: S. W. Cath, A. R. Gurwitt & J. M. Ross (Eds.), *Father and Child* (pp. 163–174). Boston: Little, Brown.

Hoffman, L. (2003). Mothers' ambivalence with their babies and toddlers: Manifestations of conflicts with aggression. *Journal of the American Psychoanalytic Association*, *51*: 1219–1240.

Hoffman, L. (2004). When daughter becomes mother: Inferences from multiple dyadic parent-child groups. *Psychoanalytic Inquiry*, *24*(5): 631–658.

James, J. (2005). Analytic group psychotherapy with mothers and infants. In: T. Baradon (Ed.), *The Practice of Psychoanalytic Parent Infant Psychotherapy: Claiming the Baby*. London: Taylor & Francis.

Katan, A. (1961). Some thoughts about the role of verbalization in early childhood. *Psychoanalytic Study of the Child*, *16*: 184–188.

Parsons, M. (2007). Raiding the inarticulate: The internal analytic setting and listening beyond countertransference. *International Journal of Psychoanalysis*, *88*: 1441–1456.

Slade, A., Grienenberger, J., Bernbach, E., Levy, D. & Locker, A. (2005). Maternal reflective functioning, attachment and the transmission gap: A preliminary study. *Attachment and Human Development*, *7*(3): 283–298.

Stern, D. N. (1995). *The Motherhood Constellation: A Unified View of Parent–Infant Psychotherapy*. New York: Basic Books.

Weise, K. (1995). The use of verbalisation in the management of feelings and behaviour: a therapeutic intervention in the nursery. *The Bulletin of the Anna Freud Centre*, *18*: 35–47.

Winnicott, D. W. (1966). The child in the family group. In: C. Winnicott, R. Shepherd & M. Davis (Eds.), *Home is Where We Start From* (pp. 128–141). London: Penguin.

Zaphiriou Woods, M. & Pretorius, I.-M. (Eds.) (2010). *Parents and Toddlers in Groups: a Psychoanalytic Developmental Approach*. London: Routledge.

CHAPTER THIRTY

"Clinician to campaigner"—fate of a missionary

Peter Wilson

I have a story about Anna Freud that I have probably told too often. But maybe it bears repetition if for no other reason than it captures something of the wry way in which she looked upon the follies about her—and upon the dangers of spreading psychoanalysis too far and wide. The occasion for the story was a meeting I had with her some thirty years ago to tell her that I intended to leave the Hampstead Child Therapy Course and Clinic, and take up a position in the Institute of Psychiatry and Maudsley Hospital, a leading teaching establishment in London, not known for its sympathies towards psychoanalysis.

I had been very involved in the Clinic for about ten years, initially for four years as a trainee and later as a part-time staff member with particular interest as consultant to the nursery school that was attached to the Course and Clinic at that time. I valued my experience there enormously but increasingly I felt in some ways constricted. The time had come I thought to move on, to simply grow up as it were beyond the bosom of my psychoanalytic family.

And so it came to pass that I found myself sitting with Anna Freud in an attempt to explain my decision to leave. This turned out not to be easy. I was always in awe of her, deeply respectful and, on this occasion, plain nervous. Words stumbled backwards and sideways and my voice wavered. It rose an octave or two like that of a child pleading to a reproving mother.

By and large, people did not leave the Clinic, other than to return home to foreign countries. And so when I had eventually exhausted myself, all I encountered was a look of sheer puzzlement on her face which left me at a complete loss to know what to say next. Suddenly, in desperation, I clutched at the idea of myself as a missionary. "Yes, Miss Freud," I said, "I have learnt so much at the Clinic that I now think I must go forward into unknown, even hostile waters to spread the knowledge … like a missionary."

There was a long doleful silence. Eventually she spoke. "Mr Wilson, I think you ought to know that missionaries very often get eaten."

And so, the question arises about my professional life since then. Have I been eaten? Has whatever understanding I had of child psychoanalysis been drawn out of me by inhospitable and alien forces? Have I adapted and applied and compromised here, there, and everywhere, to such an extent that my psychoanalytic identity had been devoured? Many I believe would think that I have, that I have strayed too far. Increasingly as the years have gone by, I have certainly spent less time in the therapy room with children or with the couch metaphorically in my mind. And I have mingled less with my brethren in the psychoanalytic world and more with other persuasions and convictions. I have even taken on a more political role, beyond the world of the clinical. And so, yes, I can see that I could be seen as having been eaten. But, I don't think so.

Setting aside for the moment any religious connotation, the word "mission" essentially means a sending. The missionary is someone who is sent to convey a message. Whilst I cannot pretend that anyone cast me in that role, I think I thought of myself, no doubt naïvely, "sent" to communicate what I thought was important in child psychoanalysis to a wider world outside that of psychoanalysis—a world that was in large measure becoming increasingly antagonistic towards it. Behaviourism, systemic thinking, empirical research were just a few of the developments that were accumulating to cast doubt on the findings of psychoanalysis and add to the general public's disinterest or derision.

Many might have said, "Why bother?" Far better to deepen one's own psychoanalytic understanding among colleagues with similar preoccupations. Far better to hold firm within a distinct conceptual framework. But for me this simply was not persuasive. It all seemed too parochial, too insular. More to my liking was the need to look outwards, to effect some broader influence. The "word" if you like needed to be spread. And in this, I saw myself in good company.

Freud, after all, despite his zealous protection of the ideas he had created, always had his eye on the fuller implications of his thoughts in the wider world. His book on *The Psychopathology of Everyday Life* was typical of his interest in the applicability of psychoanalytic ideas. And Anna Freud continued her father's broader vision throughout her life through her active interests in education and the law.

What was it that I wanted to disseminate in my broader interests? What was it in my training experience that aroused in me such a kind of passion? Well, of course, in general terms, it was psychoanalysis itself. The fundamental existence and dynamic of the unconscious, the multi-layered nature of anxiety, the inevitability of conflict, the necessity of defences, the construction of symptoms, the shaping of attitude and behaviour, the sheer complexity and energy of childhood, the power of transference, the bevy of emotions as they play themselves through the myriad of delights and complications in relationships—all of this filled the air of my training and opened my mind to all kinds of possibility. More specifically, the value of clinical supervision (the attention to the detail of the therapeutic process), the personal analysis, the experience of systematically tracing Freud's conceptual thinking, the stimulation of the diagnostic meetings and the Wednesday afternoon meetings, in which Anna Freud spoke with extraordinary clarity and perspicacity—all added up to something remarkable that needed the telling.

And so I ventured out. Initially, I, like many newly trained child psychotherapists worked in various child guidance clinics. These were not psychoanalytic institutions. They were multidisciplinary, eclectic, and under considerable pressure with limited resources. Practising intensive child psychoanalysis was not possible. Short-term assessments, once weekly psychotherapy, and meetings with parents and families were the norm—and it was this kind of work that became the bedrock of my clinical practice for many years. It undoubtedly involved an adaptation of the therapeutic approach learnt in my training. Clearly, it had its limitations compared with intensive psychoanalysis, but I was impressed by how well some children were able to hold in mind the therapeutic work and its process between the weekly sessions.

Entering into the fray of multidisciplinary teamwork, articulating the psychoanalytic perspective alongside many others was another form of adaptation. I was fortunate to benefit from the teams in which I worked. I learnt a lot from a wide range of psychiatrists, psychologists, and social workers. And they learnt a fair bit from me. Increasingly, I found myself being invited to supervise the psychotherapeutic work of other professionals from different disciplines, most notably senior psychiatric registrars in training on placement from the institute and hospital for which I had left the Hampstead Course and Clinic and in which Anna Freud had foreseen my likely end.

As things turned out, I was not extinguished. I cannot say that my "mission" conquered all, far from it, but I think I did manage to introduce to those who were half interested a way of thinking and a mode of therapeutic approach that was relatively new to them. Perhaps most important of all was the attention I paid to the underlying themes that emerged in their therapeutic work and to the feelings that were evoked in them in response to the children they were treating. This was different to their more formal training, focusing primarily on diagnosis and prescribed forms of mostly behavioural treatment. Some, not all, were intrigued and carried on their interest and respect for psychoanalytic thinking in their later careers.

Alongside this growing interest in supervision, I was spending an increasing amount of time in consultative work—that is to say, meeting with individual professionals and groups of professionals, to discuss their work and enable them to practise more effectively. This work largely came through invitation from organizations that for one reason or another needed help, in addition to whatever their own resources were to improve the quality of their work. I was chosen because of my perceived expertise in dealing with the mental health problems of children and my perceived ability to facilitate groups of staff. At different times, I consulted to groups of social workers, education welfare officers, teachers, and nursery staff. This work eventually led to a major position as consultant psychotherapist in a residential therapeutic community for disturbed adolescents, called Peper Harow. I stayed there for eleven years before it closed.

The process of consultation runs along a thin line. It is not exactly supervision for it carries with it no managerial responsibility. It is not teaching for it does not follow an agreed curriculum of any sort. And it is not psychotherapy. It is essentially an enabling experience in which the consultant collaborates with (rather than directs) staff in furthering their understanding of children's attitudes and behaviour and in finding new ways of dealing with them therapeutically. The conceptual psychoanalytic framework that I had learnt at the Hampstead Child Therapy Course and Clinic and subsequently built upon from my practice proved invaluable in helping myself and staff to make sense of the often bizarre and desperate behaviour of the children and adolescents. Of particular relevance in all these consultations was the sensitivity I had gained from my training to the compelling pressures and demands, often subtle and insidious, of transference and countertransference feelings and thoughts. Staff so often found themselves lost and embarrassed in feeling so angry, useless, aroused, and punished as they struggled in their relationships with the young people. Consultation provided a place to take stock and rebalance.

* * *

Most child psychotherapists move into management positions in the NHS once they have gained seniority and experience. I became principal child psychotherapist in the area health authority in which I worked. This entailed recruiting and supervising child psychotherapists and liaising with other members of the professional team in the Clinic. It also involved negotiating for an increased establishment of child psychotherapists in the area. I was aided in this respect by my extensive experience in the Association of Child Psychotherapists in which I spent a great deal of time negotiating with the Department of Health for improved conditions and salaries of child psychotherapists at a national level. It was one of my triumphs, assisting closely Wallace Hamilton, a child psychotherapist who worked tirelessly for the profession, to reach an agreement with the Department that actually included the word "psychoanalysis" in its formal guidance and introduced the establishment of trainee child psychotherapist posts with provision for payment of trainee analytic fees.

Whatever management and negotiating skills I had at that time could not be said to have been developed in my psychoanalytic training. If anything this training proved to be something of a hindrance. A certain ruthlessness, an unpreparedness to listen too much to the "other side", and a singular motivation to win turned out to be the virtues that were most needed—not at all consistent with those of clinical practice. However, what mattered above all else was the cause of the child psychotherapy profession—and to that end I and others got on with it.

What I think was emerging at this time was a desire to move more into the political arena, to become a campaigner, an influencer not just for the sake of the child psychotherapy profession but for all who were invested in improving the mental health of children. And it was with this idea in mind that I decided to leave the NHS and become the director of a voluntary organization, the London Youth Advisory Centre which later became known as the Brandon Centre. This was not a familiar role for a child psychotherapist, but for me it offered an opportunity that the NHS was unable to provide, namely that of leadership. Child guidance clinics suffered managerially from a clear lack of leadership. Each discipline was accountable to different management structures outside the clinics. Psychiatrists assumed leadership by virtue of their holding medical responsibility, but this was constantly challenged by the other professional groups. Rotating systems of team co-ordinators failed to work satisfactorily in most cases.

The Brandon Centre was a relatively modest organization employing a small number of administrative and clinical staff. It operated unusually as a combined family planning and psychotherapy service for adolescents, age twelve to twenty-five. It was well situated and known in an inner city area and operated largely on a walk-in basis. It clearly filled an unmet need in the community and it was busy. Two professional groups worked there: medical doctors for the family planning service, and psychotherapists for the wide range of adolescents who sought psychotherapy or counselling. All were managerially accountable to me; I, in turn was accountable to a board of trustees. This was a much simpler and more effective managerial arrangement and one which allowed me to take the lead in developing the service, expanding the building and raising funds.

Whilst I was there, I was also actively involved in the Child Guidance Trust, a small trust that existed to represent the interests of child guidance clinics. These clinics were coming increasingly under attack from NHS funders and from various statutory regulations that were requiring some professional groups to work independently of the clinics. At the same time, there was a growing concern amongst a range of practitioners and professionals about the predicament of many children and young people who were suffering the effects of neglect and abuse in a society that was placing unprecedented pressures on family life. The six-fold increase in the rate of divorce in the last thirty years of the twentieth century was but one indicator of increasing stress.

With all this in mind, the Child Guidance Trust formed itself as a pressure group to campaign for the mental health of children and for the development of multidisciplinary work which had stood at the centre of child guidance practice since its inception in the Twenties. Initially, it had very little resource to make any kind of impact, but largely due to the persistence of one or two stalwarts and the fortuitous intervention from a man in the Department of Health who arranged for some significant seed money, the Trust changed its name to YoungMinds, established a new constitution, and appointed me as its first paid full-time director.

This was a major step for me. I resigned from the Brandon Centre and embarked on what was in the beginning a very uncharted journey, taking a considerable risk in terms of my career and finances. So, why did I do it? There were of course all sorts of personal reasons, not least a kind of compulsive midlife restlessness and narcissistic pressure to stand out in some way. But, more substantially, I found myself gripped by a compelling need to "do something" about the plight of children and young people in the country in which we lived and most particularly their mental health. This need arose out of all of the experiences I had encountered so far in my work. There were just too many children growing up in very unfavourable environmental conditions, whether in the distress of their families or the poverty of their neighbourhoods. There were just too many children and young people failing at school, getting into trouble with the law, taking drugs recklessly, becoming pregnant too early, and generally being unable to make the most of their talents and abilities. And there were just too many professionals and practitioners becoming exhausted and demoralized in their efforts to help in organizations struggling against the odds with limited resources.

The fundamental issue underlying so many of these problems was the mental health of children and young people. And yet there was no organization that was specifically focusing on this issue. The major campaigning organizations were primarily concerned with poverty or general welfare or the youth justice system or sexual and physical abuse. The clear purpose of YoungMinds was to fill this gap, to raise public awareness of the mental health needs of children and young people and to campaign for comprehensive multidisciplinary child and adolescent services.

I was the director of YoungMinds for twelve years, and during this time it developed a range of activities including advocacy (e.g., contributing to government and other enquiries, responding to media requests), consultation, and training, a parent information service, and publications of various kinds. At the heart of the matter was the issue of mental health, a difficult concept to pin down, but strong enough to highlight its essential nature in children's emotional well-being. Most importantly, I and my staff constantly urged that mental health needed to be understood as much more than the absence of illness, and that services needed to be organized in terms of the promotion of mental health, the prevention of mental health problems, as well as the treatment of such problems.

At the point when I retired from YoungMinds almost seven years ago, we had succeeded in establishing a new organization in the voluntary sector that stood specifically for the mental health of children and young people. This in itself was a major achievement. We had also made a considerable impression on the political landscape in the sense that the whole issue of children's mental health rose much higher on the political agenda with more government resources being allocated to it. Needless to say, there was much more left to do. The organization was still relatively small and under-resourced to carry out the magnitude of the work that was required. The mental health problems of children in an increasingly complex society continued to prevail, particularly in the more deprived areas of the country. Satisfactory organization of multidisciplinary services had yet to be improved.

Following my retirement from YoungMinds I returned to a more consultative role as clinical adviser to another voluntary organization, called The Place2Be, that provides comprehensive school based counselling services mostly in primary schools across the country.

Conclusion

This has been essentially an account of one child psychotherapist's work following his training at the Hampstead Course and Clinic some forty years ago. It has been a long journey that has taken me through various kinds of adaptations and applications of what I had learnt during my training. These have included applied psychoanalysis in once weekly clinical work, supervision and consultation to other professionals, management and the leaderships of two voluntary organizations—one providing a clinical service, the other campaigning for children's mental health. To some extent, I was propelled in this journey by a certain kind of personal disinclination to stay confined within the familiar habitat of my training "home". But, for the most part, I was driven by a basic concern for the mental health of children and for the services that were available to help them.

In this respect, I like to think that I carried with me some of the interests that Anna Freud herself had in the external world, not only in her activities but in her theoretical writings where she emphasized (unlike Klein) the impact of the child's external world on the conscious and unconscious mind of the child. There is no doubt in my mind that throughout all the work I did, psychoanalysis gave me my steer and resolve. Of course, I did not practise psychoanalysis proper. And certainly in my work for YoungMinds, which was rightly made up of a very diverse membership, I did not pronounce my psychoanalytic background. I did not "speak" it and I avoided the use of its jargon. But I like to think that the self-awareness and the conceptual clarity that I gained from my psychoanalytic training enabled me stay on course when the going was tough, not least in the beginning. I think it helped me form a well considered understanding of what it was that constituted mental health both in children and adults. I believe too that it helped me forebear the touchy narcissisms of the many (not excluding myself) who made up the multi-professional and political world.

And so the fate of the missionary? Verdict. Not eaten. Though maybe a different shape.

PART IV

PERSONAL AND THEORETICAL REFLECTIONS FROM CLINICIANS TRAINED AT THE ANNA FREUD CENTRE

CHAPTER THIRTY ONE

Altruistic analysis

Jack Novick and Kerry Kelly Novick

We first met Anna Freud in 1965, when she was nearly seventy years old. At an age when most people are ready to retire, she was entering her most productive period, as a theoretician, clinician, researcher, and teacher. We knew her as students and then as staff and faculty members at the Hampstead Clinic, for twelve years.

Anna Freud's clinical genius had at root the simple imperative to know how children think, feel, and see the world. This demands what has now come to be called "empathic attunement", but Anna Freud did not see this as a special technical stance, requiring a different theory. Rather it was a central postulate of psychoanalysis with its assumption of the reality of intrapsychic life.

Every account of Anna Freud describes her awesome capacity for concise, clear, dynamic formulations of complex material in accessible language. All day, every day, at Hampstead she attended meetings in which clinical material was presented. Miss Freud was flexible in her analytic technique. Around the inflexible core of always being the child's analyst, many things were comfortably possible. She emphasized that analysis is a relationship between two people which encompasses both transference and reality. It was Anna Freud who pioneered the extension of analysis beyond the group of adult neurotic patients, and it was she who continued to apply analytic ideas to many other areas, from law to paediatrics.

During the Sixties and Seventies Anna Freud was at the centre of psychoanalytic history and development. When she gave her paper "On Aggression" to over 6000 people at the Vienna International Congress in 1971, it held everything known in psychoanalysis on the topic and pointed the way to future developments. She contained the past, vitalized the present, and created the future of psychoanalysis. In a survey the year before, psychiatrists and psychoanalysts were asked to name their most outstanding colleague. Anna Freud topped the list for both groups (Rogow, 1970).

Ten years after her death in 1982, for the George Klein Lecture in San Francisco, we gave a "Reminiscence of Anna Freud". We noted then how her ideas and stature had already faded out of the professional foreground, to the detriment of psychoanalytic thinking and training. At the end of that paper we spoke briefly of Anna Freud's role as an inspiration to her students. We would like to expand on that dimension and talk about the tradition of what we call "altruistic analysis".

In a 1966 paper on the identity of the psychoanalyst, Anna Freud wrote, "I would therefore advocate that, besides identification and transference and indoctrination, there also is another attribute of the training analysis which I would call inspiration" (p. 191). Anna Freud has been an inspiration for all her students, a role model in particular ways which we have only gradually realized over the years. She always worked to extend the application of psychoanalytic ideas and principles and it is striking how many of her colleagues and students have gone on to do the same thing.

In 1918, Freud presented a challenge to his psychoanalytic colleagues—to open institutions or outpatient clinics where treatment would be free. The small group of psychoanalysts rose to the challenge and, during the inter-war years, a dozen or so free clinics were opened in seven countries and ten cities from London to Zagreb (Danto, 1998, 1999). Psychoanalysts during that era felt part of a larger social sea change, a wave of radical ideas that expressed social liberalism in art, science, culture, and politics. Child psychoanalysts, only beginning to define themselves as such, played a major role in these developments.

By the early 1920s, Bernfeld, Hoffer, Aichorn, and Anna Freud were organizing groups to explore the possibility of preventing neurosis through proper parental education and the application of psychoanalysis to formal educational settings (Rosenblitt, 2005). In 1925 Anna Freud established a school in Vienna, run by Eva Rosenfeld. By 1937 she and *Dorothy Burlingham* founded the Jackson Nursery in Vienna to support the emotional health of deprived children under three. This led directly to London's Hampstead War Nurseries, founded by Anna Freud and *Dorothy Burlingham* in 1940. Immediately following the war, Anna Freud organized residential homes for concentration camp children, the amazing results of which are detailed in Sarah Moskovitz's wonderful book, *Love Despite Hate* (1983).

The experience of the War Nurseries led to the establishment of the Hampstead Clinic and training, with its cluster of services, including the free or low-cost therapeutic clinic for children and adolescents, services for parents, the well-baby clinic, the nursery for blind children, the nursery school, the borderline study group, and many more over the years.

As graduates of the Hampstead training dispersed around the world, they carried with them this tradition of service and devotion to social amelioration, through the application of child analytic knowledge to any arena that affects children's lives. Rudy Ekstein and Miriam Williams, later joined by Randi Markowitz in Los Angeles; the Katans, the Furmans, and Liz Daunton in Cleveland; Anna Freud joined Al Solnit and Sam Ritvo at the Yale Child Study Center and the Yale Law School in New Haven, later joined by Steven Marans; *Humberto Nagera* and a group of Hampstead graduates in Ann Arbor, joined later in Tampa by Frances Marton; the Laufers in London, and many more. None of this work was done for riches, academic advancement, research grants, or professional status—that is why we call the spectrum of creative applications "altruistic analysis". Danto remarks that the adult analysts, in the main, did not import the altruistic strand when they came to America, but the child analysts did and continue to do so.

In that tradition the analytic group in Ann Arbor founded the Arbor Clinic in 1982. This was a low-fee therapeutic agency for children, adolescents, and adults, staffed by recent psychology and social work graduates, with free supervision provided by the analysts. In 1994 twelve of us started Allen Creek Preschool, our multiple award-winning psychoanalytic school for children, from the age of less than one to six, and their families. Over $193,000 worth of free service is provided by child analysts every year at Allen Creek. The dividends to us are beyond measure—we are privileged to share in the details of early development in a broad spectrum of families; our theories are constantly challenged and refined; and our clinical work is enlivened by our school experience of talking with parents and teachers every day about psychoanalytic understanding of the children's development.

Another powerful influence on us all has been what we would describe as Anna Freud's theoretical style, with its emphasis on multidimensional understanding, its rootedness in psychoanalytic history, its empirical base, and its assumption that child analytic understanding is integral to the growth of psychoanalysis. When people trained at Hampstead get together, we find that what we want to do is share our work, talk about the cases we are treating and the new arenas we have discovered for applying our knowledge, help and learn from each other. This was passed on to us by Anna Freud: she inspired love for clinical psychoanalysis and facilitated identification with the historical tradition of altruistic analysis.

To be a psychoanalyst is to be immersed in history, the history of the session, the analysis, the life of the individual and his family, one's own history, and the history of psychoanalytic thought. But we know only too well in our times that history can be rewritten to suit the needs of the moment. We see this in our patients, and we spend our days combating the tendentious rewriting of personal history. We must also guard against the revision of psychoanalytic history and make sure that someone like Anna Freud does not become the Trotsky of the psychoanalytic movement. It is up to us all to define the future pathways of psychoanalysis and child psychoanalysis. The late eminent social historian and thinker Isaiah Berlin (1991) said, "Only barbarians are not curious about where they come from, how they came to be where they are, where they appear to be going, whether they wish to go there, and, if so, why, and, if not, why not" (p. 2).

References

Berlin, I. (1991). *The Crooked Timber of Humanity: Chapters in the History of Ideas.* New York: Knopf.

Danto, E. A. (1998). The Ambulatorium: Freud's free clinic in Vienna. *International Journal of Psychoanalysis, 79*: 287–300.

Danto, E. A. (1999). The Berlin Polyklinik: psychoanalytic innovation in Weimar Germany. *Journal of the American Psychoanalytic Association, 47:* 1269–1292.

Freud, A. (1966). Some thoughts about the place of psychoanalytic theory in the training of psychiatrists. In: *The Writings of Anna Freud, Vol. VII* (pp. 59–72). New York: International Universities Press.

Freud, A. (1972). Comments on aggression. In: *The Writings of Anna Freud, Vol. VIII* (pp. 151–175). New York: International Universities Press.

Moskovitz, S. (1983). *Love Despite Hate*. New York: Schocken.

Rogow, A. (1970). *The Psychiatrists*. New York: G. P. Putnam Sons.

Rosenblitt, D. (2005). Translating child analysis from the playroom to the classroom. *Journal of the American Psychoanalytic Association*, *53*: 189–211.

CHAPTER THIRTY TWO

Specifically Anna Freudian[1]

Debbie Bandler Bellman

When I trained at the Anna Freud Centre in the late 1970s, Anna Freud, though elderly, was still very much an active and influential presence. She continued to read all weekly reports and to attend meetings, and I occasionally had the privilege of learning from her comments on my work. After training, I worked in the National Health Service with Kleinians and Independents, and my subsequent adult analytic training was Independent in orientation. However, my training at the Anna Freud Centre formed the bedrock of my analytic development, and continues to inform many areas of my clinical work and thinking. These areas can be thought of as "specifically Anna Freudian". I would like here to highlight some of these aspects: aspects that do not form a coherent whole but which can be thought of as comprising—to borrow from the title of a song from a famous musical set in the Austrian Alps—a few of "my favourite Anna Freudian things" (1959).

There are several principles in an approach to clinical work that I regard as specifically—although not exclusively—Anna Freudian. These include the importance of being human, empathic, straightforward, and simple, as well as humorous and playful as appropriate. I would also emphasize the importance of listening and talking to one's patients, with interpretations being merely a form of communication rather than manifestations of the therapist's eloquence. These are principles that make up some of what I consider to be my professional, technical ego ideal.

[1]An earlier version of this contribution was presented at a Scientific Meeting of the British Association of Psychotherapists in June 2009.

The jam in the doughnut

Before training I taught in the nursery school of the Centre, and Anna Freud would often visit. One day, two particularly eminent child analysts from abroad were observing the children, along with a couple of trainees. Among the children, an overtly troubled little boy was having a snack. Anna Freud went over to the boy. The visitors, trainees, and I all waited with bated breath to catch the "brilliance" of what Anna Freud would say. Would she make some comment that would act as an interpretation and alter the course of this child's development? She sat down, commented that the doughnut looked delicious, and asked the boy which flavour jam was inside. With a big smile, the boy replied, "Strawberry!" Anna Freud knew what was important to the boy at that moment, and simply related to him through it.

Starting with the doughnut while maintaining interest in the jam inside can be regarded as a metaphor for aspects of the Anna Freudian approach insofar as it symbolizes starting where the child, adolescent, or indeed adult, is at. Regardless of whether I am interpreting the transference, countertransference, play, fantasies, affects, conflicts, or whatever, I try to start with what the patient may be able to relate to, with what is likely to have resonance, while at the same time going a bit further, moving towards the jam. As an aside, it could be said that the development of the use of countertransference is not Anna Freudian. However, during training I was able to participate in a discussion group where *Joseph Sandler* developed his concept of countertransference and role-responsiveness, which became a well-known paper (1976). I think Anna Freud was both admiring and suspicious of this idea, but it nevertheless rapidly became part of the culture of the Anna Freud Centre and opened the door for us to work in the countertransference.

Anna Freud was passionate about psychoanalysis. We could see one four times a week patient if it was unavoidable, but at least two of the three analytic training patients needed to be seen five times weekly, which was also the frequency of one's personal analysis. This latter was so that we had the best opportunity of getting to know about our own unconscious internal forces, and thus would be in the best position possible to analyse those of our patients. In regard to our patients, the greater the intensity the more possible it would be to reach the "deeper" aspects of their disturbance and facilitate a return to a more normal or usual pathway of development, which she saw as an essential aim of analytic work with children and adolescents. She also believed that one could not rush the emergence of the unconscious, that intensity and continuity were needed to allow its manifestations truly to become alive within the consulting room. Thus she eschewed simply calling all aspects of the relationship between patient and analyst "transference", and made a major contribution to the discussions that led to *Sandler* and colleagues' (1975) delineation of "transference of habitual modes of relating", "transference of current relationships", and "transference of past relationships".

Working with young children and their parents

Although I think it is not currently in fashion, it is specifically Anna Freudian to treat a child, up to age about six or seven, and simultaneously to work with the parents. The work with the parents—in practice most often the mother—is not psychotherapy but rather "parent guidance".

That is, work centred on the understanding and handling of the child's disturbance. Parental pathology and transference to the therapist are of course present. The issue is that usually these are not interpreted directly, unless interpretation is necessary to preserve the work, and transference is not fostered. Details are beyond the scope of this contribution.

This way of working has always made sense to me. While training I saw a four-year-old girl four times a week and the mother once weekly. After qualification I continued to work with parents in the National Health Service when possible, and always met regularly with parents of older children, although usually not with the parents of adolescents. There are a number of reasons for working this way. To my, Anna Freudian, mind, the degree of internalization of disturbance and psychic structure increases as development progresses, and thus many aspects of these are usually less firmly internalized in a young child than they become as the child gets older. To put it another way, there is more space for new internalizations the younger a child is, and thus the younger child is more amenable to responding to changes in the environment and parental handling, including shifts in maternal or paternal projections. I think that the therapist, who knows the child intimately from the inside, is in the best position to work with parents to facilitate changes in parental attitudes.

Issues of confidentiality are often cited as reasons for allocating different therapists to the child and parents. I have never found this to be a problem. It is possible to assure the child that that which is "private" will not be told to the parents unless it is important to do so, and would then be discussed with the child first. The rest can be taken up analytically in sessions, while at home the child feels reassured because the parents do not speak of his "secrets" because they do not know them. With the parent, the need for the child to have "privacy" can be stressed, and it can be put to them that it is the general understanding of the child that will for the most part be shared. As with the child, the parents' reactions to this become a subject for discussion.

From another point of view, the therapeutic setting is of course very different from what the child will have previously encountered, and takes getting used to. But for a young child there is no other setting where his parents (or other carers) have no contact with an important person in his life, and to do so would be, I feel, very strange indeed for the child. I have found that it is holding for children to be able to see and know that their therapist and their parents can talk to each other, and do not "hate" each other as is often imagined or at some level also wished for.

But working like this can be hard for the therapist. One learns more about external reality, which means one needs to think through where to have this reality in one's mind, when to bring it in, how to work with it, how not to let aspects of it interfere with being able to hear things from the child's point of view. It also entails being able to maintain what I think of as a dual identification: identifying with the child and with the parent(s). I feel it is important to be able to struggle with these dual identifications, and they can help the child therapist guard against the occupational hazards of feeling angry with the parent(s) and thinking one would be a better parent.

Examples

I will give a brief example of how it was helpful to be cognizant of both mother and child. When my little training patient was approaching five, her mother prepared for her birthday party with the zeal of a mother preparing for her daughter's wedding. She cleaned the house and baked for days, with the result that she had no time to pay attention to her daughter. In analysis my patient presented as increasingly withdrawn, and her play indicated she felt completely neglected and abandoned by her mother. She also felt furious: with her mother for neglecting her and with me for not coming to the party. In her sessions we spoke of these feelings, and of how she felt neither her mummy nor I was doing anything for her. The actual birthday party, I learned from the mother, was a disaster, with too much of the wrong kind of food, and my patient's fury was expressed in her rejecting all that was on offer. I took this up in her sessions as the "payback" to her mother for her mother's perceived neglect. With the mother, I suggested that next time she didn't try quite so hard, as she would then have time for her daughter.

* * *

In working with children and adolescents, Anna Freud stressed the importance of making a treatment alliance, the analytic facilitation of which I feel is important with any age: that is, the facilitation, where possible, of the child, adolescent, or adult working together with the analyst to "understand" the unconscious forces which contribute to the difficulties. I do not see analysis as an intellectual process, but it can certainly help to be interested and able to think about oneself.

A nine-year-old boy presented with a learning disturbance, and played the role of class clown. His underlying feelings of shame and embarrassment, and his narcissistic vulnerability made it very hard to approach his difficulties, and I found myself struggling to find a way of talking to him that he could bear to hear. Comments on his play, stories he told about school, his transference, his fear of criticism, his fear he was stupid, were all met by denial. One day, after he performed an exceptionally ridiculous stunt in his session, I commented that I wondered why someone who was so clever could act so stupid. This caught his interest, and he began himself to wonder why. I think he could hear my comment because it took into account his narcissistic vulnerability, was playful, and conveyed that I had another view of him to that which he himself held. He began to think it possible that eventually he could hold a more positive view of himself.

Clear thinking

Anna Freud placed enormous emphasis on the importance of clear and precise thinking. This was not about feeling one should or needed "to know", but rather about thinking through what one knew, knowing what the questions were, having a sense of what was not known. In neurotic disturbance there has been progressive development, but in the face of earlier fixation points, to which the individual regresses when confronted with what is experienced as irresolvable internalized conflicts. Developmental disturbance pertains to difficulties that arise in successive phases of development, difficulties that start in one phase and area of the personality and psychic structure and which then influence development in succeeding phases.

Thinking developmentally can be considered specifically Anna Freudian. Most disturbances contain, I feel, some degree of what can be thought of as developmental disturbance. My understanding of the manifestations of disturbance in the consulting room, e.g., developmental or neurotic, informs my technique, my communications at any given time. Anna Freud differentiated between what she called developmental help, and more classical interpretation of conflicts in child analysis. As Anna Freudians have become increasingly object-centred in our work, the concept of developmental help has become one aspect of the broader concept of the analyst as developmental object, a concept akin to Winnicott's "environmental object" (1965).

Applications in adult analysis

Sarah sought analysis when she was twenty-eight. She had had a life-long struggle with overwhelming anxiety, fears of abandonment, fears of being overwhelmed by others, and feelings of worthlessness. Although she had her share of neurotic conflicts, I do not feel such conflicts formed the bulk of her disturbance. Diagnostically, aspects of her difficulties could be considered borderline in nature, and I think that borderline disturbance can be understood as a developmental disturbance. If one thinks developmentally, then it is possible to pinpoint the specific phases and areas in which the disturbance arose, and this may include the ways in which environmental factors impinged on the development of psychic structure and object relationships.

In Sarah's analysis the transference and countertransference were characterized by anxiety, though this decreased as analysis progressed. There were a number of areas of change and development, and in addition to more analytic interventions that contributed to psychic change, there were aspects of the analytic process where my function as a developmental object was of great importance to her: despite her fears, I did not abandon her, nor did I overwhelm her with interpretations.

For the first few years there was a repeated pattern whereby any new challenge in her life—a new job, a new relationship—generated enormous anxiety and helplessness, as well as fury. At such times she would withdraw from contact with me, and I would experience her as increasingly disappearing into her anxiety and rage, calling out for my help but somehow almost beyond reach.

There were many ways in which we came to understand this pattern. On a pre-Oedipal level these included her fear that I would envy her successes, and her fear of her omnipotent rage at what she experienced as my holding her back. Her anxiety that I did not want her to develop and separate from me was also a factor. These aroused her terror that she would be abandoned, a terror that was enacted through the withdrawal that in turn left her feeling panicked and alone. These early fears reverberated in more Oedipal conflicts around competition for jobs and men. My understanding of the developmental levels of her anxieties and conflicts informed my comments, and she would eventually emerge from her withdrawn and panicked state. I also felt that my continued calm presence was an important factor in her re-emergence. However, the pattern continued to be repeated, and I felt there was more to be understood.

In the fourth year of analysis, after a period such as that described above, she came in saying that she felt better. She said she was beginning to feel she could "do it"; she could accept the new job. She spoke about her parents, how she felt they would look at her anxiously and try to protect her, and would also convey a feeling that she could not handle too much. She thought this must have started when she was just under a year old, when it was discovered there was an abnormality in the way in which the bones in her legs were developing, an abnormality that made it difficult for her to stand and necessitated an operation. She continued that she thought that even after the operation her parents treated her as if she were still fragile.

She was silent for a few minutes. Then, almost as an aside, she commented that following the operation she was immobilized for several months, and could not even be held. This historical—developmental—information made a huge impact on me. Sarah, however, seemed hardly to be registering the meaning of what she had said, and went on to speak about how she thought the new job would be even better than the one her friend had, and that this thought made her anxious. Here, I felt there was a choice of interventions. I could comment on her anxiety about surpassing her friend; I could bring this into the transference in regard to anxiety about triumphing over me. Although not wrong, neither of these felt quite right. I felt the impact of her comment about having been immobilized was present in the room, and I thus commented on the casual way in which she had told me this, that I thought the impact of it might feel too much for her to register, that the pain, helplessness, fury, longings to be held, and fears for her survival must have been unimaginably strong, and what must she have felt when no one picked her up. She said this was exactly what she had been feeling in recent weeks. In subsequent sessions it became possible to understand the cycle of intense anxiety and withdrawal when confronted by an important life change as including a large component of repetition of this early experience both of not being able to stand on her own two feet, and of not being held. For Sarah, the experience in analysis of an object who did not convey the message that she expected, i.e., that she was fragile and could not handle the next step, was also important.

I feel Sarah's early experience of immobilization, together with her experience of her parents' reactions, had a profound effect on her development in a number of areas, the two illustrated by the clinical example being the areas of object relationships and regulation of anxiety. Developmental thinking enriched my understanding of the clinical material and helped to give interpretations specificity. Interestingly, following the period discussed above, there were no further occurrences of the repetitive pattern illustrated.

Just as facilitating a treatment alliance is specifically but not exclusively Anna Freudian, developmental thinking is shared by other theoretical viewpoints. The degree to which Anna Freud and Anna Freudians elaborated on the developmental viewpoint and delineated developmental lines, such as the developmental line of anxiety drawn up by *Clifford Yorke* and Stanley Wiseberg (1976) is, however, perhaps unique.

* * *

Having begun this contribution with an anecdote about Anna Freud and the jam in the little boy's doughnut, I would like to end with another memory. When I trained it was not the norm to treat suicidal adolescents. When such an adolescent was referred to me, my supervisor, the late *Rose Edgcumbe*, and I thought it would be a good idea to ensure we had Anna Freud's support. We met with Anna Freud, and I explained that the girl was seriously suicidal and that we thought it was possible she would actually kill herself. I asked Anna Freud what she thought about my taking this girl on as a training patient. Anna Freud responded, "Is it better that she kills herself when she is not in treatment?"

In a deceptively simple way Anna Freud had, characteristically, said so much. She conveyed that one is not omnipotent, that it is better to try, that it is better for the suffering patient at the very least not to be alone. Over the years, when working with suicidal patients, I have remembered Anna Freud's question. I have also frequently told this anecdote to supervisees anxious about taking on suicidal patients.

There is of course much more that could be said, but for now my "list" of favourite Anna Freudian things is complete. Others will have different memories, and a list that is both similar and different. Although, sadly, there is not at present an Anna Freud training per se, it is through such lists, through her writings, through teaching, through supervision, and through memories, that her legacy can be communicated to new generations of child psychotherapists.

References

Rogers, R. & Hammerstein, O. (1959). Re-phrasing of "My Favorite Things". In: *The Sound of Music.*

Sandler, J. (1976). Countertransference and role-responsiveness. *International Review of Psycho-Analysis*, 3: 43–47.

Sandler, J., Kennedy, H. & Tyson, R. (1975). Discussions on transference: The treatment situation and technique in child psychoanalysis. *Psychoanalytic Study of the Child*, 30: 409–451.

Winnicott, D. W. (1965). *The Maturational Processes and the Facilitating Environment: Studies in the Theory of Emotional Development.* London: Hogarth and the Institute of Psychoanalysis.

Yorke, C. & Wiseberg, S. (1976). A developmental view of anxiety—some clinical and theoretical considerations. *Psychoanalytic Study of the Child*, 31: 107–135.

CHAPTER THIRTY THREE

Two supervisors

Ehud Koch

A neglected aspect of the child therapy training at the Hampstead Clinic was the central role of supervisors of training cases. The supervisors were a most diverse group in terms of personality and styles of teaching. All trained as child analysts, some with adult analytic training, and many with some connection to Anna Freud that dated back to the Hampstead War Nurseries. For the most part, students chose their supervisors from a roster of available supervisors. I had three supervisors for child analytic work and one supervisor for once weekly psychotherapeutic work. This memoir centres on the two supervisors who were particularly important to me.

My first supervisor was Ruth Thomas, a very tall, thin woman, probably in her sixties, whose manner and appearance was a cross between my images of a tweedy, schoolmistress/academic and a lady of a country manor house. As course tutor, she was my first contact with the Hampstead Course and Clinic: we corresponded by mail as part of the application for training process. I quickly recognized her "no-nonsense" style. In my first meeting with her, she commented, "Don't forget who you are and your accomplishments, because everyone else in the clinic will ignore them!" It was a most helpful comment in making the transition from being an American psychologist to a student in training. We met weekly in her consulting room in a maisonette flat in Swiss Cottage, London. My immediate image of the setting is of her sitting forward in an armchair, her hands crossed, or smoking a cheroot-like cigarette while sipping her coffee. She would often offer me a cup of coffee, quick to add that it was only because she was having a cup and it would be impolite to drink alone. On occasion, when her back was aching, she would listen and comment from a recumbent position.

I inherited Miss Thomas as a supervisor of my first case. My patient was an eight-year-old depressed, inhibited boy who was not achieving in school. He had started analysis some nine months before with a Swedish analyst, with Miss Thomas supervising the work. This therapist became ill and had to return to Sweden and I was asked to take on his treatment. She introduced me to him at a point when he was grieving her loss.

As it developed, object loss was a significant issue for this boy, both in terms of early carers and his mother's emotional unavailability due to her grieving when he was very young. His acceptance of me was due to his Hollywood-derived image of me being an American.

My patient was relatively non-verbal, his "communications" being countless drawings of stick figures in evolving stories of fairy-tale figures, warring cowboys and Indians, embattled knights, Norsemen, Greek heroes, all engaged in plunder, murder, and the gallant rescuing of helpless queens. What I took for Oedipal enactments, Miss Thomas would recognize as anal-sadistic and passive-active conflicts being expressed in drawings, fantasy, and in the transference. Themes of separation anxiety and castration anxiety abounded and it was difficult to tell what was primary and what was serving defensive purposes. Miss Thomas was most helpful in sorting out this barrage of enactments, in recognizing defensive and regressive moves, with a quickness at hearing the unconscious meanings of my patient's behaviour. I learned a lot about children, their development, and their psychopathology; about child analytic technique; and about psychoanalytic theory.

There were times when I thought Miss Thomas's comments were more in the nature of pronouncements rather than hypotheses, or that she drew with too broad a stroke, and there were times when I got lost in the analytic jargon. I never spoke of these reservations and suspect that this was a function of my psychology and hers.

One of the unhelpful features of Miss Thomas's supervisory style was to direct me as to what I should say to my patient, preferably at the beginning of the next analytic session. These puppet-like comments never felt good. In time, I learned to keep them in mind, and if the occasion warranted such an interpretation, to voice such in my own terms. This was another important piece of learning.

While Miss Thomas was usually supportive, there were moments when her critical remarks felt like censure. One such occasion was when she said that I had no grasp of "the whole picture", being mired in the particulars of the sessions. Another occasion was her faulting my first draft of an upcoming Wednesday presentation as a maudlin, simplistic account that showed no psychoanalytic understanding. Not only was I to rewrite it, but she inserted some long passages into my text which spoke to unconscious fantasies, in a language very different from my own. I felt only slightly consoled when fellow students in the common room at Maresfield Gardens suggested that Miss Thomas was only so critical with those students for whom she held high expectations. Ironically, this Wednesday presentation found its way into print as "The Awakening of a Depressed, Inhibited Boy" (1982).

It is true that under Miss Thomas's influence I became a better therapist, with a greater understanding of the treatment process and an enhanced understanding of psychoanalytic theory. I certainly "grew up", moving more confidently into being an independent clinician. Whatever loss I had of an over-idealized relationship, my sense of awe and respect for Miss Thomas's understanding of "the mind" has always remained with me.

* * *

I chose *Hansi Kennedy* to supervise my child analytic work with a six-year-old girl who was caught up in a sadomasochistic struggle with her mother. Prone to temper tantrums, asthmatic, overweight, and not achieving in school, she was a most challenging, tempestuous patient. She wavered in her attachment to me, I representing a rescuing and seducible prince charming, or a spoiler of any fun she might have had. After a rather profound depressed period, she showed signs of a treatment alliance and had a better understanding of her unlikeable self. After nearly two years of treatment, the work was cut short due to her father's taking a job in another country. This work was later examined in a paper entitled "Self-Observation, Insight, and the Development of 'Knowing' in a Child Analysis" (Koch, 1980).

Mrs Kennedy had been recommended by fellow students as being especially helpful in work with younger children. I had earlier been impressed by her astute observations in the context of diagnostic discussions and those of the Profile Research Group. Her language reflected her involvement with *Joe Sandler* and the Index Research Group. Her focus was often on attitudes towards the self and self-esteem and affect regulation. Her amusement at the incongruous was appealing. An attractive, forty-ish mother of two late latency boys, she welcomed me into her consulting room on the first floor of her north-west London home. By then I had two analytic patients and a once weekly psychotherapy patient, was familiar with the ways of the Clinic, and had profited from my own analysis. It was a different beginning than with Miss Thomas.

My recollection of Mrs Kennedy was that of a "participant observer and commentator" rather than a directing teacher. She made the occasional suggestion of an intervention or interpretation, but more often she would reflect on what my patient was experiencing and defending against. She was very helpful in my work with the patient's mother, who saw in her child the representation of an old, hated self. Mrs Kennedy was sympathetic and non-judgmental of my countertransference reactions, even noting Miss Freud's query, "How does he stand that child?" She was very attuned to object loss, which was a major reconstructed feature of this girl's experience, she having suddenly lost the care of a much beloved nanny at two and a half years. As I think back, I believe Mrs Kennedy's focus was much more on the ego and affective life of the child rather than on instinctual forces. It was an orientation that I came to internalize.

Some ten years later, during a sabbatical year of mine in London, Mrs Kennedy welcomed my participation in a clinical research group focusing on the role of insight in child analytic work. Her gracious, modest, and wise manner was again evident in that setting. In subsequent years, she was unfailingly welcoming when I visited London. Over tea and biscuits, we exchanged news of our lives and families. I believe there was a mutual affection and, for me, a sense of continuity with the Hampstead Clinic that I had valued.

References

Koch, E. (1980). Self-observation, insight, and the development of "Knowing" in a child analysis. *Journal of Child Psychotherapy*, *6*: 5–22.

Koch, E. (1982). The awakening of a depressed, inhibited boy. *The Bulletin of The Hampstead Clinic*, *5*: 275–295.

CHAPTER THIRTY FOUR

Anna Freud: memories and the climate of experience[1]

Ava Bry Penman

Arriving at Anna Freud's Clinic in September 1967, I now realize, turned out to be the fulfilment of a personal fantasy of coming home to an extended family. Anna Freud had been a teacher and was a Jewish immigrant who created a clinic filled with central European immigrants working with children in need. And, in a sense, I felt like a kind of refugee too, since my parents, separated from their families, had fled Hitler's Germany. I grew up around refugees and I too became a teacher of young children. The Clinic felt like and sounded like home—all those stories, those funny familiar speech rhythms, and those intense conversations! Also, for several years, Britain had been a safe haven for my parents on their way to America, and they spoke fondly and gratefully of their experience when London was their home.

As I remember the scene of my primary psychoanalytic education, Miss Freud was in her early seventies and I was in my early twenties. Skirt lengths in the 1960s were flamboyantly micro, mini, midi, or maxi, while manners of address at the Clinic were routinely formal (I was addressed as "Miss Bry …").

I can still see Miss Freud sitting at meeting after meeting, listening to Wednesday clinical papers, to discussions of diagnostic profiles, to descriptions of babies and nursery children, to discussions of borderline children, to discussions of treatment situations and technique as described on endless index cards. I still see her in the group run by Joseph Sandler, revisiting her seminal book on defences. And I continue to be deeply grateful for the chance to convene discussions *with* Anna Freud and other clinicians using details of clinical material through which basic questions and diverse ways of thinking arose naturally and fully in extended

[1] Presented at the Anna Freud Centre, London, November 2, 2007. Memorial celebration on 25th anniversary of Anna Freud's death.

conversations (in a group called "The Treatment of Atypical Children"). Anna Freud was ever present—and in the Clinic there was the ubiquitous presence of her interest.

In all discussions, I remember, Miss Freud's quiet attentiveness was punctuated by frequent sudden slight head movements—perhaps internal Yeses, Noes, Buts ... perhaps thoughts, feelings, and comments bursting forth bodily. Then, when she spoke, her thoughts were delivered clearly, steadily, and deliberately in a very slightly high-pitched girlish tone. Somehow, it was magically conversational *and* commanding—perhaps like a great story-teller. For example, after a Wednesday paper, she might say something like, "What we have heard here today is the story of a child who" ... and then she summarized, synthesized, and invigorated in a few sentences what she had heard. Soon she would continue: "And this story raises interesting issues which have the following history in our field" ... and finally she would say: "Of course there remain the questions of XX and YY ... which are open for further discussion, now, among us here today ...". It was awe-inspiring because no matter how good, uneven, or poor the presentation, Anna Freud pulled something of interest out of it, out of herself. Somehow, in this concentration of effort and economy of expression, she reduced everything to its maximum.

Ever the teacher, mindful of involving others, she was preternaturally bound and determined to bring about discussion. Meetings begat meetings, and conversations begat conversations—my memories of the Clinic are full of conversations of all kinds at all moments: in supervision, after meetings, after class, during lunch, in our common room between patients amid the great jazzy clatter of old typewriters from the 1930s and 1940s—with endless biscuits, coffee and tea, with other students and many of our supervisors. We knew and cared about our own patients and *all* patients and kept up with analytic problems and developments. We got and gave encouragement, compassion, ideas, conflicting ideas, questions, company. For me, wide-ranging conversation was the essence of the Clinic—and it all mattered a great deal. And somehow, Anna Freud "grew" this place that way: Miss Freud was the Clinic, and the Clinic was Miss Freud—at least to me.

Further, Miss Freud's dedication and single-minded devotion to clinical psychoanalysis contained a wide vision and a mission: to explore the reaches of applying psychoanalytic insight to better the lives of children within the Clinic and well beyond—through social policy and laws, in educational and medical arenas. Such issues arose for consideration in many discussions, and opportunities to act after graduation came into focus.

We all recognized, I think, that there was an inhibiting aspect to Anna Freud's allegiance to certain tenets of her father's theories. However, it became clear when she talked about the details of clinical material, that she was not so strict in practice, and when she spoke of the wider applications she was very free.

W. H. Auden wrote movingly about her father, and perhaps we may say something of the same about our Anna Freud—that to us, she "is no more a person but now a whole climate of opinion". The whole climate of experience of Anna Freud's Clinic endures: the good past is present; daily and variously, it inspires and affects life for me and for many others in many lands.

Reference

Auden, W. H. (1976). In memory of Sigmund Freud. In: E. Mendelson (Ed.), *Collected Poems*. New York: Random House.

CHAPTER THIRTY FIVE

Reflections of a child psychotherapy trainee

Laurie Levinson

To write a brief account of the impact of my training at the Hampstead Child Therapy Course and Clinic is an immense challenge. It was an experience that, although completed many years ago, is alive in my mind in some way every day.

I decided that I wanted to train there while in my second year at university. Having read Anna Freud's *The Ego and the Mechanisms of Defence*, I was so taken by her exposition of the role and functioning of this agency of the mind that I wanted to meet her and see the place where people discussed such topics. I was already studying psychology in an academic department which eschewed a psychoanalytic point of view. And so I wrote Miss Freud a letter, asking if it would be possible to visit the Clinic during my Christmas holidays. I was happily surprised to receive a reply that yes, it would be possible ... but that she herself would be away. Would I like to meet with the course tutor instead? I had absolutely no idea what a "course tutor" was, or even what the British meant by the word "course". But I agreed, as I was intrigued and curious to see what I thought was a famous clinic. I also had no idea then that the place had a full-time training programme in child and adolescent psychoanalysis. I thought I would be given a tour of an American-style clinic ....

I felt quite sophisticated as I rode into London on the Green Line bus. Staying with family friends in the countryside, I followed their instructions to get off at "John Barnes". John Barnes turned out to be a department store near the Hampstead Clinic. Having figured this out I climbed a steep little walkway to find myself in a tree-lined Victorian street with large red-brick houses and lovely gardens behind them. I arrived at number 12 Maresfield Gardens and, by now somewhat anxious, climbed the steps and asked for Miss Irmi Elkan, the course tutor.

Miss Elkan turned out to be a somewhat serious but friendly woman who, instead of showing me around as I had anticipated, began what turned out to be a psychoanalytic interview—as if I were applying to be admitted for training. Well ... I figured, I was there ... I might as well do my best to answer the various questions she asked about my life, my family, and childhood. Surprised by her directness, I was also very pleased to be taken so seriously as I was only a college second year student!

The memory of this first contact has always had a nostalgic sweetness for me. I was quite young, quite naïve; but very passionate in my conviction that this was the place where I wanted to study. Miss Elkan informed me that I was too young and too inexperienced … but that she would like me to keep in touch with her as I progressed through my studies. She would be glad to advise me as I went along. And she kept her word. When in my last year at university, the Hampstead Clinic informed me of a programme (course) in developmental psychology at London University. They thought I should apply. I did, and was accepted. One year later they found me a job for the remaining time before the next training course would begin.

Thus, my relationship with the Hampstead Clinic began long before my training did. My fellow students used to tease me affectionately that I had known what I wanted to do when I was in kindergarten! They had all had jobs, worked in the world, and felt like grown-ups already. I was a bit different in that I was younger, and still pretty inexperienced. I did not question the fact that we students were treated as if we knew very little indeed; and should just listen during discussion and … should not speak up! I figured I had come a very long distance to London to learn from these people—so why protest? I was quite aware of the hierarchical structure of the place—but willing to accept it because of the integrity of the faculty and the amazingly rich and exceedingly high level of discourse.

What stands out and what continues to be etched in my mind is the elegant simplicity with which Anna Freud described children and their problems. In any context—observing a child in her beloved nursery school; giving a formal discussion following a clinical paper; or making a comment during a meeting of a research or study group—she was a person whose confidence in her ability to understand gave her the freedom not to have to know all the answers. This atmosphere of always learning from one's patients truly pervaded my years at the Clinic. In classes and supervisions, and diagnostic meetings and case conferences, we were encouraged by our teachers to observe and to think and to *feel* … this long before the current belief in the usefulness of countertransference.

The fact of being in a full-time training allowed us the luxury of having time to "sit around" with our teachers and staff members, usually in the common room or the lunchroom. It was often during these informal moments that students and teachers would openly discuss problems, questions, clinical dilemmas, and theoretical issues. It was great to hear that everyone had their doubts and difficulties with the work—and wonderful to have the availability of a non-judgmental group of bright people to whom one could always turn with a question. Because of Anna Freud's strict policy that weekly reports be written on every patient, we all knew the details of most of our colleagues' patients—thus providing us with a wide range of clinical phenomena, diverse psychopathologies, and of course all different age groups of children.

When the annual Colloquium was created, and we former students were invited back every year for an intense weekend of study, it was in many ways a mini re-creation of our training days. We had an in-depth theoretical review of the literature on the topic of the meeting; and two case presentations—usually one adult and one child—followed by long, intense discussion groups. To this day, I look forward to the first weekend of November. The Colloquium is one of the very few professional situations I have ever participated in where one can *really* talk—with the sense that psychoanalysis is truly an exploratory process. Colleagues from all over the world and with quite different theoretical orientations come together to *talk* and to *listen* and to *learn*. It seems as if this sort of activity ought to occur more frequently—perhaps in our home societies. Perhaps it is a more special experience for those of us who trained at Hampstead—to find again that particular ambiance of easy discussion of clinical material—sharing of problems and attempts to understand and find our way through the difficulties.

All I know is that as the plane lands in London, I invariably have the pleasurable feeling that I am coming to a very familiar and welcoming place—the place where I grew up professionally, and which offers the possibility—although now we are all quite experienced—of being learners and questioners again. It is a good experience to renew each year.

CHAPTER THIRTY SIX

Fighting thoughtfully for independence

Audrey Gavshon

Much has been written about Anna Freud's fluency and clarity of thought. Her capacity to speak in public and convey complex ideas in a deceptively simple way is well known. Her fierce independence is what I remember and admired most. She fought for what she felt was right and for what she believed should be examined in greater detail before a decision was taken. I first encountered her independent spirit when I applied to train at the Hampstead Child Therapy Course and Clinic (HCTCC) in the 1960s.

I had arrived in London and was studying at the London School of Economics (LSE). Through my sister and her husband, I became acquainted with some psychoanalysts and became so interested that I entered analysis. My analyst encouraged me to apply to the HCTCC. By then I had three children and the youngest was only a few months old. I made an appointment to see Miss Freud to discuss my application, which she considered very carefully and asked, "Who will look after your youngest child?" I explained that we had a cleaner who loved children and who looked after our children when required. Miss Freud asked, "How did you find such a wonderful person?" Miss Freud had a very modern attitude towards motherhood and careers. She knew about people and the human condition. She supported my application which was forwarded to the training council. In those days, applications to any of the training schools were processed by a central training council, headed by Dr Prince. I was upset to hear that my application was rejected on the grounds that the training council believed that "A good mother stays at home and spends all the time she can focusing on the child." I continued my personal analysis which supported me through this disappointment. Miss Freud disagreed with this decision and kept me informed of the exchanges taking place between the HCTCC and the training council. In a letter dated February 17, 1961, she wrote:

> I know that you are eager to learn what further steps have been taken with regard to your position as an applicant for our Course, and therefore I am glad to inform you, and to keep you informed in future. We have now written to Dr Prince as head of the Training Council … to state the position once more as we see it …. We have also stressed in the same letter our wish to have the position of mothers of young children more fully discussed in the Training Council with regard to their suitability for training, the latter quite apart from your specific case.

I continued my analysis for about another year and was hugely relieved when a letter from Miss Freud informed me that the training council had agreed that I could start the training. Referring to the one year wait imposed by the training council, Miss Freud wrote: "Please know that this was not of my making." Her insistence that applications to the training be examined individually led to a significant change in the application process. From then on, applications to the HCTCC training were no longer submitted to the central training council, but were considered by the HCTCC's training committee.

CHAPTER THIRTY SEVEN

The Anna Freud Centre Colloquium

Steven Ablon

For the past twenty-five years I have been attending the annual Anna Freud Centre Colloquium, which brings together affiliates of Anna Freud's from all over the world. When I return to the United States, what I have learned at the Colloquium always influences my work. Although my patients did not know directly about this they must have sensed that shortly after the beginning of November there were usually changes in my approach.

The Anna Freud Centre presents a powerful ongoing oscillation between a deep understanding of analytic theory and technique and an equally deep clinical resonance with the experience of the patient. One of so many examples would be a recent case discussion in which a teenager asked her therapist to help her get a cup of water. This was interpreted productively in terms of this patient's wish for nurturing that had been absent in her early childhood. At the same time I understood that had the analyst helped to get the drink of water, this enactment would also in time have led to the patient spontaneously talking about how much she longed for this kind of help and nurturance in her life.

This is reminiscent of an experience I had with a nine-year-old patient who asked for a snack at every meeting, which I gave him. As we noticed his hunger for snacks, after a while he said insightfully: "You know Dr A, it's not the snacks that I'm so hungry for, it's love."

Analytic theory and technique has always been central to our thinking at these international meetings. This is reflected in the choice of colloquia topics. For instance in recent years:

2004: Analytic technique—is it the same as it has always been?
2005: Issues of interpretation and technique in analysis of children in difficult circumstances with specific needs
2006: Adolescence—approaches from different analytic cultures
2007: The experience of adoption: psychoanalytic perspectives

2008: Progress in genetics and progress in clinical practice
2009: Struggling with unpredictability—treating children of personality disordered parents
2010: Developmental hazards of adolescence and the move to young adulthood

At the same time there is a deep base of pooled clinical experience that takes into account where patients are at that point in the treatment, and in his or her relationship to the particular analyst. This wisdom was exemplified by "master" clinicians such as Hansi Kennedy and *Anne Hurry*. In the course of clinical discussions they would often add a sentence or two about how they saw the situation. This illuminated the issues in a very helpful and powerfully human way. An instance I remember hearing about was when a very anxious adolescent girl started her meetings at the Centre. She could hardly talk and a senior clinician offered her some tea with sugar (a "grown up" beverage and very English!). Clearly this had great meaning for the patient who settled and was able to proceed steadily with very difficult and painful work.

When Anna Freud wrote *Normality and Pathology in Childhood* in 1965, the technique of child analysis was based on Freud's model for the analysis of the neurotic adult. This included the importance of analysing defences, clarification and interpretation of the transference, and verbal insight. Influenced by her developmental viewpoint, Anna Freud introduced some modifications in the technique for child analysis. Subsequently at the Anna Freud Centre the experience of analysing children, including those with developmental difficulties, made apparent the importance of relational factors, play, action, enactment, symbolic expression as well as words, the centrality affect, and the countertransference and the transference-countertransference matrix. In time these technical shifts also came to be incorporated into adult analysis in terms of concepts such as object relations, self-psychology, and relational and intrasubjective approaches.

In this way Anna Freud's pioneering contributions were elaborated and extended in many directions. These, like Anna Freud's subsequent transformations, are not a matter of either/or but rather yes/and, providing a valuable rich palette with a hierarchical mobility. Today, along with changes at the Anna Freud Centre, analytic principles are increasingly utilized in treatments of much less frequency, and with children whose lives have included great dislocations and trauma.

It has been noted that nothing is constant—and the one sure thing is that there will always be change! Ability to change is therefore crucial for any organism, or any system of inquiry that attempts to remain theoretically and clinically germane. The Anna Freud Centre's flexibility, yet retention of traditions like the Colloquium and its questioning attitude, exemplifies this resilience.

APPENDIX

Biographical cameos[1]

Marion Burgner (1930–1996), née Chasek, was born into a Russian Jewish immigrant family and grew up in east London. She won scholarships to grammar school and then to the University of London, obtaining an honours degree in English from Birkbeck College and later also qualified in psychology. She trained at the Hampstead Child Therapy Course and later qualified as an adult psychoanalyst, becoming a training analyst at the British Psychoanalytical Society in 1984. In addition to clinical practice she worked for various organizations including the Hampstead Clinic and the Child Guidance Training Centre. She worked with an early HIV/AIDS research group at the Tavistock and Portman Clinics, and taught for many years at University College Hospital. She also was involved in research participating in the Young Adult Research Programme led by Anne-Marie Sandler at the Anna Freud Centre (members of which were Julia Fabricius, Dr Luigi Caparotta, Rose Edgcumbe, Hansi Kennedy, Rosemary Davies, Dr Rosine Perelberg, Dr Duncan McLean, Anne Harrison, Dr Anne Zachary, Professor Maria Tallandini, Dr Sally Weintrobe, and Dr Brian Martindale). Over the years, Marion was a member of numerous other study groups including the Clinical Concept Research Group (chaired by Humberto Nagera), the Profile Research Group, a study group she co-chaired with Audrey Gavshon, and the Hampstead Index Committee chaired by Joseph Sandler. She applied her intellectual rigour

[1]Many important figures at the AFC are among the contributors to this book, and hence their biographical details appear at the beginning. Due to limitations of space those presented here are but a small selection of the many who gave of their talents and time to consolidate the Anna Freud Centre's reputation as a centre of excellence. The bulk of this appendix was researched and written by Christiane Ludwig-Körner, largely on the basis of her personal interviews. Entries for Dorothy Burlingham, *Marion Burgner*, Rose Edgcumbe, Kate Friedlander, Anne Hurry, George Moran, Humberto Nagera, Joseph Sandler, and Clifford Yorke were assembled by the editors from archival records and/or obituaries.

to integrating Anna Freud's developmental perspective with newer ideas emerging from the Hampstead Clinic (e.g., teasing out aspects of the representational world, such as "object constancy" in terms of relationship, as Peter Fonagy noted in her obituary), and reconciling classical theory with findings from her wide clinical experience with severely disturbed children, adolescents, and young adults. Her prescient contributions included several papers written with Rose Edgcumbe, reconceptualizing different phases of development (1972a, 1972b, 1975) while emphasizing early object relationships. In a paper which became a classic in its own right, they elaborated on Anna Freud's concept of the "phallic-narcissistic phase", delineating early pre-Oedipal narcissistic construction of body self-representations from Oedipal acquisition of sexual identity in the context of an intimate threesome. Exploring phallic development in both girls and boys, they saw penis envy and exhibitionism as a complicated compromise formation involving aspects of gender identity, pathological object relations, defences, narcissism, and self-esteem. A later paper (1980), written with Hansi Kennedy, focused on the early family origins of sadomasochistic behaviour in children, linking sadism not to the anal phase but to a phallic-Oedipal configuration and search for gratification through omnipotence, control, domination and denigration of the object, safeguarding the integrity of the self-representation. She also wrote on the effects of paternal absence (a repeated theme in the clinical papers of this volume) based on discussions in a group co-chaired with Audrey Gavshon, including Carla Elliott, Susan Vas Dias, and Irene Wineman. In later years, based on research at the Brent Consultation Centre, she published a paper on adolescent breakdown, suggesting that major psychiatric problems indicate a failure in negotiating psychic separateness from internal primary objects. [Compiled from Anne-Marie Sandler, *Bulletin of the British Psychoanalytical Society*, *32*(11): 19; Fonagy, P. (1997). Marion Burgner. *Psychoanaytic Psycho-therapy*, *11*: 173–176.]

Dorothy Burlingham was Anna Freud's lifelong companion and co-founder of the War Nurseries and the Hampstead Clinic. A member of the famous Tiffany (glass) family, she moved from New York to Vienna with her young children after the early death of her husband. She became closely identified with the psychoanalytic movement, had a short analysis with Theodor Reik, which ended with his move to Berlin, and then with Sigmund Freud. Seeking nursery education for her young family and for other American children, she decided to found a school, in which Erik Erikson and Peter Blos were teachers. Together with Anna Freud, she also founded a crèche for twenty deprived pre-nursery school children, financed by herself and Edith Jackson. The City of Vienna invited her and Anna Freud to organize a course of lectures for nursery school teachers; and to institute the first seminars in child analysis. Among the distinguished analysts who attended those seminars were Anny Katan, Jenny Waelder-Hall, Siegfried Bernfeld, Richard and Editha Sterba, and August Aichhorn.

Arriving in England after the *Anschluss* with the Freud family, she too became a member of the British Psychoanalytical Society. In addition to her interest in mothers and infants, and especially blind children and twins, she devised and founded the Hampstead Psychoanalytic Index, and was active in many groups at the Hampstead Clinic, including the educational unit or the group for the study of adult psychosis. She died in 1979, aged 89. [Source: Yorke, C. (1980). Dorothy Tiffany Burlingham (1891–1979). *International Journal of Psychoanalysis*, *61*: 560–562.]

Gertrud Dann (1908–1998) trained as kindergarten and infant's nurse and worked in children's homes in Munich, Hamburg-Blankenese, and Deisenhofen, before she established her own kindergarten in her parents' home in Augsburg. In the War Nurseries, she was also responsible for the infants. After caring for "Bulldogs Bank Kinder" (who with the exception of one child were ultimately all adopted), she too worked with Alice Goldberger in Lingfield House, a home for children from concentration camps. When this home, too, was dissolved, like her sister Sophie, Gertrud helped from 1958 in the library of the Clinic or the Freud house. She died on April 2,1998, also in Horncastle House, Sharpthorne, Sussex. [Interviews with Gertrud Dann: 14.7.1996, 20.11.1996, 21.11.1996, 18.9.1997.]

Sophie Dann (1900–1993) was the eldest of five daughters of the merchant Albert Dann and his wife Fanny Dann, née Kitzinger, from Augsburg, Germany. When she began her work in the War Nurseries she brought with her professional experience in heading various social services: a Jewish kindergarten in Munich; a mothers' school (*Mütterschule*) of the City League of Women and Home Care Associations of Augsburg; welfare care for the Jewish community, and a mothers' school courses for Jewish girls who had to emigrate. In December 1940 Anna Freud was looking for a nurse for her sick aunt, Minna Bernays, but Sophie and her second youngest sister Gertrud (see below) were involved in obtaining conversion of their work permits into those for nursing, and had to change residence from Essex to London, so could not begin work for Anna Freud right away. Meanwhile Minna Bernays was transferred into hospital. Sophie and Gertrud had just taken up a new job with an old lady (Sophie as nurse and lady's companion, and Gertrud as cook and housekeeper) when they received a telegram from Anna Freud, telling them that they could immediately start working in the newly opened War Nursery. With heavy hearts they had to turn down the offer for the moment since they felt obliged to first find a substitute for their employer. They joined Anna Freud when another children's home was opened six months later. Sophie Dann was responsible for the care of the infants, the mothers, and the milk kitchen—and later also for the infirmary. After the closing of the War Nurseries, from October 1945 until September 1946 together with her sister Gertrud she cared for the "Bulldogs Bank Kinder", the group of young children who had survived Theresienstadt. After this, she worked in a home in Lingfield, likewise with children who had survived concentration camps. Yet time and again, she was solicited as nurse for Anna Freud or the grandchildren of Lady Betty Clarke, the generous benefactress who had made her house Bulldogs Bank in West Hoathly available. From 1969 on, she helped with cataloguing Freud's library, and subsequently establishing the index. She died on December 18, 1993 in the old people's home Horncastle House, Sharpthorne, near West Hoathly, Sussex. [CLK interviews with Gertrud Dann: 14.7.1996, 20.11.1996, 21.11.1996, 18.9.1997.]

Rose Edgcumbe was connected to Anna Freud's project in more ways than one. Born in London, like so many of Anna Freud's young charges, she was evacuated (to Yorkshire) with her mother during the Second World War. On her return to London, she attended South Hampstead High School for Girls in Maresfield Gardens, a few houses down from the Anna Freud Centre. In the mid-1950s, after completing her undergraduate studies in psychology at University College London, she continued her studies in the USA under the auspices of a Fulbright scholarship. Rose worked there as a clinical psychologist in a hospital for children with special needs. She became both intensely interested in child development and disillusioned with academic psychology. On her return to England two years later, she went to Manchester, working with children at Booth Hall Hospital, before beginning her training in child analysis at the Hampstead Child Therapy Course and Clinic in 1959, qualifying in 1963, and joining the staff. In 1971 she began training in adult psychoanalysis at the Institute of Psychoanalysis in London. A frequent observer in the HCTCC nursery (established in 1957), her early writings reflected the range of her interests from the border between therapy and education (1972), aggression (written with Joseph Sandler in 1974), and sexuality, and several co-authored papers with Marion Burgner, on changing needs and need-satisfying relationships during the early developmental phases (1972), and a much quoted 1975 paper which became a classic. Anna Freud is said to have responded to their presentation of Oedipal, and early pre-Oedipal narcissistic phallic manifestations in both girls and boys by saying: "Well! To think we have been so wrong for so long." Edgcumbe's interest in gender issues continued with a paper on negative Oedipal issues in the gendered three- to five-year-old girl's changing sexuality (1976). She also wrote on pre-linguistic interactions (1981) and different somatic and verbal modes of communication, focusing on the two person psychology of the caregiver's attempts to achieve understanding of their pre-verbal baby's communications. (This paper derives from discussions of a study group at the Hampstead Clinic on Language Development chaired by Humberto Nagera. Members included Pauline Cohen, Carla Elliott, Barbara Grant, Jill Hodges, Elizabeth Model, George Moran, Doris Wills, and Irene Wineman. She also belonged to the Clinical Concept Research Group, whose members included Huberto Nagera (chairman), Anna Freud (consultant), Sheila Baker, Alice Colonna, R. Putzel, W. Ernest Freud, Ismond Rosen, and Anne Hayman.) Edgcumbe's early paper on Anna Freud (1983) grew into a book, which she published in 2000, on her view of Anna Freud's formulations of "development, disturbance, and therapeutic techniques", with an emphasis on object relations. It was fitting that she wrote the book. Clifford Yorke (2001) mentioned that Anna Freud once asked him: "Why can't we have more students like Rose Edgcumbe and Hansi Kennedy?" After George Moran's tragic death in early 1992 (see below), Rose agreed to become acting director of the Anna Freud Centre for fifteen months until 1993 when the post was taken by Anne-Marie Sandler, and then Julia Fabricius in 1996. [Source: Rose Edgcumbe: obituary in *The Guardian*, written by Clifford Yorke, September 1, 2001.]

Dr Kate Friedlander (1895–1949) was instrumental after the war in convincing Anna Freud to organize the Hampstead Child Therapy Clinic and Course, where she later worked as teacher and training analyst. Like Anna Freud, she was dedicated to making sure that psychoanalysis was not a therapy for the rich and that its applications were tied to progressive educational and child guidance institutions. Dr Friedlander's book, *The Psychoanalytic Approach to Juvenile Delinquency* (1947) was a pioneering effort to explore the applications of psychoanalytic theory to outreach interventions, and a wonderful example of her contribution and commitment to the field of applied child psychoanalysis. Dr Friedlander developed the initial training scheme that Anna Freud presented to the training committee and British Psychoanalytical Society during a joint meeting in 1947, and supported Anna Freud during her struggle to get the creation of a clinical training at the Hampstead Clinic approved. She died at the age of forty-seven from an inoperable brain tumour. Her death left Anna Freud at a crossroads as she had to take over the implementation and administration of the future training course. [Young-Bruehl, 2004.]

Manna (Martha) Friedman(n), née Weindling, was born in 1915 in Cologne, Germany as the second oldest of seven children. Emigrating in 1939 in the nick of time to London, out of her large family, only her sister and oldest brother survived the Holocaust. Like many of the Jewish immigrants, she worked first as maid and was then accommodated by remote relatives. In London, she completed her training as a kindergarten nurse, and began training as a social worker. From 1942 to 1946 she worked in a War Nursery in Birmingham as head of the kindergarten, where she also trained prospective kindergarten nurses. Together with Alice Goldberger, and the Dann sisters, she too worked in Lingfield House, Surrey, caring for children and youth from the concentration camps. Initially, she wanted to participate in this work just for two years, as she had decided to emigrate to Israel to her sister. Yet she spent three years there as it was difficult for her to separate from her protégés. And when she was in Israel from 1949 to 1955, she maintained close contact with Alice Goldberger and the children, through weekly letters (which Alice collected, and later on returned to Manna). Today, they are with the daughter of one of those girls from the home. For many of these children or young people, she became a substitute mother or grandmother. While in Israel, she directed a kindergarten on a kibbutz and brought her training as a social worker to an end. It was her love for Oscar Friedmann (see below) which made her return to London where she married him after his divorce. (In contrast to her husband she writes her surname only with one 'n'.) From 1957 until her retirement in 1978 she led the HCTCC nursery school group. [Interviews with Manna Friedman: 21.11.1996, 26.11.1996, 12.7.1996, 23.4.1997, 19.3.2000.]

Oscar Friedmann (1903–1958) worked as social worker and teacher in Düsseldorf where he was born, before becoming director in 1932 of an institution for juvenile delinquents in Wolzig close to Berlin. Together with these young people he was taken to the concentration camp Sachsenhausen. As a result of mistreatment there he suffered an ear injury and had a permanent hemiplegic paralysis in his face. In his analysis with Ada Müller-Braunschweig in Berlin, he tried to overcome the psychic harm. When in 1938 he brought a big group of Jewish children to England, he initially wanted to return to Germany, yet was persuaded to stay in England. Thus his first wife, two children, and sister were saved. After the end of the war, he worked together with the committee of Bloomsbury House in London, which cared for children and young people saved from the concentration camps. On August 14, 1945, over 300 children and youth landed in Crosby-on-Eden. Flown out by various military airplanes to England, they were brought to a reception camp in Windermere. Oscar Friedmann regarded his task as the psychic care of those children and youth. After his training as psychoanalyst at the British Psychoanalytical Institute (his analyst was Katja Levy), he had his own practice in London. He participated in a Hampstead Child Therapy Clinic research project on the simultaneous analysis of mother and child, and wrote and published on that subject. He died on December 28,1958 in London following a heart attack, three years after his marriage with Manna. [Interviews with Manna Friedman: 26.11.1996, 19.9.1997, Gilbert, 1996).

Alice Goldberger (1897–1986) came from Berlin, where before emigrating she had worked inter alia as educator and group nurse in the Mossestift orphanage; as director of the War Nursery of the commune Grunewald; as kindergarten nurse in the city shelter (district office of Berlin-Charlottenburg); as youth leader in institutions of the Pestalozzi-Fröbel-Haus, and, respectively, since 1934 as director of the kindergarten home of the Jewish Community. After her emigration in 1939, she was put into the internment camp on the Isle of Man, where on her own initiative she established a kindergarten. Anna Freud, who was attempting to liberate her nephew Ernst Halberstadt and the housekeeper Paula Fichtl from internment in this camp, got to know about her work and invited her to join her team. When following the increasing bomb attacks it became necessary to evacuate the children into the countryside, Alice became the director of the home New Barn', in Essex. After dissolution of the War Nurseries, she cared for the children who had been saved from the concentration camps. In 1947, at fifty years of age she was among the first group of the War Nurseries colleagues who received their training as "Child Expert" (Liselotte Frankl was her training analyst). She found she worked particularly well with blind children and Anna Freud often assigned her very difficult children for therapy. After the dissolution of the children's homes she lived with Sophie Wutsch and some of the children who had not yet found a home, in an apartment in West End Lane, in north London. On the occasion of her eightieth birthday, a film of her life was shown on the English television programme *This Is Your Life*, instigated by some of her protégés from the concentration camps. She died on February 22, 1986 in London. [Sources: interviews with Manna Friedman; Anneliese Schnurmann, Gertrud Dann, Entschädigungsakten 21 WGA 395/55, TV programme: *This Is Your Life*.]

Dr Ilse Hellman(n) (1908–1998) was the youngest (two older brothers) of a Viennese industrial family. After her studies in social work, she worked from 1931 in a home for juvenile delinquents near Paris and subsequently in Paris itself with children from multi-problem families. In parallel, she started her studies in psychology at the Sorbonne, which she continued from 1935 in Vienna, as her French work permit expired. She became an assistant to Charlotte Bühler, who at that time was researching newborn babies and infants. Other assistants were Esther Bick, Liselotte Frankl, and Lotte Danzinger. In Vienna, she had made the acquaintance of René Spitz, who showed great interest in Charlotte Bühler's infant research and came there several times to attend lectures. According to Robert Emde, Spitz was inspired by Charlotte Bühler for much of his own research (personal communication on 25.9.1999). In 1935, Charlotte Bühler was invited to London to build up a private Child Guidance Clinic ("Parents' Association Institute"). Two years later, Charlotte Bühler asked Ilse Hellman to support her in her work in London, as she could only stay for several months at a time. Hellman accepted in order to escape the Nazi regime. With the beginning of the war, Bühler's Institute in London was closed down and Ilse Hellman worked as a developmental psychologist caring for evacuated children, who, due to the war, were rapidly assigned to foster families. Moreover, she was responsible for those women and children who had been evacuated at the beginning 1941 from Gibraltar. This PhD awarded psychologist, who was initially rather sceptical towards psychoanalysis, found herself convinced step by step by Anna Freud and Josefine Stross to start an analytical training. Susan Isaacs arranged an additional income for her answering letters to the editor of the *Nursery World*—so that she could begin training at the British Psychoanalytical Institute (her training analysis was with Dorothy Burlingham till 1945). In 1952 she became a member of the British Psychoanalytical Society and in 1955, a training analyst. Together with Dr Rowley, for a while she directed the vocational training committee of the British Psychoanalytical Society.

She was friends with Liselotte Frankl, Sylvia Payne, and Paula Heimann, and belonged to the "Middle Group".

In addition to her own clinical practice, she collaborated in research projects at the Hampstead Child Therapy Course and Clinic, such as with an idea of Dorothy Burlingham's—the simultaneous analysis of mother and child. (Treatment material of these two totally independently working analysts was evaluated by a third colleague, a "coordinator", and she was one of the evaluators.) Another study focused on the treatment of young people. Her publications cover these and other subjects. She married Arnoldos Noak, a professor of art history from Holland with a professorship in Leeds, who died suddenly at the age of sixty-six from cardiac insufficiency. Ilse Hellmann herself worked until over seventy years of age in a cancer hospital, where she supervised doctors. In addition to intensive analysis, she was one of the first involved in short-term therapy and counselling work, continuing to treat patients until she was eighty. Until the end of her life, she maintained contact with some of the children from the War Nursery. In old age she lived in the immediate neighbourhood of her only daughter and granddaughter. [Sources: telephone calls with Dr Ilse Hellman, 6.6.1997, 7.6.1997; interview with her daughter Maggy Williams, 21.11.1997.]

Anne Hurry is a graduate of the Hampstead training, and worked at the Centre as a member of staff as child psychotherapist, supervisor, and inspiring teacher in the training. She also provided a discussion group in her home for self-selected AFC/UCL master of science students in psychoanalytic developmental psychology. She was the founding chair of the child psychotherapy training at the British Association of Psychotherapists, where she was also a supervising and training therapist for the adult psychoanalytic psychotherapy section. Anne is past editor of the *Journal of Child Psychotherapy* and has published widely on both clinical and theoretical topics. Above all it is as an experienced clinician that Anne has become known and much admired. On the basis of extensive analytic work with severely disturbed children, she built on Anna Freud's dictum that although interpretations suffice in work with neurosis, child analysts must modify their clinical strategy when their young patient has deficits in their capacity to relate. Thus, in a clinical chapter she wrote for a book edited by the Laufers (1989), Anne demonstrated her remarkable resilience in continuing to work affably in the face of a youth's extreme aggression, and providing a "new developmental experience" through her capacity to survive his attacks and bear his affect. In recent years her buoyancy has also seen her through personal adversity. In 1998 she edited a remarkable book, *Psychoanalysis and Developmental Therapy* (widely referred to, as reflected in this volume), where she expanded further on Anna Freud's concept of developmental help. Here too, she cogently advocates that the therapist assume a developmental-relational technique to supplement interpretative interventions, especially when early models of relating prevail, that are inaccessible to conscious representation. This is in keeping with the project set by Anna Freud in 1978: "To the extent to which developmental harm can be undone belatedly, child analysis may accept it as its next duty to devise methods for this task" (p. 197). In her own clinical chapter, the direct simplicity of her words to her patient illustrates her belief that *procedural* transformations can occur in therapy as the child internalizes the new experience of a relationship which offers recognition and hope while containing despair and rage.

Hansi (Hanna) Kennedy, née Engl (1923–2003), was born three years after her sister in Colonia, near Vienna. Her first encounter with psychoanalysis occurred when she was a child through her neighbours, the Lampl family, with whose children she played. As a young girl she absolutely wanted to become a kindergarten nurse and went to Hedy Schwarz, who was director of a Montessori kindergarten in Vienna, to get experience. Hedy Schwarz was just preparing to emigrate to London and advised her to do the same. Her father, who had business contacts with London, succeeded in emigrating with his family in time. She belonged to the first group of colleagues who received the child analytical training from Anna Freud. In the evenings and at weekends, she took additional courses at the university and studied psychology. When the children's homes were disbanded, she had just received her diploma in psychology. Kate Friedlander invited her in 1947 to work as a psychologist in the Child Guidance Clinic in Chichester, West Sussex, which she had founded. She worked there for four years as a child therapist. In the mornings, she went five times a week to London to Dorothy Burlingham for analysis before going to Chichester to care there for her patients. In 1951 she married the merchant Gerhard Helmut Kahn, who as a soldier took the name Kennedy. With him, she had two sons (born 1952 and 1955). From 1952 she worked as psychoanalytical child therapist in the Hampstead Child Therapy Clinic and in her own practice. In addition to child psychoanalysis she participated in research, wrote numerous publications, and was engaged in her psychoanalytical training. In the first phase, while building up the Sigmund Freud Institute, Alexander Mitscherlich invited Hansi Kennedy regularly to Frankfurt for control analysis (supervision) and seminars. From 1977 up to her retirement 1987 she was the co-director of the Hampstead Child Therapy Course and Clinic, which was renamed the Anna Freud Centre in 1984. [Interviews with Hansi Kennedy 11.7.1996, 23.4.1997, 5.6.1997 and her curriculum vitae.]

Dr George Stritch Moran trained at the Hampstead Clinic. When he was appointed director of the Anna Freud Centre from October 1987 he brought both continuity and innovation until his tragically early death from motor neurone disease in January 1992. Early on in his career he participated in the HCTCC Diagnostic Study Group in collaboration with Stanley Wiseberg, Hansi Kennedy, Cliff Yorke, and others, and the Developmental Disturbances Study Group (members of which also included Hansi Kennedy (chair), Pauline Cohen, Geraldine Fitzpatrick, Audrey Gavshon, Barbara Grant, Steven Marans, Turid Nyhamar, Sarah Rabb, and Janet Szydlo). His ouvre is in keeping with his reputation as a brilliant thinker (as well as risk-taking explorer and athlete). His conceptual work included expositions on the rationale for adaptations of technique necessary to accomplish intermediate aims and strengthen the therapeutic alliance; towards achieving the long-term aim of intrapsychic structural change; and on the relevance of observations of interactive constitutional, environmental, and maturational factors in early childhood to psychoanalytic formulations and practice. In addition, he made a remarkable contribution to practical medical management of juvenile onset diabetes and other chronic physical illness in childhood, through a series of clinical studies at the Anna Freud Centre on the interrelatedness of psychological and biological processes. These paid close attention to links between self-damage and low self-esteem, and the intensification of anxiety related to aggressive impulses by the fear of death, deriving from the real danger inherent in the illness. Importantly, he conducted the first randomized controlled study of psychoanalytic treatment of unstable diabetes in children. Illustrating the effect of fantasy on emotional regulation, these studies found that unconscious uses of the body to represent psychological states can lead to self-damaging acts with irreversible long-term consequences (Moran, 1984; Moran & Kennedy, 1984; Moran et al., 1991; Fonagy & Moran, 1993). (Also see chapter Twenty Eight, this volume). Furthermore, these fine-grained empirical studies had practical applications in providing verification of the efficacy of child psychoanalysis, and demonstrating how analytic treatment can profoundly influence an ill child's perception of his/her own body and the illness, thereby significantly improving outcome of physical treatments. Later, George Moran became chair of the Young Adults Research Group studying the efficacy of psychoanalysis with this age group, which continued after his death under the clinical direction of Anne-Marie Sandler.

Although Anna Freud remained deeply involved in the Centre until her death in 1982, from 1978 to 1987 the Centre was jointly directed by Clifford Yorke and Hansi Kennedy. After this, George Moran was appointed as director of the Anna Freud Centre, a post he held until his untimely death. He had been involved in preparing a manual of child psychoanalytic technique for purposes of outcome research.

Dr Humberto Nagera was born in Havana, Cuba, in 1927. He holds a BSc from the University of Havana and an MD from Havana Medical School (1952). He joined the staff of the Hampstead Clinic in 1958 just before the Cuban revolution. In the words of Anna Freud's biographer Elisabeth Young-Bruehl: "Nagera arrived at a time when Anna Freud was offering her staff preliminary formulations of the Developmental Profile and emerged as the Profile's most eager champion. In the Profile, he saw the psychoanalytic equivalent of basic diagnostic procedure in medicine and he joined Anna Freud in her conviction that the scientific rigor of psychoanalysis depended on innovations like the Profile" (p. 367). His participation and leadership on the Concepts Research Group at the Hampstead Clinic led to the publication of a series of three volumes edited by Nagera, published in 1969, consisting of a wonderful synthesis of Freudian theory and its evolution. In the words of one of the Concepts Group participants: "His leadership and organizational skills made this effort a wonderful learning experience for all trainees involved, we really learned our Freud and hoped that future generations would benefit from our effort" (Pat Radford, personal communication, 2011). He left the Hampstead Clinic in 1968 to become professor of psychiatry at the University of Michigan in Ann Arbor where he worked from 1968 to 1987. Most recently, he has been professor of psychiatry at the University of South Florida since 1987. In 2002, he founded the Carter Jenkins Center in Tampa, Florida, an organization dedicated to providing educational and clinical services to the community from a psychoanalytic developmental perspective. Dr Nagera remains a spokesman for the Anna Freudian tradition in his role as director of the Carter Jenkins Center, which houses amongst other things training for psychoanalytic candidates and numerous live seminars and internet interactive opportunities to learn and discuss Anna Freud's work both in English and Spanish. His own work and legacy is reflected in his numerous publications, dealing with a broad range of problems of developmental theory and basic psychoanalytic concepts of the libido theory, instincts, metapsychology, conflicts, anxiety, female sexuality and the Oedipus complex, and developmental psychopathology, including obsessional neurosis and a book on Vincent van Gogh. [Sources: Young-Bruehl, and www. cgi.marquiswhoswho.com.]

James Robertson (1918–1988) came from a working class family in Glasgow and had five siblings. He was a Quaker and as a conscientious objector looked after the victims of bomb attacks. His task after the end of the war was to reintegrate those children who had been cared for in the War Nurseries in their families or respectively to find foster families for those children who could not return to their families. Extra-occupational, he gained a diploma as social worker at the London School of Economics. In 1948 he accepted a position at the Tavistock Clinic in a research project of John Bowlby on reactions upon separation of small children, where he stayed until 1975. The psychoanalytical training, which he had started parallel to this work, was supported by Anna Freud. After retiring, together with his wife he created the Robertson Centre with the aim of making available over fifty years of professional experience on the issue of attachment and separation beyond the circles of experts to a wider public. Alongside Dorothy Burlingham and Anna Freud, the psychoanalysts Ruth Thomas and Claire Winnicott became founding members. The manuscript of the joint work of James and Joyce Robertson "Separation and the Very Young" was finished three weeks before he died in December 1988 and was published after his death 1989. [James and Joyce Robertson, 1989; interview with Joyce Robertson, 25.4.1997.]

Joyce Robertson was born 1919 in London into the emotionally well functioning network of a big working class family. Having grown up in a close family collective where there was always someone to cuddle a baby, to respond to needs, to console or to feed him or her, it was obvious to Joyce and her husband that small children needed an attachment figure, whom they love and who is sensitive to the pains provoked by separation. Joyce Robertson loved working with the very young children, whom she could easily calm down, and soon became an expert in questions concerning the mother-child relation. Interviewed by Dorothy Burlingham and Anna Freud, she was admitted to the training courses and later also conducted some child therapies. After both her daughters (born 1944 and 1950) had grown up a bit, Joyce Robertson continued from 1957 to work again with Anna Freud, first in the Well-Baby Clinic, later in the kindergarten of the Hampstead Child Therapy Clinic. In 1965 she switched to the Tavistock Clinic, helping with John Bowlby's attachment-separation research. The Robertson couple became known worldwide through their films on the reaction of small children on separation. [James and Joyce Robertson 1989; interview with Joyce Robertson, 25.4.1997.]

Professor Joseph Sandler (1927–1998). Gifted with an extraordinary capacity for theoretical conceptualization, and a clarity which enabled formulation of complex ideas in simple language, Sandler worked closely with Anna Freud, and rose to become a leading figure of modern psychoanalysis. He was born and grew up in Cape Town, where having matriculated at fifteen, he earned a BA in psychology from the University of Cape Town at eighteen, completed his master's degree in 1946 and left for London, receiving his PhD from University College in 1950. (This was supervised by Sir Cyril Burt, who was later exposed as a fraudster, falsifying data to prove that intelligence was inherited.) He then embarked on medical training at University College Hospital, working as a clinical psychologist at the famous Maudsley Hospital, which had given refuge to many professionals fleeing Nazi Germany and Austria. Simultaneously, he trained as an adult psychoanalyst, qualifying in 1952 at the age of twenty-five. He also became the youngest editor of the *British Journal of Medical Psychology*, and later of the *International Journal of Psychoanalysis*, founding the *International Review of Psycho-Analysis*. In 1968, he was appointed to the chair of psychoanalysis applied to medicine at Leiden University, and in 1979 became Sigmund Freud professor at the Hebrew University in Jerusalem, and then Freud Memorial professor of psychoanalysis, University College London 1984–1992. In addition he held twenty-four visiting professorships, was president of the European Psychoanalytic Federation and of the International Psychoanalytic Association—and yet still found time to write forty-four books and 200 papers spanning fifty years of innovative scientific work reformulating psychoanalytic theory in a contemporary conceptual framework. At Anna Freud's Hampstead Clinic he directed the Hampstead Psychoanalytic Index Project, a unique initiative which pioneered the classification of clinical material according to simple theoretical concepts. He also established and led research teams there and at the Sigmund Freud Centre for Study and Research in Psychoanalysis in Jerusalem, the Sigmund Freud Institute in Frankfurt as well as at the Psychoanalysis Unit at University College London. His wife Anne-Marie, who trained at the Hampstead Clinic and later became its director, co-authored many papers with him. [Adapted from Joseph Sandler: obituary in *The Independent*, written by David Tuckett, October 12, 1998.]

Dr Anneliese Schnurmann (1908–2009) was born into a wealthy manufacturer family in Karlsruhe, Germany. She did not know her father, who died shortly after her birth from a riding accident. In her sixth or seventh year, her mother fell severely ill from TB and died in 1915. She was cared for inter alia by her sister who was eleven years older. When Anneliese was fourteen her sister married, and the young couple accommodated her with them in Berlin. She was there, when her two nieces Hannah (1922) and Julia (1926) were born. Engagement with them awoke a lifelong interest and joy in the development of children. Until her death, there was a close relationship with these families. When in school in Berlin, she became friends with Susanne, the youngest sister of Dietrich Bonhoeffer. Anneliese Schnurmann was interested in social issues and the suffering at that time, particularly of young people, aggrieved her. She wanted, as far as it was possible, to offer assistance. At one meeting with the Bonhoeffer family, Paula, the mother of the numerous children, proposed to address the issues of nutrition and youth occupation. Thereupon, Dietrich Bonhoeffer and Anneliese Schnurmann created the "*Jugendstube*" (youth room), a day shelter for young people. As colleagues they could obtain help from the handicraft teacher Hanna Nacken and the youth warden Nore Astfalck, with whom Anneliese Schnurmann later became friends. When in 1933, the "Frankfurter Schule" at the University of Frankfurt, where Anneliese Schnurmann studied sociology with Karl Mannheim, was dissolved, she continued her studies in Geneva, where in 1935 she completed her doctorate as *Licenciée en Sciences Sociales*. After this followed studies in psychology and pedagogy at the University of Basel. In 1936, she briefly taught in Haslemere, Surrey at a boarding school, Stoatly Rough, for Jewish child emigrants. This home was directed by Hilde Lion, Emmi Wolf, and Nore Astfalck, who had to leave Germany for political reasons. In 1939, Anneliese Schnurmann herself emigrated to England when, shortly after the war broke out, she just stayed on with her friends in Haslemere. She registered with the Women's Voluntary Service and was assigned as "assistant nurse" to a paediatric clinic in Shottermill. Through her friend Nore Astfalck who lived close by, she got to know Anna Freud. From November 1942 until the closure of the War Nurseries in 1945, Anneliese Schnurmann worked alongside Ilse Hellman and Sophie and Gertrud Dann in the service for infants and toddlers at 5 Netherhall Gardens. From 1945 to 1949, she was in analysis with Kate Friedlander. She was among the first six participants of the Hampstead Child Therapy Course (1947 until 1950). From 1948 on, she was employed as a child therapist at the East London Child Guidance Clinic, and in 1951 she became the successor of Hansi Kennedy at the Chichester Child Guidance Clinic (until 1956). From 1961 until 1965 Anneliese Schnurmann trained as adult psychoanalyst at the British Psychoanalytical Institute. Konrad Gomperts was her training analyst and Dorothea Ruben and Joseph Sandler were among her supervisors. From 1952, she worked at the Hampstead Child Therapy Course and Clinic, conducting child psychoanalyses, and became a training analyst and supervisor in the training of psychoanalytical "Child Experts". She also had a private practice, where she carried out psychoanalysis and psychotherapies until her retirement in 1983. Until her death, she kept in close contact with some of the children formerly in her care. [Interviews with Anneliese Schnurmann 24.11.1996, 26.4.1996, 8.6.1997; curriculum vitae.]

Sydney Clifford Brookfield Yorke (1922–2007) was born in Rotherham, south Yorkshire. His medical studies at King's College Hospital in London were interrupted in 1945 when medical students were sent to help those suffering from starvation in Holland, and in his case, to Belsen, the Nazi concentration camp in Germany. Resuming his studies, he subsequently did his national service as a medical officer in the Royal Navy aboard an aircraft carrier. After the war he specialized in psychiatry at the Maudsley Hospital in London where he first met Anna Freud. After working at the Cassell Hospital, he trained at the British Institute of Psychoanalysis (analysed by Dr Ilse Hellman). In 1967, during the heyday of the Hampstead Clinic, when trainees and visitors from around the world flocked to attend the famous diagnostic and clinical meetings on Tuesdays and Wednesdays (respectively), Anna Freud asked Cliff to be psychiatrist-in-charge at the Hampstead Clinic. Then, in 1978, after he had completed his training as a child psychoanalyst, Anna Freud invited him to take over from her as director of the Clinic, a post he shared with Hansi Kennedy until 1987, four years after Anna Freud's death, when George Moran took it over; then Rose Edgcumbe held the fort while awaiting Anne-Marie Sandler's return from Jerusalem, where her husband Joe was Sigmund Freud professor of psychoanalysis at the Hebrew University until 1985. Later Julia Fabricius and finally Mary Target, Peter Fonagy, and Linda Mayes became joint directors. Clifford Yorke continued to practise, teach, and supervise at the Anna Freud Centre, also playing the piano and singing with colleagues in cabaret presentations; and in 1995 he gave a series of talks on Radio 3 called "Childhood and Social Truth". [Adapted from Clifford Yorke: obituary in *The Guardian*, written by Ken Robinson, July 17, 2007; and Luis Rodríguez de la Sierra, obituary in *The Independent*, July 10, 2007.]

References

Burgner, M. (1985). The Oedipal experience: effects on development of an absent father. *International Journal of Psychoanalysis*, *66*: 311–320.

Burgner, M. & Edgcumbe, R. (1972). Some problems in the conceptualization of early object relationships—Part II: the concept of object constancy. *Psychoanalytic Study of the Child*, *27*: 315–333.

Edgcumbe, R. (1976). Some comments on the concept of the negative Oedipal phase in girls. *Psychoanalytic Study of the Child, 31*: 35–61.

Edgcumbe, R. (1981). Toward a developmental line for the acquisition of language. *Psychoanalytic Study of the Child, 36*: 71–103.

Edgcumbe, R. (1983). Anna Freud—child analyst. *International Journal of Psychoanalysis, 64*: 427–433.

Edgcumbe, R. (2001). *Anna Freud: a View of Development, Disturbance and Therapeutic Technique.* London: Routledge.

Edgcumbe, R. & Burgner, M. (1972). Some problems in the conceptualization of early object relationships—Part I: the concepts of need satisfaction and need-satisfying relationships. *Psychoanalytic Study of the Child, 27*: 283–314.

Edgcumbe, R. & Burgner, M. (1975). The phallic-narcissistic phase—a differentiation between preoedipal and Oedipal aspects of phallic development. *Psychoanalytic Study of the Child, 30*: 161–180.

Edgcumbe, R. & Sandler, J. (1974). Some comments on "aggression turned against the self": a brief communication. *International Journal of Psychoanalysis, 55*: 365–367.

Fonagy, P. (1992). A one day scientific meeting. *Psychoanalytic Psychotherapy, 6*: 136–136.

Fonagy, P., Moran, G. S., Edgcumbe, R., Kennedy, H. & Target, M. (1993). The roles of mental representations and mental processes in therapeutic action. *Psychoanalytic Study of the Child, 48*: 9–48.

Fonagy, P., Steele, M., Moran, G., Steele, H. & Higgitt, A. (1993). Measuring the ghost in the nursery: an empirical study of the relation between parents' mental representations of childhood experiences and their infants' security of attachment. *Journal of the American Psychoanalytic Association, 41*: 957–989.

Hurry, A. (Ed.) (1998). *Psychoanalysis and Developmental Therapy.* Madison, CT: International Universities Press.

Kennedy, H. & Moran, G. (1991). Reflections on the aim of child analysis. *Psychoanalytic Study of the Child, 46*: 181–198.

Kennedy, H., Moran, G., Wiseberg, S. & Yorke, C. (1985). Both sides of the barrier—some reflections on childhood fantasy. *Psychoanalytic Study of the Child, 40*: 275–283.

Laufer, M. & Laufer M. E. (Eds.) (1989). *Developmental Breakdown and Psychoanalytic Treatment in Adolescence: Clinical Studies.* New Haven, CT: Yale University Press.

Nagera, H. (1970). *Basic Psychoanalytic Concepts of Metapsychology.* London: Karnac, 1990.

Nagera, H. (1975). *Female Sexuality and the Oedipus Complex.* New York: Jason Aronson.

Nagera, H. (1981). *The Developmental Approach to Childhood Psychopathology.* New York: Jason Aronson.

Sandler, J. (1976). Countertransference and Role-Responsiveness. *International Review of Psychoanalysis 3*: 43–47.

Sandler, J. (1983). Reflections on some relations between psychoanalytic concepts and psychoanalytic practice. *International Journal of Psychoanalysis, 64*: 35–45.

Sandler, J. (1990). On the structure of internal objects and internal object relationships. *Psychoanalytic Inquiry, 10*: 163–181.

Sandler, J. (2003). On attachment to internal objects. *Psychoanalytic Inquiry, 23*: 12–26.

Sandler, J. & Freud, A. (1983). Discussions in the Hampstead Index of the ego and the mechanisms of defense. *Journal of the American Psychoanalytic Association, 31*: 19–146.

Sandler, J. & Sandler, A. (1994). The past unconscious and the present unconscious: a contribution to a technical frame of reference. *Psychoanalytic Study of the Child, 49*: 278–292.

Yorke, C. (2001). Anna Freud: a view of development, disturbance and therapeutic technique by Rose Edgcumbe. *Journal of Child Psychotherapy, 27*: 218–220.

Young-Bruehl, E. (1988). *Anna Freud: A Biography.* New York: Summit.

SUBJECT INDEX

AUTHOR INDEX

PERSONAE

For Product Safety Concerns and Information please contact our EU representative GPSR@taylorandfrancis.com Taylor & Francis Verlag GmbH, Kaufingerstraße 24, 80331 München, Germany

Batch number: 10731077

Printed by Printforce, the Netherlands